Praise for

"An antidote to feeling overwh... *The Trying Game* is a compassion... and ultimately empowering guide t... every imaginable step on this journey."

—Lori Gottlieb, *New York Times* bestselling author of *Maybe You Should Talk to Someone*

"I believe every woman doing fertility treatments needs her Amy Klein. Find yours! It's too scary and confusing to go it alone."

—Alyssa Shelasky, *The Cut*

"Infertility can be incredibly difficult to navigate emotionally and physically. As an IVF veteran, Amy Klein does an exceptional job of tapping into the emotional aspects of the infertility journey while also providing readers with helpful information about various fertility treatments from medical experts."

—William Schoolcraft, MD,
founder and medical director of CCRM Fertility

"Amy Klein's *The Trying Game* is just what our fertility community needs right now. Unlike other fertility books, this is a real book for the real woman, written by a woman who has been there before. I'm thrilled to be able to provide this as a resource to my patients."

—Natalie Crawford, MD, MSCR, *As a Woman* podcast

"Amy Klein's writing on fertility is candid, warm, and honest. She pulls no punches, and the result isn't just informative—it's empowering. If you're struggling to create the family you imagined, Amy's is the voice you want in your head, and your heart."

—KJ Dell'Antonia, former editor of the *New York Times* Motherlode blog and author of *How to Be a Happier Parent*

THE TRYING GAME

Get Through Fertility Treatment and Get Pregnant Without Losing Your Mind

Amy Klein

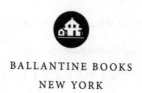

BALLANTINE BOOKS

NEW YORK

This book contains general information and advice relating to fertility problems. It is not intended to replace personalized medical advice, and should be used only to inform patients and supplement the regular care of a physician. We strongly recommend that you consult with your doctor about questions and concerns specific to your fertility concerns. The authors and publisher expressly disclaim responsibility for any adverse effects that may result from the use or application of the information contained in this book.

For the real Solomon

In the end, everything will be okay. If it's not okay, it's not yet the end.

—*Fernando Sabino*

CONTENTS

Section II: Let's Get Physical (and Technical)

Section III: Emotionally Speaking . . .

THE TRYING GAME

PROLOGUE

Drip, drip, drip.

I watch the pink drops plunk into the toilet, seeing all my hopes and dreams go down the drain with them.

I'm not injured. It's just my period.

JUST.

I'd never been a big fan of my monthly menstrual cycle—the terrible cramps, the raging hormones, my bloated stomach, and, let's face it, all the mess—but when trying to conceive, my period meant one thing: I wasn't pregnant.

There were many, many months I wasn't pregnant. And it wasn't pretty.

Staring down at the stained toilet water as salty tears tumbled down my face, the pain overwhelmed me. Stabbing jabs from my stomach reminded me, *No, you're not going to be a mom yet.*

I felt so alone. My friends who were mothers told me to "keep trying" and "relax" and "have patience" because it took them an incredibly long time to get pregnant (three months!!?#@!). Sure, I had a husband, but he didn't want to talk about this subject 24/7. (Yes, I would have talked about it for 247 hours if there were that many in a day.)

I didn't know where to turn.

At the bookstore, I eyed pregnancy books longingly, hoping I'd "Expect to be Expecting" soon, but I couldn't find much on the subject of Trying to and *not* getting pregnant.

Online, I found a ton of fertility boards with WHLA—Women Who Love Acronyms, something I *just* made up to show you how annoying it can be when they talk about TTC (trying to conceive) with DH (dear husband) and their 2WW (two-week wait) after their BD (baby dance = sex) before they POAS (peed on a stick, i.e., took a pregnancy test) hoping for "magic baby dust." These women had a *lot* to say with excellent emoticons and cutesy GIFs, but no real helpful tips.

On the other end of the spectrum, I found incredibly technical scientific information online about fertility, such as the study "Mutations in an Oocyte-Derived Growth Factor Gene (BMP15) Cause Increased Ovulation Rate and Infertility in a Dosage-Sensitive Manner." Yet even with my health and science journalism background, I couldn't always decipher what all the studies meant or what their practical applications were—if they had any at all.

I just wanted someone to tell me how ovulation strips actually worked (did they?!), when it was time to go to a fertility doctor, and how to react to my friend's in-your-face pregnancy announcement (do not throw Tupperware at your partner, trust me). That's why I started writing about my quest to get pregnant for *The New York Times* Motherlode blog.[1] I couldn't find anyone discussing the process in a straightforward, acronym-free manner. (I also couldn't find someone objective, who wasn't shilling a product or program like, "Get Pregnant with Maca Wheatgrass Royal Jelly in Three Easy Steps!")

Here's an embarrassing confession: When I started writing the "Fertility Diary" column, my *New York Times* editor and I thought I'd write about trying to get pregnant for a bit and then transition over to "regular pregnancy" issues. "Probably three to six months," she said. HA! How naive we both were about fertility treatment.

There are so many different ways to be Not Pregnant: You can be younger with endometriosis or older with not enough eggs; your husband can have slow sperm (don't tell him that, though), or you may not have a partner involved at all. You can get pregnant and not *stay* pregnant, you might have a kid already but have trouble conceiving another, or you might simply not know what is wrong—*if* there's anything wrong at all—except for the fact that you are still Not Pregnant.

I wasn't one of those women who always knew she wanted to be a mother—especially after leaving my traditional Jewish community, where most of my friends had kids by age twenty-five. It was only after I married Solomon at forty-one and found myself pregnant a week later that I realized I really wanted to have a child. Over the next three years, I had ten doctors, nine rounds of IVF, four miscarriages, three acupuncturists, two rabbis, one Reiki healer, five insurance companies, two egg donors, thousands of pills, shots, supplements, and Band-Aids, an amazing repeat pregnancy loss specialist . . . and one real, live baby. One beautiful baby.

Don't worry, this is not a book about how I got that baby. Everyone thinks that what *they* did to get pregnant is what *you* should do, but there's no *one* way for all of this to work. I've eaten dozens of pineapple cores, immersed myself in a Jewish ritual bath, and had so many pins in me I thought I'd entered a bloodletting clinic instead of an acupuncturist's office.

I'm not going to talk about the "one" way to get pregnant, or flood you with statistics that you can find on every clinic's website. I just want to help you.

I myself didn't have much help. I didn't know which doctor to see, what tests to have done, and why I should seek outside support. I messed up along the way, choosing the wrong type of treatment, starting a supplement regimen too late, telling too many people when I was pregnant, and not trusting my own instincts or my husband's (yes, Solomon's right sometimes, but don't tell him I said that!) when we went down the wrong road.

That's why I'm writing this book. I want to share with you all that I've learned. I don't want you to make the same mistakes I did and I want to save you from some of my trial and error.

I may not have done every single treatment (egg freezing, surrogacy) or had every diagnosis (endometriosis, PCOS), but I've *been* there. I've been through it all emotionally: from starting off as an optimistic woman, blissfully ignorant about my own fertility, positive I would get pregnant as soon as I started Trying (which I did! but to no avail), to becoming someone who quickly got a med school–like education in reproductive endocrinology (which is what fertility doctors practice).

I went from being someone who could picture every detail of her own labor to a despairing woman who didn't even know if she would ever have a baby, from feeling lucky in love to wondering if my marriage would even survive this endless roller coaster, from believing that I was #blessed to begrudging every other pregnant woman on the street.

Look: I'm not a doctor, an embryologist, an acupuncturist, or a healer, but I know all types of experts in the field, people I trust and have worked with personally or as a journalist asking for advice. When I don't know something, I let them tell me the answer—or "an answer," since there is no one answer, and you have to do what works for you.

Still, this is not a medical textbook. While I will discuss some procedures you may need to look into, supplements you may want to ask your naturalist about, or diagnoses you may want to investigate, in *no way* can I give medical advice. But I can guide you through the overwhelmingly technical and excruciatingly emotional process of Trying. And hopefully, I can point you in the right direction so you can get the best medical care without too much confusion, frustration, or isolation.

The truth is, most people won't understand what you're going through. If they've never struggled with getting pregnant, or never wanted kids in the first place, they may make you feel like you're being overly emotional, overwrought, over*something*. "At least you can get pregnant," someone told me after a loss. I wanted to punch her in the face and tell her, "Well, at least you know you have blood in your body since it's coming out your nose." But I didn't. I complained to another friend, who said, "Nobody will say the right thing right now." And somehow that made me feel better.

Really, I just want to make you feel better. Of course I want to make you a parent, but since that's not in my power, I want to make you feel less alone. I want you to know your options every step of the way and I want to help you to feel more informed, and therefore more sane. I may not always have the answers, but at least I know the questions to ask. I'll talk to experts, I'll tell you stories about women in the trenches. I'll tell you my story—when it helps.

First comes love, then comes marriage, then comes baby in the baby carriage. That's what we've been taught to expect. But life doesn't always turn out the way we hoped. Sometimes we get *what* we want but not *how* we want it. Let's face it, no one ever says, "I dream of having my eggs extracted and mixed with my husband's sperm in a test tube to create a baby."

I hope to be able to get you through this without losing your mind, your friends, your partner, and your entire life. No one wants to be Trying, but I hope I can at least make this stressful time a little less trying.

Section 1

GETTING YOUR EGGS TOGETHER

Chapter 1

Oh Shoot, Am I Infertile?

When my husband and I were trying to have a kid, a lot of people were like, "*Oh my God that's so hot,* you guys doing a lot of f*****g?"

—Ali Wong, *Baby Cobra*

You know you're not expecting if:

a) You only feel "in the mood" about two weeks after your period, hoping that's when you ovulate.

b) During sex, you start fantasizing about the sperm racing inside you rather than the joystick inside you.

c) You're counting down the days till your period and for the first time in your panicked life, you desperately hope you don't get it.

d) You get it. And you cry.

Don't cry. And don't panic. That's probably the best piece of advice I can give you—the one I wish someone had reminded me of every step of the way. "The hard thing about this is that I don't know if I'm at the beginning, middle, or end," says Kara, a teacher, who, at thirty-two, spent a few months "casually" trying: having sex every other day after her period ended, not really making a big deal of it. Still she kept getting her period, month after month. "Am I ever going to get pregnant?" she lamented.

Maybe you're like Kara, and you've been kinda sorta trying for a while. Or maybe you're more like other women, who get that positive pregnancy test only to find themselves bleeding a few days later. That's what happened to me. A week or so after my wedding, I noticed that I hadn't gotten my period. *Stress,* I figured. A few days after *that,* I popped into a drugstore to buy a pregnancy test or three. Six pink lines later, I was shocked to find I'd tested positive! A few days later, the morning I was supposed to go to the OB/GYN, it was over. Had I not taken the tests, I would have thought it was a very late period.

Many women who aren't paying attention experience these early misses, called "chemical pregnancies," and they don't even know about them. But my doctor confirmed it: I was pregnant, and then I wasn't.

I wasn't concerned. Solomon and I took the doctor's advice and took a month off to go on our planned honeymoon to hike Machu Picchu. (Am I a good wife or what?) The following month, I got pregnant again, another miracle! But that one didn't stick, either.

That's when I started going into what Solomon calls "Kitchen Sink Panic," where you throw everything you ever worried about into this one moment: *What if I waited too long? What if we're going to have fertility problems? Will we have to do IVF? What the heck is IVF anyway? Do we have the money for it? Do we have the patience? The time? What if we never have a baby after all??!! Am I infertile?*

Kitchen Sink Panic

I know it's easier said than done, but try not to spin out of control. Remember: Just because it hasn't happened yet does not mean that it's not *ever* going to happen. It could happen any day now—any moment, actually. One day you're just going about your business and the next, after a night of passionate (or even practical) lovemaking with your partner, his speedy sperm could be getting ready for a hot blind date with your eggs, booking a room in Hotel l'Uterus for the next ten months.

And so you never know. And maybe that's the most frustrating thing of all. You *never* know how long this is going to take. Maybe next week you'll be like that elated woman in that annoying commercial, where she's waving around her positive home pregnancy test singing/dancing "I'm pregnnaaant!" Or it may take you a minute. But we don't know anything just yet, so there's no need to jump to any dire conclusions.

"My whole life, I thought I was going to be a mom," says Maria, who was twenty-eight when she got married and twenty-nine when she started Trying—without immediate success. "I have a career I love and care about, but if you grow up so focused on becoming a mom, you want it to happen right away," she says.

We've all been led to believe that conceiving is the *easy* part. The cheap part. Two bottles of beer and a cigarette afterward. Most of us have spent a good portion of our lives trying *not* to get pregnant. I thought all you needed was a night of passion (more like an hour), and voilà!—you'd be knocked up.

And you're not—not yet, anyway. So yeah, it blows.

It sucks that you even have to think about any of this. That you might have to understand how baby-making works, how your own body works (or doesn't work), and how to get it working in order to have a baby. It all feels so unfair—especially when millions of women around the world can skip this part and go straight to being "Pregnnaaant!"

Consider this though: Some 10 percent of women in America (about 6.1 million) have difficulty getting or staying pregnant, according to the Centers for Disease Control and Prevention (CDC).[1] So you're not alone, even if it feels that way.

When Trying Is *Trying*

What the heck does it mean to "try to conceive"? (Acronym Alert: TTC is the first of many acronyms we will find in the fertility community.) I can tell you this: Trying is the opposite of sexy. Sexy is spontaneous, whimsical, free, hot, and passionate. It doesn't usually include looking at the calendar, counting the days since your last period, and scheduling a rendezvous with your partner according to your ovulation schedule. "Honey, I'm taking my basal body temperature!" does not scream "sexy" the way "I'm so hot for you!" does (although they *literally* mean the same thing).

"Trying to have a baby turned sex into a have-to instead of a want-to," says Leena, who started trying at thirty-two and thought it would be easy because her childhood best friend had had no problem. "I've never been good at have-tos. It turned sex into broccoli when it should be ice cream."

At its most basic, trying to get pregnant means having unprotected sex. Let's just assume that you have that part down correctly. Next, make sure you've stopped all birth control, removed all IUDs, and aren't using any lubes with spermicide, and that your partner has *not* had a vasectomy. (True story: I met a woman who wasn't aware her boyfriend had done this!)

Speaking of birth control, don't worry about the pill ruining your fertility forever. A comprehensive review of seventeen studies in the aptly named journal *Contraception* showed that pregnancy rates in women one year "after discontinuation of contraception"—both the pill and IUD—"are broadly similar" to those of women who used no contraception at all.[2] (People who took oral contraceptives might have "some delay" in conceiving, another meta-study found, but it's temporary, "typically limited to the early months following cessation" of birth control.[3]) So give it a couple of months before you start worrying.

After you go off birth control, you can start Trying before your period comes. But you do need to make sure your period returns eventually. It helps to know that your period has returned and is back to its regularly scheduled 28- to 30-day monthly programming. This is a good indication that you are ovulating—which is a necessary condition for getting pregnant. (Menstruation is not a guarantee of ovulation, which you'll learn more about in chapter 2.)

"Understanding ovulation is the key to conception," advises the American Pregnancy Association's "Essential Guide to Getting Pregnant,"[4] explaining that ovulation is when the ovary releases an egg so it can travel down the fallopian tube and become fertilized by waiting sperm. The uterine wall lining (the endometrium) thickens so that a fertilized egg can implant, and voilà! Pregnancy.

Duh. I always thought I understood the basics of ovulation, menstruation, and conception, but like many women, I didn't have much of an idea how my body worked. I had no idea that there was only one egg released per cycle—usually from alternating ovaries—and millions of sperm vying to impregnate it (finally, some good odds for women!).

This much I'm sure you know: Women conceive when a man's sperm fertilizes her egg. When is that, you say? That's the $100,000 question.

When Should We Have Sex (and How Much)?

Fun fact: Did you know that there's only a short window every month when you can actually get pregnant? I wish someone had told me this

Scientifically Speaking: An Annotated Guide to the Birds and the Bees

"A man pees inside a woman" is what my best friend told me when we were six. I suppose that wasn't *that* far off from what I later learned in biology class: that the man's sperm meets the woman's egg and makes a baby. Sounds simple.

As you may already suspect, it's not that easy—a lot has to occur to make that destiny happen.

After ejaculation, the sperm[i] enter high up in the vagina near the cervix, the opening of the uterus. Some of the millions[ii] of sperm battle through the cervical mucus to make it into the uterus, swimming toward the fallopian tubes,[iii] where the ovulated egg awaits[iv] (or where the sperm hang out until ovulation).

The egg sends out a signal to attract the sperm.[v] Usually, only one sperm penetrates the egg's shell (the zona pellucida) to fertilize the egg and create an embryo. The embryo moves toward the uterus, dividing into more and more cells.[vi] Some three to four days after fertilization, the embryo reaches the uterus, and attaches to the uterine lining a couple of days later. This is called implantation,[vii] and that's when pregnancy officially begins.[viii]

Hopefully it will end with a baby.[ix]

[i] Just because a man has semen doesn't mean there's sperm in it. That's why a man's semen should always be tested.

[ii] Most men have millions of sperm in their semen, but not everyone's sperm are motile, or fast movers, another thing that needs to be checked out.

[iii] Some say only 1 in 14 million sperm makes it into the fallopian tubes.

[iv] The egg waits 12 to 24 hours after ovulation, but the sperm can hang out there (just chillin') surviving up to five days.

[v] "The Sperm's Siren," a new book that should be written?

[vi] We will discuss the stages of embryo development in the IVF chapters, where you're waiting on edge for reports on their progress.

[vii] Many people falsely call an IVF embryo transfer an "implantation," which drives sticklers like me crazy.

[viii] NOT when life officially begins—which is up for debate, depending on whom you ask.

[ix] We will discuss this in later chapters.

when I was younger. I was always frantic when I was late, not realizing that it is highly unlikely to conceive the day right before and after my period.

Lemme explain: We usually ovulate—i.e., one of our ovaries releases a mature egg—somewhere near the middle of our cycle, though not *in* the middle. Our "fertile window"—the point in our cycle when sex can result in conception—can start anywhere from five days before ovulation until the day of ovulation. And the best time to conceive is right *before* ovulation.

Sperm can survive in your body for up to five days, but your egg can only be fertilized for 12 to 24 hours after its release. That's why it's better to have sex closer to ovulation, so the sperm can "catch" the egg as soon as it's released.

Many people obsess over *how* to have sex. But "there is no evidence that coital position affects fecund-ability," research has found about fertility.[5] You just gotta get that sperm near the cervix. Hello, missionary . . . and doggie style! Also, men, listen up: Studies have found that "female orgasm may promote sperm transport."

As funny as it might look on a TV sitcom, there's also no research supporting putting your legs in the air over your head to get the sperm in place, or as I call it, postcoital yoga. (Inverted plow pose does help you relax, though.)

It's not *how* you do it, it's how *often*.

"Sex is like pizza—it's never really bad and you can never have too much," my husband, Solomon, likes to say. "Like pizza for *men*," say I, who has had plenty of bad, um, slices, and knows that there *is* such a thing as too much.

When you're trying to get pregnant, is there such a thing as *too much sex*?

In the movies, when a couple decides to start trying to have a baby, they go at it passionately 24 hours a day, seven days a week. But now you know that sex only works if it's during the fertile window.

For men with normal semen quality, daily ejaculation is fine, a recent study found.[6]

The List: Some Fertility Acronyms

Here are some nonmedical acronyms you might find in fertility groups.

2WW: The Two-Week Wait, while trying to find out if you're pregnant.

AF: Aunt Flow, or your period.

BCP: Birth Control Pills.

BD: Baby Dance, or sex for conception purposes.

BFN: Big Fat Negative (or the "F" word, if you must) on a pregnancy test.

BFP: Big Fat Positive (or the "F" word, if you must) on a pregnancy test.

DH: Dear Husband, who, in this process, doesn't always feel so dear.

DD: Dear Daughter.

DE: Donor Eggs.

DS: Dear Son.

OPK: Ovulation Predictor Kit.

Frostie (not an actual acronym): Frozen Embryo.

PG (also not an acronym): Pregnant.

POAS: Pee On a Stick.

PUPO: Pregnant Until Proven Otherwise (i.e., before the test).

RE: Reproductive Endocrinologist, i.e., a fertility doctor.

SO: Significant Other.

TTC: Trying to Conceive, or as I like to say, "Trying."

But a long abstinence of more than five days can hurt sperm. In fact, for patients with male factor infertility, frequent ejaculation may *improve* their semen.[7]

The optimal amount of sex—and ejaculation—is every other day during your fertile window. In fact, when it comes to getting pregnant, there's no difference between having sex two times a week or three times a week, provided you're doing so during the fertile window. (That said, having sex only once a week may decrease your likelihood of conceiving.) So if you ovulate on day 15, start Trying on day 11.

Ways to Track Ovulation

Did you know some women can actually feel when they're ovulating? The Germans have a perfect word for it: *mittelschmerz,* which literally means "middle pain" and is the mild discomfort you feel in one ovary when your egg drops.

But don't worry: Most women have no clue when they're ovulating.

That's why there are a number of ways to track ovulation—and let me say they are *all* pains in the neck.

"Charting is relatively easy and inexpensive," one website counsels about keeping track of your cycle.[8] HA. Define "easy."

So why track ovulation? Simple: If you're not having sex during your fertile window, you cannot conceive.

First, you'll want to know *if* you're ovulating, then *when* you're ovulating, and finally, how regular your ovulation is, so you get a feel for it over a few months.

WHAT: Basal Body Temperature (BBT)

WHY: Your resting body temperature goes up for a few days after you ovulate.

HOW: Buy an accurate basal body thermometer, take your temperature at the EXACT same time each morning the minute you wake up (before bathroom or coffee), and write it down every day for a few months to see your pattern of ovulation. (The BBT shows that you *already ovulated,* so it's better for finding out your fertile window for future cycles than to tell you when to have sex.)

WHO IT'S GOOD FOR: Architects, actuaries, accountants, and people who like to make graphs or do connect-the-dots puzzles.

WHAT: Cervical Mucus

WHY: Cervical mucus is a barrier to your uterus—and it also helps transport sperm. The mucus increases and changes in consistency before ovulation.

HOW: Manually. (Fingers. Vagina.)

WHEN: After your period ends. Mucus will go from dry and sticky to wet and loose to creamy (ugh!) before ovulation to stretchy like egg drop soup during your most fertile window. DROP EVERYTHING NOW AND HAVE SEX. After ovulation, cervical mucus becomes dry and sticky again.

WHO: Chefs who can differentiate between roux, béchamel, and hollandaise.

WHAT: Cervical Position

WHY: Your cervix—the narrow necklike passage forming the lower end of the uterus—changes position four times during your cycle, rotating from closed, near your rectum, after menstruation to open and vertical near ovulation.

HOW: Stand with one foot up or squat, insert your fingers into your vagina, and assess the position.

WHO: The types of people who would hire midwives and doulas when pregnant.

WHAT: Ovulation Prediction Kits (OPKs)

WHY: These over-the-counter pee sticks measure the surge in your luteinizing hormone (LH), which happens a day or two before ovulation—signaling it's go time.

HOW: Buy a lot of these sticks in bulk and pee on them a week after your period ends. Wondfo sells One Step ovulation strips in bulk. There are also electronic reusable tests.

WHO: My motto is, "Why do something yourself when there's technology for it?" Caveat: It only predicts your LH surge, not *if* you ovulate. A new at-home test, Proov, can confirm that ovulation has taken place.

How Long Should You Be Trying?

"My mom always told me she got pregnant as soon as she started trying—and it's true, my sisters and I are so evenly spaced apart," says Maria, who was freaking out after two months of not getting pregnant. "So I had this level of anxiety when it didn't happen right away."

How long is it "supposed" to take to get pregnant?

According to the study "Increased Infertility with Age in Men and Women,"[9] (shoot me now?), when having sex twice a week:

- 92 percent of 19- to 26-year-old women will be pregnant within a year.
- 86 to 87 percent of 27- to 34-year-old women will be pregnant within a year.
- 82 percent of 35- to 39-year-old women will be pregnant within a year. (The age of the man—yes, the creatures who contribute half the DNA but don't always get discussed—doesn't affect much until age 35, after which the male factor becomes "more pronounced," rising 10 percent in men over 35.)

A word about age and fertility: I hope you're not one of those people who is uncomfortable with her age, because it's about to become a central part of the discussion.

I was forty when I went to an OB/GYN to get a pre-pregnancy checkup. I wanted to know if I needed to be off birth control for a few months before we started.

"I wouldn't wait—not at your age," the young woman said snidely.

I was shocked. No one had ever spoken to me like that about my age. In the years to come, I would have to get used to it, because, "The age of the female partner remains the *single most important factor in predicting success with [fertility] treatment*,"[10] according to the *Journal of Human Reproductive Sciences*—and every reproductive endocrinologist you'll ever meet.

But listen, I've met twenty-eight-year-olds who have trouble conceiving and forty-five-year-olds who have had babies with no medical intervention. I myself conceived *twice* at the age of forty-one without medical intervention and likely would have given birth at forty-two had I been with the right doctor.

The world's oldest woman to conceive naturally had a baby at fifty-nine (!), according to *Guinness World Records*. The world's oldest (so far) IVF patient to have a baby with her own eggs was forty-nine, and with donor eggs, seventy-four.

Age is a crucial criteria, but it's not the only one. The older you are, the more time it may take to conceive, the fewer good eggs you may have, and the greater risk you have for miscarriage. But all these age-based statistics and the stats themselves are an average, a guide, if you will, often based only on people who had trouble conceiving, and not always applicable to you and me. So don't ignore them, but take them with a grain of salt, the seasoning that is one part of the fertility sandwich.

Doctors love to talk about age—but we can't help how old we are when we start Trying. (I couldn't, anyway, since I only wanted to have children with a partner.) What is a bit more under our control is time to conception: How long is it going to take you to get pregnant and have a baby? That's why I'm here: I want to get you there faster.

Maria didn't know she should give it six months before starting to worry. Her husband, who is significantly older, was worried about his meandering sperm doing their job. "Our level of anxiety was so high, he came with me on a work trip across the country and that's when we conceived," she admitted. It only took them *four months*.

But for others, the prescribed time—a year if you're under thirty-five, six months if you're over thirty-five—is too long, too stressful.

"I can't imagine waiting a year, *then* finding out we'd have trouble," says Kara, the teacher who started at thirty-two after getting married to her boyfriend of four years.

In the beginning she thought, *It's fine, it's normal, it doesn't happen right away,* but she was getting more and more frustrated. "There was tension; I got into fights with my husband," she says. She soon started

---

TIP: Can Cough Syrup Help You Get Pregnant?

While some fertility advice sounds like old wives' tales, others are backed by scientific evidence.

Here's an inexpensive one: cough syrup.[11]

Yup, regular over-the-counter Robitussin—or any expectorant—taken before ovulation can do the trick. When you have a bad cough, guaifenesin, the active expectorant ingredient in cough syrup, loosens the mucus in your lungs—and your entire body. It can help thin the cervical mucus, the fluid our cervix produces during our cycle that helps transport the sperm to the uterus and fertilize our eggs. Too-thick cervical mucus can prevent sperm from reaching the uterus.

In one of the first studies using cough medicine on women who had a problem with their cervical mucus, three-quarters showed marked improvement and 40 percent became pregnant.[12]

But cough medicine can have side effects, and is not considered safe for those already pregnant. Talk to your doctor about which cough medicine to take, what dosage, and when to take it to help the sperm have a speedy ride.

charting with ovulation kits and realized she actually wasn't ovulating, so she went to a doctor for further testing.

It was a good thing she did, because she got a health diagnosis that would affect her fertility, then had to start treatment, enduring lots of failures. She finally got and stayed pregnant at thirty-five. Kara is so glad she took charge of her reproductive health when she did: "If we'd waited a year, we would have depleted our emotional reserve before we started."

The first couple of months you're Not Pregnant, you don't need to rush to a doctor. But there are a whole bunch of other things you can be doing to get you closer to your goals.

No One Said It Would Be This Hard

Now that we all have a PhD in Our Bodies, Ourselves, I want to take a step back and acknowledge the elephant in the room: the disappointment.

It's disheartening that this *might* not be as easy as you thought.

"I wasn't even trying," my friend told me when I started asking my mom friends how long it took them to get pregnant. "I forgot to take the pill for *one* day," said another, probably exaggerating. We've all heard countless stories of accidental pregnancies, and we all thought it would be us starring in that cute soft-focus movie montage, where one scene has you kissing and the next has you patting your belly and then all of a sudden you're in the hospital holding your sweet little cherub.

There's a famous Yiddish saying my grandmother loved: "Man plans and God laughs." (For my wedding, the saying should have been "Woman plans outdoor picnic wedding, God makes it rain the day before.")

The stakes are much higher with babies than weddings. When I realized it would take longer than I thought to have a baby, I felt sucker punched in the gut—right where my baby should be. That state of shock can last awhile. Eventually I had to stop singing the sad "How Things Are Supposed to Be" refrain.

Yes, I had a vision of what my ideal pregnancy and birth would look like. But it was time to tuck it away so I could get down to the business of making my dreams a reality.

Chapter 2

Woman, Know Thyself: What You Can Do Before Starting Treatment

Had I been too busy to notice the ticking of my biological clock? Had I taken fertility for granted, assuming I had all the time in the world? Had my body stopped sending me signals because I'd ignored them for so long?

—Elisabeth Rohm[1]

After my wedding, I had two failed pregnancies, and decided it was time to go to a fertility clinic. I still believed I'd have a baby soon . . . I just needed a little help. Maybe a doctor could speed things along.

The clinic ran a bunch of tests—I couldn't tell you exactly which ones because at that early stage, I simply put my trust in the doctor and nodded along without asking too many questions. They told me not much was wrong with me except my age (of course) and that I needed to take some extra folic acid. We started with intrauterine inseminations (IUIs), like a turkey baster that places the sperm inside you. (We'll discuss IUIs in chapter 9.)

Three exciting rounds resulted in . . . drumroll, please!! . . . nada.

I was about to turn forty-two, and even though I wasn't yet well versed in fertility statistics, I knew that wasn't good.

"Why don't we have your tubes checked?" the doctor said after the failed IUIs, like it was an afterthought. "Although," he added, "you *did* already get pregnant twice on your own, so I'm sure your tubes are *fine*."

Apparently, he didn't know the meaning of the word "fine," because that's not what showed up on my hysterosalpingogram. One of my tubes was blocked. I had been operating at half capacity and my doctors didn't even know it. Sure, I got pregnant twice—but that was from *the same ovary*. No wonder the IUI baster wasn't cooking my turkey!

During my years of infertility, I had many tests done. Some days it seemed like all I was doing was scheduling tests and/or calling for their results. But the tests weren't done all at once, and certainly not before I began treatment. It was as if a new lightbulb switched on at each new doctor—like, "Hey, have you done X?" or "Why don't we try Y?" If only there was a standard checklist I could have gone through before starting fertility treatment . . .

But there actually *is* a checklist—one that should be done before starting *any* treatment.

"People are going through cycle after cycle and being told they have unexplained infertility yet even the most basic testing hasn't been done," says Dr. Aimee Eyvazzadeh, a San Francisco-based reproductive endocrinologist. I can't tell you the number of women I've spoken to who have been rushed into an invasive treatment without a preliminary evaluation first. (Myself included.)

At thirty-seven, Phoebe was just out of a long marriage that "thankfully" hadn't resulted in kids. After attending an egg freezing seminar Phoebe had a gynecological exam, which revealed a fibroid, a noncancerous growth in the uterus. "It's no big deal, but we should keep an eye on it," Phoebe's gynecologist told her.

Phoebe forgot all about the fibroid until a few years later when she married her dream guy. Before starting fertility treatment, she had to undergo surgery to have that "no big deal" fibroid removed. It took her out of the Trying Game for six months! And she was forty-one years old.

"When you're a hammer, everything looks like a nail," Solomon loves to say, pinpointing the moment when the doctor rushed us into IVF without properly assessing us as the moment where we went horribly astray.

That's why Dr. Aimee, as she likes to be called, is promoting diagnosis *before* treatment. Ensure all systems are go—before you get your car on the racetrack. She's created the TUSHY method, which is a (catchy?) acronym for basic testing that every OB/GYN can and *should* do before rushing people into expensive and invasive treatment.

- "T" is for testing the fallopian **tubes**.
- "U" is for an ultrasound of the **uterus**.
- "S" is for **semen** analysis.
- "H" is for **hormone** testing.
- "Y" is for **your** genetic profile.

If doctors took the basic steps in examining us, Dr. Aimee notes, our health care costs would not only go down, but we'd get pregnant faster. "Decrease heartache and increase joy."

Where to Begin: Hormones

If you're trying to get pregnant, or if you simply want to assess your current fertility for self-knowledge or fertility preservation, i.e., egg freezing, get your hormones tested.

There are two main hormones tested to evaluate your fertility potential:

- Anti-Müllerian hormone (AMH), which assesses your egg quantity, and can be tested on any day of your cycle.

- Follicle-stimulating hormone (FSH), which stimulates ovarian follicle growth and may predict your egg quality. Not all doctors measure this. It should be done on day 2 to 4 of your cycle. (The first day of your period is when you have a full flow, not just spotting. If you get your period late in the day, consider the next day Day 1.)

"When they go low, we go high," Michelle Obama said, totally *not* referring to fertility, but that's my mnemonic device to help you remember that your FSH should be lower (under 10) and your AMH should be higher (over 1). These numbers will assess your fertility potential for your age, within a range. A low AMH at a young age could be a sign of trouble. A high AMH at an older age could mean your eggs are great.

In a study of three thousand women, 10 percent of thirty-year-olds were found to have a low AMH (like those of a forty-year-old) and 10 percent of forty-year-olds had a high AMH (like those of a thirty-year-old).[2]

In other words, age isn't everything.

So, where should you start? You may be able to get these hormones tested with your OB/GYN—tell her you want your fertility panel blood work done.

As a late-twentysomething working in private equity and then at 23andMe, Afton Vechery went to her OB/GYN to get her hormones tested to assess her future fertility. The doctor pooh-poohed her. "Oh no, you don't need that," she was told. She insisted . . . and was shocked when the bill came back at over $1,500. That's why Vechery cofounded Modern Fertility, a home-testing hormone kit company. She's spoken to lots of women who've said, "I wish someone would have told me I could have checked on these tests sooner!"

Now they can. Modern Fertility and other companies like Kindbody can assess your hormones, and explain what it means vis-à-vis your fertility (and they can even assess if you might be nearing menopause). Experts like Dr. Aimee can do this for you, too.

But should we be testing our own fertility? Should we be taking our diagnoses into our own hands?

"I think it's great that ovarian reserve testing is available—it provides essential information," says Dr. Eric J. Forman, medical and laboratory director of Columbia University Fertility Center. "Unfor-

Does Birth Control Affect Your Fertility?

Although birth control has been shown to have no effect on future fertility, many women blame their fertility problems on the pill.

Long-term birth control use "might mask something else, like if a woman has PCOS or hasn't ovulated—something she does not realize until she comes off the pill," says Dr. Forman. For ten years, I was on continuous birth control—I got only about four periods a year—so until I went off it, I had no idea if my periods were still regular (they were) or if I had other problems with my cycle.

Although some doctors say you don't have to go off birth control to test your fertility or freeze your eggs, some research shows that being on hormonal birth control can affect your fertility. A 2013 study found a "decrease of serum AMH levels during the use of all combined contraceptives," and after nine weeks, AMH was affected "independently of administration route," meaning, regardless of the type of birth control. Another study found that while AMH was not affected, the antral follicle count—how many eggs you might produce in a medicated cycle—was affected.[3]

"If you have a low AMH, you might want to reassess it," Dr. Forman says. Going off the pill for two or three months might produce better results, he said. One friend considering egg freezing called me in a panic when her AMH test produced an undetectable number. She went off birth control, and two months later that number almost tripled!

tunately, it's frequently misinterpreted or misused, causing unnecessary anxiety."

Anxiety is the *last* thing you need when you're trying (there'll be plenty of that during pregnancy and parenthood) and there is always the danger of too much information.

Hormone assessment predicts how someone will respond to *stimulation*. AMH "is a quantitative assessment of the pool of available follicles that might be able to grow. It's still not proven that it has any predictive value on the quality of the eggs or fertility in general," Dr. Forman says. Meaning, if you want to get pregnant, these tests might not prove a thing.

In fact, a 2017 study of 750 American women age thirty to forty-four years old with a low AMH who had been trying to conceive naturally found that both groups took the same amount of time to conceive.[4] The researchers noted, "Biomarkers indicating diminished ovarian reserve compared with normal ovarian reserve were not associated with reduced fertility." Meaning, the tests had no correlation to "natural" fertility.

"There are women who are unaware that their numbers are abnormal, because they were able to become pregnant," Dr. Forman says.

That's what happened to Tai. When she decided to freeze her eggs at thirty-seven, her hormones were so low, they were "undetectable." She was inconsolable. But after marrying a year later and trying naturally, she found herself pregnant and now has a healthy toddler. Now she is trying again—and this time, at age forty-one, those numbers do matter, since she's doing IVF. The hormone levels can predict how you will do in fertility treatment—how many eggs you might get—but when trying naturally, you only need one.

Does all this mean you shouldn't test your hormones? No.

"I think the idea of women educating themselves is beneficial, but it should be coupled with counseling," Dr. Forman says. "Our goal is not to scare people," but we also don't want to "leave them complacent, thinking, *Oh, my AMH is good, I don't need to do anything for five years*."

So get your hormones tested, especially if you're headed to a fertility clinic. But take the results with a grain of salt—and gather the rest of your medical history.

Next Up: Your Genetic Profile

Children who know the stories of their parents, grandparents, and other ancestors showed higher levels of emotional well-being, according to the study "Do You Know? The Power of Family History in Adolescent Identity and Well-Being."[5] Of course, happy families may be more apt to pass on the stories of their past—as well as healthy self-esteem.

Maybe that's why I don't know much about my family history. I don't know how my (now divorced) parents met, where their first date was, or even the stories of how their respective parents met and married. Sure, I know where they're from, but not much beyond that (except for the story of how on the boat from Poland to America, my grandfather ate a banana with the peel on it because he'd never seen the fruit before). Suffice it to say, I did not know *anything* about my family's reproductive history except what age my mother was when she had me and my siblings: twenty-three, twenty-seven (me), thirty-one, and thirty-three. I didn't know if she tried for a long time, if she had any miscarriages, if she was taking any medication, or if my father had any sperm problems. (Ugh, just writing that sentence creeps me out!) Only after I was in the thick of it did I take note of my mom's compression stockings—yes, she had blood clotting problems—the same ones I found out I had after a few failed pregnancies.

Forget knowing my family's history and genealogy: I'd have been better off with my family's actual *health* history. If your parents had problems conceiving, you might face a similar struggle. Some hereditary conditions that are linked to infertility include early menopause, endometriosis, and low sperm count. Male factor infertility, for example, can be passed down from grandfather to father to son.

And a woman whose mom went through early menopause may be at risk for the same. People with a familial history of autoimmune disease should get tested for these diseases, too.

TIPS: Family Reproductive History Questionnaire

QUESTIONS A WOMAN SHOULD ASK HER MOTHER:

1. Did you have any trouble getting pregnant? How long did it take?
2. Did you ever lose any pregnancies/babies?
3. Do you have any conditions like PCOS or endometriosis?
4. Do you have conditions like thyroid disease or blood clotting? Or any autoimmune disease?
5. At what age did you reach menopause?
6. Do any genetic syndromes run in your family?

QUESTIONS A MAN SHOULD ASK HIS FATHER:

1. Do any of your family members have cystic fibrosis?
2. Have you or your brothers had infertility?
3. Do any genetic syndromes run in your family?

But don't bank on your family history.

After her marriage failed, actress Sarah Fazeli decided to freeze her eggs at age forty. The doctor asked her some questions about her relatives, like how old her mother was when she reached menopause. "She had my youngest sister at age forty; my eldest sister had also given birth at age forty, and my other sister has four children, including a set of twins," Sarah says. The doctor seemed confident Sarah would be a good IVF candidate—until her numbers came back undetectable. "I cried for a week straight. I kept kicking myself—if only I'd frozen my eggs at age thirty, when I was ready but my husband wasn't. Or age thirty-three. Or thirty-five."

Your genetic profile is not only about your family's history, it's about your own sexual past. Sexually transmitted diseases like chlamydia and gonorrhea can affect your fertility. An estimated 2.86 million cases of chlamydia and 820,000 cases of gonorrhea occur annually in the United States, according to the CDC.[6] About 10 to 15 percent of women with untreated chlamydia will develop pelvic inflammatory disease (PID). PID can cause permanent damage to the fallopian tubes, uterus, and surrounding tissues, which in turn can lead to infertility.

The CDC recommends routine screening for gonorrhea and chlamydia for women under age twenty-five, but many doctors screen older women, too.

"I offer and recommend STD screening for everyone, regardless of age," Dr. Aimee says.

ST(F)U: Semen, Tubes, Uterus, and Freaking Out

It's not just our sexual history that can come back to haunt us, but our reproductive one. I can't tell you how many women have just casually mentioned to me as an aside, "Oh my god, I have the most painful period!" or "I never know if I'm going to even *get* my period."

For each of the six months Karen Jeffries was trying, she thought she was pregnant because she wasn't getting her period, but every pregnancy test was negative. Then at twenty-nine, she finally went to her OB/GYN, who diagnosed her with polycystic ovary syndrome (PCOS)—a hormonal disorder affecting some 10 million women around the world and a leading cause of infertility, often categorized by irregular periods, excess androgen, and enlarged ovaries or an excess of eggs (although sometimes it is symptomless).[7]

"I had no idea. I didn't really remember if I got my period regularly—in high school I was an athlete, I was really skinny, and I wasn't tracking it," says Jeffries, author of the book *Hilariously Infertile* and a website and social media accounts of the same name dedicated to

Emotionally Speaking: Is Infertility Funny?

When Karen Jeffries first went to the fertility clinic and the doctor discussed her husband's "donation," the couple looked at each other in disbelief. "Did he just refer to your sperm sample as a '*donation*'?" the then twenty-nine-year-old cracked up. They were even more tickled when the results came back and the doctor referred to her husband's sperm as "clean and buff."

"We both were picturing Oompa-Loompas," she says. That's when she decided that infertility *was* funny—and a few years later, after the birth of her two daughters she created a social media account and wrote a book about it.

"My uterus is in a bad mood," one T-shirt reads. "I think my unfertilized eggs are cuter than your offspring," quips an e-card.

"You *can* have humor in infertility," Jeffries says. "I always had an inappropriate outlook on things—that really did help me. I've had women from all over the world tell me, 'OMG all I did was cry and now I found your website and I'm crying from laughing now.'"

Some of her most popular posts and memes are about unsolicited advice ("Thanks for telling me just to have sex if I want to get pregnant. I've spent thousands on fertility treatments and never thought of that"), and other people's pregnancy announcements ("If everyone could just stop getting pregnant that'd be great").

And maybe it's easier for Jeffries to laugh because she's long out of treatment. But she still wants to help people.

"It's such a somber and emotional time, it's so hard—if you can add levity to it, it makes it easier."

showing the lighter side of infertility. "Then in college I was on the pill, which kept me regular. I had PCOS the whole time and I didn't know."

Andrea Syrtash *did* know early on she had endometriosis, a chronic disorder in which the tissue lining, the inside of your uterus (the endometrium), grows outside the uterus—but didn't realize how much it would affect her fertility. When she was fourteen, the relationship expert and founder of Pregnantish, an infertility lifestyle website, was hospitalized for painful and heavy menstrual cycles because of the endometriosis. The disorder affects some 7 million women in America, according to the Endometriosis Research Center, and is a leading cause of infertility. It's often symptomless, and it can cause scarring of the fallopian tubes and make it harder for sperm to reach the eggs—*and* can also impact egg quality. Adenomyosis, another disorder of the endometrial tissue, is when the endometrium grows *inside* the uterus, and can affect fertility, too.[8] (For more on these conditions, see chapter 22.) Had she known, Syrtash says, "I might have seen a specialist sooner." Syrtash had years of fertility trouble, and finally had a baby with the help of a gestational carrier (see chapter 23).

After Trying for six months, my friend Ken and his wife went to a specialist. "There's no reason you shouldn't be pregnant," the doctor said. (How helpful is *that*?) I asked Ken if his wife's cycle was regular. "Well, she spots a few days before her period," he said. A simple online search showed that it could mean her menstrual cycle was too short to carry a baby. "Please bring it up with your doctor," I told him. After a few months of acupuncture, her cycle regulated and she got pregnant.

Do I Need to Worry About All This Now?

There are many lifestyle choices that *may* affect our fertility: smoking (stop!), drinking (bring it down to moderation!), exercise (no more than five hours of biking a week for men[10] or more than three to five

Prove You've Ovulated

There was "no way" Amy Beckley would do IVF for a second child. The pharmacologist had spent "quite a bit of money" conceiving her son with IVF, and with her expertise in hormone signaling, she wanted to go back to the drawing board. At the lab, she tracked her own hormone levels and found she had low progesterone, which had likely caused her years of infertility and multiple miscarriages.

After ovulation, progesterone rises in order to prepare the uterus for pregnancy. Unlike the LH surge, though, the increase in progesterone is the only way to confirm that you've actually ovulated.

Some 46 percent of women did not ovulate even though they thought they had because their LH levels were increasing, according to one study.[9] "Conditions like PCOS cause a false surge—they'll get a positive on the ovulation strip but they won't actually ovulate," Beckley says.

That's why she helped create a home progesterone test, Proov, which confirms ovulation (but only after the fact, so it's not a good way to help you with charting). It can let you know if you need progesterone supplementation after ovulation to help you get pregnant. (Cost: $39.99 for a pack of seven test strips or $99 for twenty-one test strips.)

"The progesterone levels need to be elevated during implantation," Beckley says, referring to when your embryo burrows into your uterine lining for the long haul—typically seven to ten days after ovulation. (If you're doing IVF, you likely receive progesterone supplementation.)

Trying for a year before going to a fertility specialist can be very frustrating, Beckley says. "We're targeting people earlier on in their journey and advocating for them to have their physician monitor them and/or do it at home."

Three years after having her son, her daughter was born.

hours of vigorous aerobic exercise for women), weight (get yourself
to a healthy BMI—not too over- *or* underweight!—so it doesn't affect
ovulation).[11] I don't want to scare you. I just want to lay it all out on
the line to save you from my own haphazard "hmm, let's see what we
have here" medical diagnosis.

"There's no single test where you can look in the mirror and say,
'I'm fertile, everything's fine, have a glass of wine.' That's very damaging," says Dr. Aimee.

You know what else is damaging? Not knowing your own cycle.
Do you know how long your cycle is, how regular you are, if you have
painful periods or other menstrual idiosyncrasies? How about what
your PMS feels like? Do you know your own PMS symptoms, like
sore breasts or fatigue and headaches? Trust me, you'll want to start
paying attention to these things now. Because when you're really Trying, waiting eagerly for your period *not* to come, wanting to know if
you just "feel" pregnant, you're going to want to know how it felt
when you . . . weren't. Know thyself.

"Our fertility is such a precious commodity and we cannot take it
for granted," Dr. Aimee says. "We have to shift things for women and
doctors so women can understand their full fertility picture."

Chapter 3

Mind/Body/Soul/Baby: Is the Alternative Route for Me?

> It was a long road. I would go to the doctor in Beverly Hills every day at five in the morning to get tested to see if I was ovulating. I was trying everything: I did acupuncture and got a nutritionist to eat healthier, thinking that was an issue.
>
> —Kim Kardashian West[1]

Now, I know I just sent you to a few doctors, but before you bring out the big guns, let's talk about complementary and alternative medicine (CAM) and if it will help you get pregnant. Because let's face it: If it ain't gonna help you have a baby, you can probably save it for another time, a time when you have money to burn.

Should you try these methods before starting fertility treatment or while you're in treatment? Is there any proof it will work? And do you *have* to add alternative treatment, supplements, dietary changes, and mind/body work if you want to get pregnant?

I want to tell you about two of my own very different alternative experiences: when I was in my mid-thirties, I was hit with searing stomach pains. I stopped eating, so I lost twenty pounds (yay!) but hadn't slept in months (boo!). The gastroenterologist wanted me on heartburn medicine . . . forever. Someone in L.A. referred me to Dr. Marc LeBel, an acupuncturist who specialized in auricular medicine—a microacupuncture technique using tiny needles that stay in the ear, which holds a microsystem of the body. It was weird in a thousand different ways, but it worked. I left his office each week feeling as if my stomach were unclenched and as if I'd gotten a surge of dopamine that lasted for days.

Flash forward a decade: I was living in New York and went to a highly recommended fertility acupuncturist in Chinatown. With barely a workup or a diagnosis, he needled me in my knees, stomach, wrists, and ankles. YOWZA! It hurt like hell, and I lay there immobile, terrified that moving would exacerbate the pain. I didn't feel any different after the treatment, my IVF cycles did not improve, and his pungent teas made me gag. Still, I continued to go, twice a week, for months at a time. I was lured by the successes, the wall of baby pictures. Half a year later, I began skipping appointments, dreading the needles, which were draining me and my bank account.

I tell you these two stories to prove nada.

Yeah, nothing.

That's because it's really hard to "prove" that alternative medicine works, since it doesn't use the same standards as Western medicine: a standard licensing practice or uniform treatment, the studies, the scientific hypotheses, the control groups, the success stories. For every study that proves acupuncture or diet or alternative medicine is helpful, I can show you five that prove it isn't.

Researching alternative modalities and their effectiveness on getting pregnant is also hard because studies show that most people use more than one alternative treatment at a time—acupuncture and herbology or supplements and Reiki, for example. Who's to say which treatment worked?

If you're like my cynical Israeli husband and want a dozen scientific studies to prove everything and you only believe in Western medicine, then you'll probably agree with the *Nature* editorial "Hard to Swallow,"[2] which describes Traditional Chinese Medicine (TCM) as "largely just pseudoscience, with no rational mechanism of action for most of its therapies," and, well: NEXT.

But if you're more like me and have learned the hard way that there are limits to Western medicine and science ("unexplained infertility," anyone?), and you're willing to try nontraditional medicine, then step right up.

Instead of proving anything, I am going to guide you through some of what's available, how it works, who it might work for, and when it may be a good time to give it a shot.

So, how alternative is alternative? Once you start down this road, there seems to be no end to treatments (shamans clearing chakras?). Let's focus on the most mainstream, from acupuncture and herbs to diet and supplements to environmental and mind/body work.

Acupuncture for Infertility

Traditional Chinese Medicine (TCM) is based on thousands of years of Chinese medical practices. Some believe a form of acupuncture was practiced as early as the Stone Age, when knives and sharp tools were used to relieve pains and disease, as well as constipation due to the diet of the time. (Take that, Paleo dieters!)

TCM includes acupuncture, herbal medicine, massage, and dietary therapy. Unlike Western medicine, which works on curing ailments and fixing problems, "Traditional Chinese Medicine is preventative—it's about optimizing your overall health," says Dr. Angela Le, an integrative reproductive health expert, acupuncturist, and founder of Fifth Avenue Fertility Wellness in New York. "Women should use TCM to support their reproductive health as early as possible. It really can make a difference for your fertility and overall health to address any imbalance you might have before trying to conceive."

Fertility acupuncture places needles at points believed to influence reproduction, like regulating hormones and endocrine function, reducing contractions to help implantation, and improving blood flow to the uterus. Acupuncture can "help regulate your endocrine system," says Daoshing Ni, a California licensed acupuncturist who works at Tao of Wellness, which offers acupuncture, herbal therapy, massage, and nutrition guidance for wellness. Dr. Dao, as he's known, who is also the author of *The Tao of Fertility*,[3] says that not only can acupuncture balance your hormonal system—so necessary for fertility—it can help make your system more sensitive to IUI and IVF medications, so your body needs less of them and will respond better. He says acupuncture can also improve circulation, which is essential, especially for older women: "It helps increase circulation to the ovaries and helps them have better egg quality."

I think that acupuncture can be most beneficial to women who have irregular cycles—or no cycle at all, especially before starting more invasive fertility treatment. And Dr. Dao says he has the proof: "We can get someone who has a thirty-five-day cycle closer to a twenty-eight-day cycle, getting her ovulation day closer to fourteen," Dao says, referring to the fact that a woman needs a long luteal phase—enough time after ovulation—to allow embryo implantation. He also says acupuncture can improve "vaginal discharge," which aids sperm getting to the eggs.

"We look for a lot of objective symptoms," says Dr. Dao, who works with gynecologists and IVF docs to come up with a patient's diagnosis. Sometimes he might send her to get her tubes checked, sometimes he sends her to get her uterus looked at, and sometimes he'll send her to a fertility doctor to get her blood work done.

"If someone is much older, we'll send her straight to a fertility doctor because we don't want to waste time," he says, noting that they'll concurrently do TCM. On the other hand, if a person is younger, he tells her, "Let's work together for three to six months, and if you're not pregnant by then, let's do something different."

Of course, Dr. Dao would like to help women get pregnant naturally, with acupuncture and herbal supplements, both of which, he says can also reduce inflammation. "IVF is really rough: There's a lot of hormones and injections and it's expensive. We want to make sure our patients can do everything they can before they go: Once you start IVF, you're not looking back anymore. You're pushing forward."

Herbalism and Supplements

I admit it: I was not strong enough—dedicated enough, perhaps?—to handle the herbal teas given to me by the Chinatown acupuncturist.

Herbalism—botanical medicine, herbology, phytotherapy, whatever you wanna call it—is the traditional medicinal or folk medicine practice of using plants and plant extracts for overall health and specific conditions.[4]

The tea I was given by my doctor in Chinatown, a leafy green-brown mix that was stored in a plastic packet that reeked when opened, tasted like grass trampled by a thousand piglets. So . . . no. Definitely not twice a day. I told him this, and he gave me a pill instead.

Turns out, both options were wrong.

"The purpose of herbs is to customize [to an individual]," says Mike Berkley, a fertility acupuncturist and certified Chinese herbologist. He might see two women with PCOS, but one is a twenty-two-year-old weighing 185 pounds, and the other is forty years old and weighs 125 pounds. "They're completely different presentations," he says, and they need different prescriptions for a tea—never a pill. He sends his prescriptions to an herbal pharmacy that has the actual plants and makes customized tea packets.

What's in the packets? Berkley could tell me, but then he'd have to kill me. No, just kidding—he could tell me, but I wouldn't understand. "There are over a thousand herbs—it's like food, there are thousands of different kinds. Each herb has its own flavor, nature, temperature, and function." On his thorough intake interview, he'll ask about everything from your bowel movements to your sleep patterns to the state of your cervical mucus. He says a TCM doctor assesses a patient's tone of voice, complexion, eyes, overall demeanor, and how they walk, sit, and stand, to arrive at a diagnosis. "Before the patient says one word, the doctor already has some idea of who this person is, merely by observing them."

He'll design a "decoction" of two to thirty herbs to be brewed into tea and drunk twice a day.

The big question: To tell your fertility doctor, or not to tell your doctor?

Consult with your RE first—but know that your doc may not be into it. Some say they don't believe in it "but it can't hurt," while others don't want you taking anything that could interfere with the treatment.

Berkley says he wants total transparency with your fertility doctor, but if a cycle (or two or three) doesn't work, he recommends taking the herbs—after informing your doctor. "They're trying to protect you; their heart is in the right place," he says.

Angela Le agrees. "It's important to let your doctor know what you're taking," she says. If they don't approve, she'll skip the herbs and use other tools, like diet and supplements.

Supplements—or "nutraceuticals," a sector of dietary supplements made from whole foods and used to augment health[5]—are first and foremost intended to improve egg quality.

It's often said that women are born with all their eggs and there's nothing to do to improve it. But that's not exactly true, says Rebecca Fett, author of the must-read book *It Starts with the Egg: How the Science of Egg Quality Can Help You Get Pregnant Naturally, Prevent Miscarriage, and Improve Your Odds in IVF.*[6]

"The conventional thinking is that women are born with all the eggs they will ever have and that the quality of those eggs declines drastically with age. But this isn't the whole story," she says, noting that for most of our lives, our eggs are actually in a state of "suspended animation as immature cells," and that in the three to four months before ovulation, the egg has to undergo a transformation: It has to grow and start producing more energy, as well as separate and eject chromosomes. And if that process goes wrong—which it often does, especially the older you are—the egg will have chromosomal abnormalities. "These chromosomal abnormalities are the *single most important* cause of early miscarriages and failed IVF cycles, as well as the reason it takes older women so much longer to conceive," Fett says.

"Many women are told there is little they can do to improve egg quality, but the latest research defies that old assumption," says Fett, whose book is based on some five hundred studies, proving that there are things that can help the eggs grow—or harm them—before ovulation. "There is a brief window of opportunity in which you can make a difference to your egg quality."

Fett, by the way, put together her own supplement regimen and improved her diet and environment, and on her first retrieval, despite a dire initial prediction—had twenty-two eggs retrieved, nineteen of which became quality embryos. Two of those became her children.

You have to be careful when looking on the Internet for supplement suggestions, Fett writes in her book. "As just one example, research has clearly demonstrated that melatonin supplements improve egg quality and are thus often recommended for women undergoing IVF. But the problem is that taking melatonin supplements long term could potentially disrupt ovulation."

Lifestyle: Can Your Environment Harm Your Fertility?

Supplements aren't the only way to improve egg quality. The industrial chemicals BPA (bisphenol A) and phthalates—the toxins found

It Starts with the Egg
Supplement Recommendation

WHO: Anyone with diminished ovarian reserve or hoping to improve their egg count and quality—i.e., everyone?—as well as women with a history of implantation failure or recurrent pregnancy loss. "There's a huge variation in egg quality in women of different ages," Fett says. "There's no answer to when is 'too late'—a woman may have a good chance at forty-five, you never know."

WHEN: Improve your egg quality three to four months before retrieval. If you're limited on time, you can take the supplements during your treatment or while trying to conceive naturally, but if you're limited on funds and only have enough for one or two more rounds, it may pay off to take a break and let the supplements do their work. "There's no reason to wait. If someone is over forty, they shouldn't delay IVF, but if that round fails, they have a few months to prepare for a second round," Fett says.

HOW: Fett recommends CoQ10. Coenzyme Q10, an antioxidant that occurs naturally in our bodies, helps our cells with growth and maintenance.[7] Levels of this coenzyme, which helps our body unlock the energy in nutrients, decrease as we age—yes, even our cells slow down! Scientists are hailing the supplement—often sold as ubiquinol,[8] a form of CoQ10 that's more easily absorbed by the body[9]—as a supplement that can improve everything from heart disease to ALS and Parkinson's.[10] Fett notes that because CoQ10 increases energy production in mitochondria, it's important for egg and embryo development. "You would have to eat about three pounds of sardines every day to get the same amount of CoQ10 found in a typical supplement dose." It may also help men with fertility issues.[11]

As always, check with your doctor to see if it's right for you.

in everything from plastics to cleaning products to perfume—can alter hormones in the body. Even flame retardants found in carpeting and certain types of mattresses can adversely affect fertility.[12]

"Avoiding toxins is critical to egg quality," says Fett, who offers a detailed outline on how to clean your home environment of the worst offenders. There are also numerous reputable websites that suggest ways to eliminate common household toxins. For example, you can peruse the Environmental Working Group's online Skin Deep Cosmetics Database, which has reviews of eighty thousand personal care products.

I didn't.

Truthfully, I'm a terrible environmentalist. I use tons of Tupperware and disposable water bottles, and who knows what's lurking in my inexpensive drugstore makeup? Even the *thought* of greening my house makes me want to crawl onto my (probably toxic) bed and hide under my (probably toxic) covers.

Look, I've watched *The Handmaid's Tale:* I *know* that the increase in chemicals in our environment is blamed for declining fertility—especially sperm quality. More recent studies show how even a little BPA injected into mice can affect egg implantation and the uterine environment.[13]

But there's only so much a person can reasonably do. Right?

"IVF is a stressful process," Fett agrees. "If it's all too much," she says, referring to adding supplements, cleaning up your environment, *and* changing your diet, "choose one or two aspects to focus on." She stresses the first two, and points out that you can go through your plastics, cleaning products, fragrances, and other products once, and then you're done. "It doesn't need to be a source of ongoing stress," she says, noting that you might as well do it now because "when you're pregnant or have a newborn, it's really important to reduce chemicals. Try to clear your house of the worst offenders. You don't need to eliminate chemicals from your life—the goal is to rescue what you can."

Phew.

Your Diet and Fertility

Show me a woman who doesn't have issues with food, and I will show you a woman who was raised on a desert island.

Yes, that's why I saved diet for last. Food feels like the last refuge. You can take away my coffee, you can limit my drinking *and* my running, but when you touch my tuna bagel, I might just lose it.

There are many, many fertility diets out there. Some eliminate meat, others dairy, some are vegetarian or vegan, some are all organic, others have no carbohydrates or include only low-glycemic-index foods. Most will eliminate processed foods and sugar—which is never a bad thing. (Tell that to my secret Cheez Doodle stash.) Some doctors swear by keto; others eschew it and swear by Paleo. Some promote vegan. The Nurse's Health Study, of more than 18,000 women over eight years, suggests everything from whole milk to slow carbs, less animal protein,[14] and no trans fats.

Picking a fertility diet is kind of like picking any other diet: You have to choose one that works for you and not cherry-pick from a bunch of different approaches. Also, do keep in mind that there *are* different diets for different fertility diagnoses: If you're not ovulating or you have irregular menstruation, you might need a different diet than someone who has endometriosis or PCOS, or someone like me who had recurrent miscarriages. (See chapter 22 for Aimee Raupp's inflammation diet.)

"I'm not going to lie: It was a little stressful," says Renata, who, after numerous failed rounds of IUI and IVF, including a miscarriage at thirteen weeks, had acupuncture treatments with Angela Le and followed Le's elimination diet (no dairy, eggs, gluten, soy, or meat except organic chicken and wild-caught fish, etc., etc.).

"It was more challenging to shop for everything and cook," she says, not to mention *expensive.* "But we're spending so much on fertility, what's an extra $200 on our grocery bill?" On the other hand, it gave her something else to focus on—especially since she found herself socially isolated during her infertility, not going out with friends and drinking. "I found comfort in researching and cooking—it was my therapy."

Her sixth IVF worked—she now has a healthy baby boy—which she attributes in part to the acupuncture and diet. She's not following the diet so closely anymore, but kind of wishes she were. "It sounds super cheesy, but I felt cleaner and better about myself; my body felt better."

I went on a gluten-free diet for my last pregnancy. But when my doctor told me to go organic, I balked. You do what you can do.

Humor: Your Fertility Diet

1. No grains except those eaten by twelfth-century poets.
2. Milk is allowed if it's from a pregnant emu (second trimester).
3. Vegetables harvested in the late afternoon—preferably dusk—are good for egg quality. (But not when it's cloudy out.)
4. You can have meat on Thursdays, but only the animal's sex organs.
5. Eat as much butter as you want—good luck finding something to put it on!
6. Cook with hand-drawn well water.
7. The only oil you can use is the most expensive one.
8. If you see a carb, say something.
9. If you find out what a legume is, can you call me?

Body Work for Pregnancy

There are a number of body work therapies for pregnancy (under these or other names).

Yoga for Fertility

"Yoga can help balance the endocrine system in general," says Lynn Jensen, a certified yoga therapist who developed Yoga for Fertility in 2002 after her own fertility struggles (IUIs, endometriosis, surgery, three rounds of IVF) twenty years ago. Yoga for Fertility (including a book,[15] video, and online and live classes in her Seattle location) is a gentle yoga that supports the reproductive system as well as the endocrine system. Every gland can impact fertility if it's out of balance—especially when you're throwing more hormones into your system, she says. "Yoga can help move those excess hormones out of the body once you're finished with them."

After her own fertility struggles two decades ago, Jensen ended up adopting, and although many of her thousands of students get pregnant, she wants to remind students to always be open to other paths. "The more paths you're open to, the more the universe can help you: It leaves you more open for opportunities that might arise to be a parent."

Mayan Massage

Nurse practitioner Diane MacDonald was horrified when doctors wanted to remove her uterus to solve the issue of her painful periods. Then she met Rosita Arvigo, a doctor of naprapathy (which focuses on connective tissue and ligaments) and an ethnobotanist who studied with healers in Mexico and Belize and created the Arvigo Techniques of Maya Abdominal Therapy™, one type of Mayan massage. After doing the massage for three months, MacDonald's pain disappeared. She apprenticed at Arvigo's center and is now the program administrator there.

The gentle abdominal massage focuses on aligning all the organs functioning in the lower pelvis. "If the uterus is not in an optimal position, it could be restricting blood flow. By improving overall circulation to these organs, it only enhances fertility," MacDonald says. The therapy is good for women with a tilted uterus, endometriosis, fibroids, and chronic miscarriages, and men with sperm issues.

Physical Therapy for Infertility

A ten-year study of almost 1,400 women with various infertility diagnoses at one physical therapy center had the women undergo manual physical therapy, including techniques to reduce blockages and minimize adhesions, as well as manipulations to restore organ function.[16] The study found that there was a 60.85 percent rate of clearing occluded fallopian tubes, with a 56.64 percent rate of pregnancy in those patients. Patients with endometriosis experienced a 42.81 percent pregnancy rate. The success rate was 49.18 percent for lowering elevated FSH, with a 39.34 percent pregnancy rate in that group, and 53.57 percent of women in the study with PCOS achieved pregnancy. Patients who underwent IVF after the therapy reported a 56.16 percent pregnancy rate. "The manual physical therapy represented an effective, conservative treatment for women diagnosed as infertile due to mechanical causes," the study concluded.

Hypnosis for Infertility

I'm a believer in hypnosis, because over the years, my father has used it on me (to help me study better for tests in high school, run marathons after college, and most recently to help find my keys). I've never used it for fertility, but research shows an interesting effect. A small study of almost 100 women doing IVF also had them do hypnotherapy before embryo retrieval.[17] Some 53.1 percent achieved clinical pregnancy compared to 32.1 percent in the control group. The study suggests that hypnosis relaxed the uterus and reduced "uterine contractions," which are known to decrease implantation.

"We can hypothesize that hypnosis relieves the sensation of stress and thereby reduces the uterine activity and improves the interaction between the embryo and the uterus while increasing the chances of embryo implantation."

Hypnotherapist James Schwartz, founder and director of the Rocky Mountain Hypnotherapy Center in Lakewood, Colorado, and author of the book *The Mind-Body Fertility Connection: The True Pathway to Conception,*[18] says you should start hypnotherapy *before* fertility treatment, if you can: "It can sometimes enable women to conceive on their own." He says that you can do both Eastern and Western medicine at the same time, as "Mind-body healing never replaces traditional medicines; it is a complementary modality to be used in conjunction with a woman's primary practitioners."

So, Should You Find an Alternative Therapist?

First let me say that if time is of the essence—if you're older, or if you have premature ovarian failure—you might only try alternative therapies *in conjunction* with traditional medicine. If you're young and want to explore more natural modalities first, you may have some time to spare before turning to medical intervention. Conversely, many women have turned to these therapies when Western medicine had failed them.

"You have to find the right fit," Angela Le says of finding any kind of healthcare practitioner, noting there's "a lot of variation" in both the medical and wellness worlds. "It's essential to feel comfortable and safe," Le says about finding care with an experienced practitioner. "This is a very vulnerable market. Because of this, it's critical to listen to yourself."

Chapter 4

I Did It My Way: Single Mothers, LGBTQ Paths to Parenthood, and Freezing Future Fertility

> Many people ask why I didn't adopt. Would they ask a heterosexual couple that same question? Why wouldn't I want to have my own biological children? While I don't rule out adoption in the future, for me it was important to have kids with my DNA. My dad passed away when I was 15 and having my children is a way of him living on through them—literally. My family is definitely unconventional and that's awesome!
>
> —Perez Hilton[1]

I, of all people, know that life is not a storybook romance. Man can meet man, woman can meet man, woman can meet woman, a person can meet no one, and any of these combinations can have a baby: The desire to be a parent transcends gender and heteronormativity. And when it comes to fertility, nothing is normal.

There are particular challenges for people who are not Mr. and Mrs. Smith (or "Mr. and Mrs. Klein," as my conservative religious high school alumni organization insists on addressing its consistently unanswered donation request form). What does it take to have a baby on your own? What are some challenges for gay and lesbian singles and couples? If you are transgender or transitioning, what are some things you need to know about your fertility? And regardless of your sexual orientation or gender identification, how should *anyone* go about preserving their fertility?

The more different we are, I guess the more we're the same. What I've found talking to single mothers and LGBTQ and nonbinary people is that although there are some unique issues—no uterus, no eggs, no sperm, no hormones, no partner—in the end, once you go through the fertility ringer, you're equal in the eyes of bureaucracy, frustration, disappointment, and hope for achieving parenthood.

Single Motherhood by Choice

I was never sure I wanted kids, but I was pretty sure I wouldn't be able to do it on my own. The few women I knew who did, either had a lot of money or very close parents, and at the time, I had neither. I didn't have enough of a salary to afford full-time childcare while I continued to work, or a mom who would come with me to every doctor's appointment.

That's what Alyssa Shelasky's mom did. Shelasky, author of the memoir *Apron Anxiety: My Messy Affairs In and Out of the Kitchen*, *New York Magazine* columnist, and freelance writer, among other things, lived down the hall from her parents and her sister's family in a New York apartment building. "Coming from a helpful, close family—and by that I mean emotionally close and geographically close—is what ultimately made the decision a no-brainer for me."

How does a woman decide to be a single mother by choice? ("By choice" means "a single woman who decides to become a mother knowing, at least at the outset, that she will be the sole parent of her child," says Jane Mattes, founder and director of the organization Single Mothers by Choice, which has some thirty thousand members.)

Shelasky always wanted to be a writer and a mother, "but I never had the traditional, 'first comes husband, then comes babies' dream. In fact, I'd called off three engagements by the time I was thirty-five. Marriage always freaked me out for some reason I've yet to explore in therapy." After a bad breakup, she asked herself, "WHAT DO YOU WANT?!" Her answer? To be a mom.

For her, the hard part was worrying that others would pity her. But after meeting these "sexy, empowered single moms by choice," she realized, "Ohhhh, it's not like they couldn't get a man . . . it's that they didn't NEED a man." She bought sperm from California Cryobank, the largest sperm bank in America. (For more on how to choose a donor, see chapter 23.) At thirty-seven, she got pregnant with her daughter on her second IUI. "Would I have continued if there were complications? It depends. I had my mother with me at every single doctor's appointment and a village of friends supporting me all the way through. With them behind me, I think I could have handled anything emotionally or physically."

While breastfeeding her six-month-old daughter, Shelasky swiped right on Tinder . . . and found love. Now he's her daughter's father. While meeting a man was "lovely," she says, and no single mom should rule it out, "I'm not sure I can still call myself a single mom— and it's such a tribe I was proud to be part of . . . I don't want to let it go." Looks like she'll have to—after one failed round of IVF, she and her new beau got pregnant naturally, when she was forty-one. "Single moms are incredible, they are superwomen. I'll always feel emotional about the days when I made the biggest decision of my life. All those feelings are still so warm and joyful and celebratory and I see that same magical spirit every time I look at my daughter."

But not everyone is so gung-ho about single motherhood.

"That was the *only* option," says Emily, who'd never planned on being a single mother but realized in her late thirties that her dating life did not look promising. "I didn't want to leave this world without being a mother."

Emily didn't have an easy go of it, either. It took her four years, three clinics, six IUIs, five rounds of IVF, and two miscarriages—not to mention one myomectomy removing a fibroid—before she had her daughter at forty-two.

Was it difficult doing fertility treatment on her own, especially given all she went through?

"I don't have anything to compare it to," Emily says, noting that she wasn't alone because she had friends who wanted to come with her to every appointment (including a gay couple who later became her daughter's godparents). "I saw other couples go through it—they all seemed like they were having a very hard time." She often thought, "'At least I don't have anyone to put pressure on me,' and so in some ways it felt easier to do it alone."

Is it lonely being a single mom? Emily calls it an honor. "It's given me so much more than I ever dreamed of. I knew it would be great, but I didn't know it would be this fulfilling," she says. "For me it was lonelier to be single. At least with a child you have a little partner. She made me into a 'we.'"

How to Inseminate at Home

If you want to avoid the clinic, you can inseminate sperm at home with intravaginal insemination. (Some mistakenly refer to this as intracervical insemination [ICI], which is actually another in-office procedure that places the sperm near the cervix.) Here's what you should know:

1. **Make sure you are good to go:** Talk with your gynecologist to make sure everything is in working order (see chapter 2).
2. **Time your ovulation:** Chart for a couple of months and use the best ovulation predictor kits (OPKs). You need to inseminate during your fertile window.

3. **Do genetic carrier testing** with the sperm donor to make sure you are genetically compatible. (More on that in chapter 8.)

4. **Have the sperm ready and waiting in a sterile environment:**

   a. If you're using frozen donor sperm, you need to bring it to body temperature and inseminate within one hour.

   b. If you're using a known donor, sperm also must be warmed to body temp and inseminated within the hour. Make sure you have an STD report from your donor, as well as a legal agreement in place.

5. **Choose your insemination method:** You can buy cervical cap or syringe-and-soft-cup insemination kits on Amazon, or order from new companies like Mosie Baby, a syringe designed by a woman and for a woman specifically for insemination. You can also get a needleless syringe from the sperm donor clinic.

6. **Assume the position:** Lie down on a towel or on a pillow to elevate your hips. Locate your cervix and insert the sperm, following the instructions on the kit or from your donor clinic.

7. **Keep still:** Remain elevated for 15 to 30 minutes. Some say an orgasm (without penetration) will help the sperm move into the cervix.[2]

8. **Try and try again:** If you have enough sperm, two inseminations a cycle are more effective, but that's it—three inseminations have shown the same efficacy as two.

Are Two Uteri Better Than One? Lesbian Reproduction

Whether using an IUI like Alyssa or IVF like Emily, lesbians also need donor sperm to get pregnant. But in addition to questions like,

- Whose sperm to use?
- How to inseminate it?

For lesbians, it's:

- Whose eggs are being fertilized?
- Who is carrying the baby?

The simplest way to do artificial insemination is using the same woman's ovaries *and* uterus, thereby avoiding invasive and costly IVF. For Tammy and Frankie, that was a no-brainer. "I always dreamed of being pregnant, and Frankie had no interest," says Tammy, a lawyer.

In couples where both women want to experience pregnancy, childbirth, and the works, choosing who gets to be pregnant often comes down to age, health, and reproductive capabilities. "I was sad and frankly a little bit jealous that my partner got to do this," says Sandra, who, at forty-one, just didn't have good enough egg quality to do IUI, and couldn't justify (or afford) expensive IVF when her wife, seven years her junior, had seemingly perfect fertility.

There's often an emotional loss for people who need to use donor sperm or eggs. "Somehow it really just hit me: I cannot physically conceive a baby with my future wife," one woman wrote on Offbeat Home & Life, a website devoted to the nontraditional life.[3] "As much as we love each other, our physical love can never translate into a new addition to our family. We could never have a 'happy accident,' as it were."

That's why some lesbian couples decide to do reciprocal IVF (also called co-maternity or co-IVF[4]), fertilizing one partner's eggs to transfer to the other's womb. "Reciprocal IVF was perfect for us because it allowed us to both participate in the way we valued most: Katie really wanted to carry a baby, and I really wanted a biological child," Christina Bailey says of her partner, Katie, who uses the Instagram handle @babybaileymamadrama and is the purveyor of Bold

Look Apparel, which produces T-shirts printed with sayings like "My Bun" and "My Oven."

Reciprocal IVF "made sure no one was left out," Christina says about their decision to use her eggs and Katie's womb to have their two daughters. Things didn't go exactly according to plan: The donor's sperm didn't fertilize her eggs so they had to choose another one, spending a lot more than they had planned—none of it covered by insurance, of course. The biggest challenges were actually the changing emotional roles they played, with Christina taking a secondary role when Katie was pregnant and nursing.

"As babies, both girls were more attached to Katie, probably because of breastfeeding, so that can be hard for me," Christina says, noting that this might be how a father feels.

On the other hand, after the births of their two daughters, the dynamic shifted when Katie got offensive comments like how she should have her "own" baby, i.e., with her own eggs. "We know that the girls are very much Katie's, so we don't take these comments too seriously," Christina says. "We love that we both had a physical part in the journey."

Men Having Babies

For gay men, the challenges are somewhat different.

"All my patients have obstacles. Gay men have an obvious obstacle. They don't have a uterus or ovaries," says Dr. Guy Ringler, a reproductive endocrinologist at California Fertility Partners, who was one of the first fertility doctors to help gay men become parents.

The good news is that fertilizing donor eggs (with one or both partners' sperm) and transferring the embryo to a (costly) gestational surrogate (who has no genetic relation to the baby) "provides the highest pregnancy rates available," he says, estimating it at a whopping 75 to 80 percent. That's because they're selecting high-

Legally Speaking: Establishing Parentage

A birth certificate is not an establishment of parentage, says Bill Singer, Esq., partner at Singer & Fedun, a firm specializing in the creation and protection of families of all configurations. "A birth certificate is only a record of birth; it doesn't create or terminate parentage," he says, noting that laws differ by state. He says there are only a few ways to be a parent in his state: to gestate a baby, contribute genetic material, or adopt.

Legal parentage can be challenged in matters of inheritance, getting government benefits like Social Security, or traveling abroad. It can also be problematic in times of divorce. (A Florida lesbian couple doing reciprocal IVF—one woman provided the egg, the other carried the baby—were in court for years fighting over parental rights, with the birth mother claiming the genetic mom "just donated" an egg.[5])

He advises all couples using third-party reproduction to establish legal parentage either by adoption or a birth order establishing parenthood. They should make sure the donor's parental rights are terminated, he says.

People doing fertility treatments under medical supervision—IUIs, IVF, etc.—are usually protected, but for those doing at-home insemination not under medical supervision, a donor's rights may not be terminated. "The infertile person must make sure rights are properly formalized. Just because the single mother only lists her name on the birth certificate doesn't mean the sperm donor is not a [legal] dad," he says.

Although it may cost a few thousand dollars to hire a lawyer, it's better to establish parenthood in advance, he says.

quality eggs from a young woman coupled with a proven in-utero environment (professional guidelines recommend that surrogates should have already given birth).

Dr. Ringler says that as opposed to in the hetero fertility world, where IVF couples are getting older, gay couples are getting younger. "When I started twenty years ago, they were in their late forties and fifties when they had the resources to make this happen," he says. (They also might have been waiting for it to become available.) But today, with more awareness of treatment options, greater acceptance of LGBTQ issues, and greater access to resources ("I have patients whose parents are supporting them to have babies and bring grand-children into the world," he noted), his gay patients are getting "younger and younger."

Dr. Ringler says for HIV-positive men, clinical studies have estab-lished the safety of using semen samples that have been processed with a special sperm wash to separate sperm from semen and the components of semen that contain viral particles. "The sperm pro-viders should be on antiretroviral medications and have an undetect-able viral load in their serum when providing the semen specimen to be washed."

But with both gay and hetero couples, when one partner is HIV positive, "the decision of how to go about trying to conceive is going to be different for every couple," says Dr. Matthew Scherer, an infec-tious disease specialist. "If the HIV-positive person has a suppressed viral load long term, many studies have now shown that there is probably no risk of sexual transmission, so many heterosexual cou-ples are comfortable with trying timed condomless intercourse." Of course, he adds, "It always has to be an individualized decision."

Despite all these advances, it's not always easy—or cheap—for a gay couple to have a baby. Anthony and Kirk, a married Portland couple who have been blogging about their pursuit of parenthood at Two Beards and a Baby, hit a lot of hurdles since they started. First, they wanted to use a friend as an egg donor, but their clinic discour-aged it because she was over thirty. Then, none of the twenty-eight eggs retrieved from the clinic's donor became viable embryos. "We don't understand what happened—we were totally unprepared for that," Kirk says. (Welcome to the club.)

Thankfully, their clinic gave them another donor gratis, and they fertilized half the eggs with Anthony's sperm and half with Kirk's so they'd each have a biological baby, although they plan to only transfer one embryo to their surrogate at a time.

Then came the most difficult part: finding a gestational surrogate. "We knew we wanted to be a part of the pregnancy process," says Kirk, who is a therapist and is well-versed in attachment theory and how important the in-utero environment is, even from "the very first moment where the embryo connects to the human body for the first time." But when the couple's first surrogate match came through, "We weren't prepared for the costs," Kirk says, explaining that they needed to have the $60,000 in escrow to pay the surrogate fee, and didn't. With the help of two crowdfunding campaigns (which I'll talk about in chapter 7) and the nonprofit Men Having Babies, they waited for a less expensive option. "The financial piece is huge: IVF is expensive regardless, and surrogacy is expensive because you're asking someone to carry a child for nine months!"

The emotional part is also difficult. "We don't have a lot of control—we can't do anything," he says, echoing a feeling expressed by many people who go through IVF. But for them, it's worse. "While we're waiting, the world is changing dramatically," Kirk says. As LGBTQ rights change, the couple can't know how laws may affect them in the future. "That is painful."

Paving the Road to Trans Parenthood

Five years after transitioning, thirty-year-old Kaci Sullivan started trying to get pregnant with his husband. He had had a son with his first (now ex-) husband while living as a woman (his birth gender). Before he transitioned, medical professionals in Madison, Wiscon-

The Art of Co-parenting

Stewart Lewis always knew he wanted to be a father, some way, somehow.

"Obviously I wasn't going to do it conventionally," says the singer-songwriter and young adult author, who is gay. When he was thirty-six (and single), he was talking about it backstage with Katrina, a groupie-turned-friend, who offered to have his kid. "Katrina's gift is being with children, she works with children, she has children," he says. On their second at-home insemination, she got pregnant.

They both went into it with naïveté, he says—no legal agreement, nothing signed. She didn't realize how it would impact her relationship (her boyfriend left), and he didn't realize he shouldn't verbally commit to a strict lifelong visitation agreement of three weekends a month. After he got married, his husband needed to move for his job, so Stewart had to work out a new visitation agreement (summers, winter break, long vacations, etc.).

"There were some rocky parts, but it's turned out to be pretty great," he says of their teenage daughter, who he thinks is "pretty lucky" to have an unconventional family. "I think nowadays there are so many different ways to have a family."

If you're considering co-parenting, Lewis advises picking someone whose character you know deeply, who you know is "good people," so that person will inherently instill that in your child. He also suggests going into it with your eyes open, and having some sort of legal agreement in place. "You never know what life's going to throw at you."

sin, told him to freeze his eggs, but he couldn't afford it. "I also really needed to transition," he says.

The biggest misconception about transitioning, he says, is that "if we do choose to take hormones, we are told from day one that it will make us infertile. That's a blatant lie that is not backed up by science or facts."

Sullivan stopped taking testosterone for three months before he started Trying, and got pregnant six months after that. He stayed off hormones throughout his pregnancy.

As a YouTuber who has vlogged about his experience, Sullivan says he's heard from people that it can take anywhere from three months to a year off hormones to conceive.

The full effect of hormone replacement therapy on fertility is unknown, says Dr. Johanna Olson-Kennedy, medical director of the Center for Transyouth Health and Development at Children's Hospital Los Angeles. "As long as you've undergone your first, endogenous puberty, you likely still have reproductive capacity," she says.

A number of studies have shown that after stopping hormone replacement therapy (HRT) for a few months, trans women (male-to-female) can impregnate a biological woman, and trans men (female-to-male) can produce eggs and carry a pregnancy (as long as their reproductive system is intact)."On average, patients were off testosterone for four months before starting their cycle," found one study of twenty-two trans men (female-to-male).[6]

But it's not easy to stop HRT. "Let's not forget—when people make a decision to stop hormones in order to either experience pregnancy or impregnate a partner, they are likely to experience gender dysphoria," Dr. Olson-Kennedy says.

Sullivan did. "Going off hormones is always a lot harder than going back on them again. On them, everything runs better. It's like a mood stabilizer, like the brain fog has lifted. We wanted that baby, but it was a brutal pregnancy, in general," he says, noting that he didn't leave his house toward the end of the pregnancy because he was stressed out about people's reactions to seeing a pregnant man. But he viewed it as something necessary to get what he and his husband wanted. "Even though it's not the organs I'd like to have, I was still grateful: My body is so amazing, look what it's doing!"

Trans men who had babies were at increased risk of postpartum depression because of a lack of gender-sensitive resources, according to the "Men Having Babies" study.

Sullivan faced discrimination as a pregnant man—that's why he wanted a home birth. "I was trying to prevent myself from the awkwardness of gendered spaces," he says. But after a few days of labor (!!), he had to go to the hospital, where he was treated terribly. "But where's the mom?" one of the nurses said, seeing him with his new baby. "There is no mom, it's me and my husband," he told her. "She couldn't possibly process it."

Because stopping HRT can be so disruptive, many recommend fertility preservation *before* initiating transition. The World Professional Association for Transgender Health (WPATH) and the Endocrine Society recommend that all transgender people be counseled about the effect of treatment on their fertility and their options for fertility preservation before they undergo transition.[7] "Providers should offer fertility preservation options to individuals before gender transition," advises the ethics committee of the American Society for Reproductive Medicine (ASRM) in their recommendation for Access to Fertility Services by Transgender Persons.[8]

But that's not as simple as it sounds.

"If they're initiating transition in adolescence or early adulthood, reproduction is usually a lower priority than physically changing their body," says Dr. Olson-Kennedy, who counsels children and young adults from ages two to twenty-five. "At those ages they don't want to think about not starting hormones for something they feel ambivalent about in the future." The egg retrieval process is quite invasive, and even sperm retrieval can be complicated for a young person.

She says sometimes the concern over a young patient's future fertility—"What if the child changes their mind about biological children?"—is put forth as a "big obstacle" to prevent young people from transitioning.

Which is a shame, she says.

"We're trying to protect people's capacity for reproduction as well as putting a barrier in front of people before they receive services," she says. "I don't want to minimize the importance of reproduction, but I want to make sure we're not saying something that's not proven."

Sullivan says to take into consideration "that when the medical profession tells us we can't have family, that's coming from the heteronormative lens that families aren't for queer people. Right now, the majority of homosexuals struggle to adopt children."

"There's no harm in freezing sperm or eggs if you can afford it," he tells people. But he wants them to know there are always options. "I would say it's safe to trust your body a lot more than people are telling you," he says.

"Families are for everyone. Families are for queer people. And if you want a family, you should try to have one: Chances are that you can."

Fertility Preservation: Should You Freeze Your Eggs?

If you're a woman even *thinking* about getting pregnant, you've probably heard a lot about your age. When it comes to fertility, it's the age of the eggs, not the uterus, that counts. In other words, it's not *you*, it's your oocytes. Essentially, your eggs' age is the highest determining factor for a successful pregnancy. And when you choose to do "cryopreservation," you are freezing your age, is the thinking.

What is it like to freeze your eggs? It's the first half of the IVF process, so see chapter 11—but stop before the transfer.

Why do it? There are many reasons: Maybe you haven't met your partner yet and are worried about egg quality; perhaps you're with the *wrong* partner, someone who doesn't want to be a parent or wouldn't be a good one; maybe you're sick, or you're transitioning; or you simply need to postpone parenting because of school, work, or another situation (dealing with family, travel, etc.).

So should you do it? There's a long answer and a short answer. The long answer is that it depends on:

1. **Your age:** The best age to freeze your eggs is between thirty and thirty-four, according to a recent study,[9] and is most cost-effective until age thirty-seven; after that, egg quality may be a problem. "Younger is better," says Dr. James Grifo, director of the NYU Langone Fertility Center, which has birthed more than two hundred babies using frozen eggs and embryos. "I think there's an age where it's too young—the chance of using the eggs is low and the cost is high—storage cost is a factor."

2. **Your hormone level:** As mentioned in chapter 2, your hormone level (along with your antral follicle count) may predict how you'll respond to medication, how many eggs you'll get, and how many rounds you might need to do. You can also find an online egg freezing calculator that assesses, based on your age and hormone levels, how many eggs you might need for one baby.

3. **Your financial situation:** One round of egg freezing can cost over $10,000, though some companies dedicated to egg freezing like Kindbody can offer it for less. Storage can run up to $1,000 a year. Can you afford this investment? Will your company or insurance pay for any part of it? Would your parents or grandparents? (Now's the time to guilt them . . .)

4. **Your physical/emotional state:** You need about two months (they can be nonconsecutive) to do the work-up and then the egg freezing. Can you be in one place for that long? Can you do it by yourself and deal with all the emotions it might evoke? Can you handle the health risks that come with taking too many meds or something going wrong?

Two other things to consider:

    a. **Consider freezing embryos, too:** Frozen embryos (eggs inseminated with sperm) have a better success rate than frozen eggs. So if you already know who your sperm donor might be, you might consider freezing embryos.

    b. **Consider where to freeze:** There are many new companies dedicated solely to egg freezing, which might offer the procedure at a lower cost than a full-blown IVF clinic. Be sure to ask about future costs, those you might incur after the eggs have been harvested and frozen: Do they fertilize the eggs? Transfer them? How much will it cost to move them to a regular IVF clinic?

And the ultimate caveat: It might not work. Your frozen eggs may not result in a baby. There's limited data available on women using frozen eggs successfully: Some conceived naturally so they didn't need the eggs (for the first kid, anyway); others haven't tried because they're not ready; and some women who did try to conceive using frozen eggs were unable to—especially if the women were older when they froze their eggs. (The average age at which women freeze their eggs is about thirty-eight years old.[10])

"With 'fertility preservation,' I thought I could have children on my own timeline. I was wrong," Ruthie Ackerman wrote in her *New York Times* "Modern Love" column essay called "Don't Put All Your (Frozen) Eggs in One Basket."[11] The Brooklyn writer, who froze fourteen eggs in her mid-thirties, tried to use them at forty-one, to no avail.

Some women believe there's a lot of pressure—too much—on young women to freeze.

"I see mixed messages everywhere," Natalie Lampert writes in *The New Republic*. "We are told to lean in. We are told to recline. We are told we should want to have it all. We are told we cannot. We grow up using various forms of contraception, and then, when we're 'launched' into fledgling careers and relationships, we are besieged with warnings about our fading fertility and urged to consider freezing our eggs—yesterday," writes Lampert, who is writing a book on egg freezing and femtech. "If ovaries could talk, I think it's safe to say that many would be muttering in exasperation."[12]

There are plenty of people who will tell you egg freezing is anxiety-producing, a scam, hype, antifeminist, a corporate ploy to devote your life to your frozen eggs—"a bogus bribe," as an article in *The Guardian* says.[13]

Maybe it's expensive, maybe it won't work, maybe you'll never use those eggs. But still. Provided the aforementioned conditions (age, hormone level, finances especially) are right, I say, unequivocally, YES, freeze 'em.

Ask *any* woman who has had to do *any* fertility treatment, and she'll say she wishes she had frozen her eggs. Had she frozen eggs years ago, she'd have younger eggs to work with. Because a younger egg is almost always a better egg. A forty-one-year-old using eggs she froze at thirty-six is much better off than she would be using her own forty-one-year-old eggs.

Miriam froze her eggs at thirty-seven (we'll hear more about her in chapter 16). Four years later, after she got married and had a failed IVF attempt with her husband, they defrosted her eggs—and she had a baby.

Many women who ultimately don't use their frozen eggs still say they're happy that at least they did everything they could.

"As twenty- and thirtysomethings, we thought we had many years to make the decision; we went skiing, we traveled, we went to parties, we felt very young, everyone told us we looked young. You don't realize your body's not so young," says Ziva, who went back to Israel before her forty-first birthday so she'd be eligible for egg freezing. For her, the procedure was a wake-up call, and after freezing her eggs, she returned to Israel for good to have a child on her own. She didn't use her frozen eggs, but did an IUI to have her daughter. When Ziva tried to have a second child using her frozen eggs, it didn't work. Still, she doesn't view egg freezing as a failure. "It worked for me because it encouraged me to have my baby right away," she said. "If I didn't do it, I would still be waiting for Mr. Right to come."

So I say: If you can afford to freeze your eggs, do it.

Plus ça Change . . . The More They Stay the Same

Yes, we may have different genders, different sexual preferences, different partnership arrangements, and different equipment, but we are all equal in the eyes of . . . the fertility clinic.

We all have to find a way to deal with our fertility challenges: to find a good doctor, pay for treatment, deal with nosy family members and friends (without alienating all of them), manage our disappointments through setbacks—and I don't care who you are or how much money or clout you have, you are almost always going to have a setback! So before we start the nitty-gritty of treatment—where to go, how to pay for it, what to expect from it (besides a baby)—let's prepare ourselves emotionally.

Chapter 5

Regrets and All the Feels: Getting Your Emotional House in Order

> As a woman, you just think things happen naturally and
> I felt like I was damaged. . . . I felt like I was broken. I felt
> like, oh well, maybe I'm not good enough.
>
> —Emmy-winning rapper Eve

There was always a loop repeating in my head that I tortured myself with while I waited for blood work/pregnancy tests/insurance approval:

This is all your fault. This is all your fault.

Usually by "your" I meant *my.*

See, three months into our relationship, Solomon said to me, "Let's just get pregnant." In New York dating time, this was monumentally fast. But in Israeli time, it was normal.

Still, I was intrigued. I was thirty-nine (*not getting any younger,* as my religious father liked to periodically point out) and didn't like to think of myself as uber-traditional. Wouldn't it be *amazing* to walk down the aisle at my younger sister's Orthodox Jewish wedding and flaunt my big pregnant belly in the rabbi's face with *no ring*? That would show them.

In the end, my anxieties (or latent traditionalism) won out: *What if Solomon is only with you because of the baby? Don't you want him to commit his everlasting love to you first?*

I didn't go off birth control, and it took Solomon more than a year to propose, and then another three months to wed and start Trying. And then our first two natural pregnancies ended in miscarriage. I couldn't help but think, *What if that was the year that my eggs expired?*

What if we'd started trying at 39½ and not 41¼, and I had gotten pregnant then? I would have had a baby by now and no damn IVF, I thought. And:

It's all your fault, it's all your fault, it's all your fault.

On bad days, "your" also meant *his. If you hadn't waited so long to propose, we wouldn't be in this position*, I thought on those days. (TBH, I might have said it out loud once or twice.)

Strolling Down Memory Lane

We all have our spirals of self-blame. For some women, it's about not taking care of that crazy period pain sooner; for others, it's about The One That Got Away; and for a few women I've spoken to, it's an abortion in the past that keeps them up at night.

Clarissa was in graduate school and got pregnant by a guy she was casually dating. She terminated the pregnancy early on. "The timing wasn't right—was this something I wanted with a stranger?" she says. Still, after she married later in life, she "leap-frogged" over her own eggs and had a long journey with donor eggs, and she couldn't help but ruminate on the pregnancy she had terminated. "I look back on that choice and I know it might not have been a healthy baby, but I also feel like, if I hadn't done that, I'd already have a kid." It's ironic, she says: "You get pregnant when you don't want to, and when you want to, you can't."

When every doctor, nurse, and insurance rep talks about your age, it gets you thinking about all your young, unfertilized eggs, all the potential fathers you didn't marry (or let impregnate you), all the things that *might have already made you a mother* so you wouldn't be in this damn position.

When my self-flagellation about not getting knocked up at thirty-nine wasn't searing enough, I dug deeper and brought out older regrets: *What if I had slept with that guy in the bar when I was thirty-five? What if I'd married my first true love at thirty?* What if? What if? What if?

The more I tried and failed, the bigger my regrets became. *I shouldn't have gone to* that *doctor who forced me to start IVF. I shouldn't have taken* that *low-dosage medicine that wasted my eggs. I shouldn't have gone running while pregnant. I should have found out what exact genetic testing technology they used. I shouldn't have thrown out my "bad" embryos.* And on and on and on.

(If I were to perform a lobotomy on Solomon, these are the regrets I might find: *I should have slept with that woman who wanted me when I first started dating Amy. I should have ordered the pizza . . .*)

I have driven myself mad with regret. With the song of *"what if's."*

"Every feeling serves a purpose," my aunt, a therapist and also a maternal figure, loves to say.

As a Jew, I am quite familiar with guilt (and its Catholic cousin, shame), but what in God's name is the purpose of regret? To distract me from my pain? To punish me for my past sins (thanks, rabbi!)?

Just Give Me a Reason

"Regret is so cruel," says Ellen S. Glazer, a clinical social worker who specializes in infertility counseling and the author of *The Long-Awaited Stork: A Guide to Parenting After Infertility*.[1] "Sadness is horrible, anger torments—especially for people angry at themselves," she says. With other emotions accompanying infertility, like envy or helplessness, Glazer listens with compassion and sees people move forward. But regret is the most painful and debilitating. The feeling of "I should have tried ten years ago" keeps people frozen, she says.

Does it serve a purpose? I asked her.

"There's something about looking back and feeling like one has made the wrong choice," she says, "and with infertility, people have so little control, so magical thinking sets in; maybe regret serves a purpose: 'I do have some control, I somehow caused this.'"

Regret is blaming the victim: yourself. "Infertility is hard enough, and then for people to put it on themselves, that you somehow *did* it to yourself?"

It's not like the regret comes out of nowhere. There are people who delayed childbearing. There are reasons behind our feelings. But there are also *reasons* why we did what we did.

When she encounters this line of *what if* thinking, Glazer may go back in time with the person who says "I should have started ten years ago" and have them examine their thought process. She might say, "Really? But I thought you only met your husband five years ago," showing the person that if they had to make the same decision in the same circumstances, they might make the same choice all over again. "I think we all make the best decisions we can in a given time," Glazer says.

Right. Because when we imagine making a different decision, we also imagine the circumstances being different, too, and therefore, we'd have different results.

For example, what if three months into my relationship with Solomon, I *had* stopped using birth control—and gotten pregnant? If I still had my same reproductive health, I'd have miscarried twice. Then what? Would my burgeoning relationship have been able to handle the weight of *that*? I doubt it. He might have been thinking, *Why should I do this with someone who can't have children? She's too old for me, I'm outta here!* (He later told me he did have some fleeting mean thoughts of, *What have I gotten myself into?* but they passed. Besides we were married. He was *stuck*. Sucker!)

Going back further, if I'd gotten knocked up by a rando at a bar, I probably would have done what Clarissa did. And if I'd married my first love at thirty, maybe I'd have a couple of kids, but I'd likely also be divorced, stuck in the suburbs, without a career.

In other words, I'd have made exactly the same choices.

So the path down regret lane is filled with dead ends.

There is one way regret can help, Glazer says: in the case of "future regret." She remembers a couple where the woman wanted children and the man didn't, an impasse if ever there was one. One day the husband shocked the both of them and said he would have a child. "If I say no to this, there's no way our marriage could survive, and I'll always regret that. I know my wife will be a wonderful mother and there's a chance it will be fine for me." The couple went on to adopt three children. And he was overjoyed.

If you can think of something *now* that you might regret in the future—starting IVF, freezing more eggs, having a baby on your own, this is the moment to take action.

Stress and Fertility

While we're on the subject of self-blame, let's talk about stress and fertility.

Forget about the people who say, "Just relax and you'll get pregnant." I mean, literally *forget they ever existed*. Like, if that's their starting gambit, it won't get any prettier. They'll regale you with stories of their best friend's veterinarian's aunt's lover's niece who had been trying forever—*She did forty-five rounds of IVF! Drank witches' blood! Took a vow of celibacy!*—and when she stopped everything, stopped thinking about it, lo and behold, she got pregnant.

When someone said, "just relax," I thought: *Now you're telling me that my own stress is causing this lack of a baby? Are you saying this infertility is* my fault? *That if I weren't so GODDAMNED STRESSED OUT ALL THE TIME I WOULD BE @#$@# PREGNANT????* (They usually ran for the hills at that point, planning not to return till I gave birth.)

Listen: When I was interminably single, people kept telling me to "stop focusing on finding the one and it'll happen . . ." You know what happened when I stopped focusing on dating? I got off all the dating websites, hung out with my girlfriends, read lots of books, and grew cobwebs down there. It was only when I decided to leave Los Angeles and move to New York in order to find a husband that I met Solomon.

So I don't buy that simply "not focusing" on conceiving is the magic pill.

Still, I want to investigate the science behind stress and its relationship to infertility.

"The relationship between stress and infertility has been debated for years," begins a study in *Clinical Neuroscience*.[2] "Women with infertility report elevated levels of anxiety and depression, so it is clear that infertility causes stress." DUH. The study goes on to say that women who struggle to conceive are twice as likely to suffer from emotional distress than fertile women.[3]

"What is less clear, however, is whether or not stress causes infertility," the authors note, saying it's impossible to prove the causality because it's based on people self-reporting, and also because people feel really optimistic at the start (as you should!). So is the stress causing the infertility or is the infertility—and its failure—causing people to feel disappointed . . . and stressed?

Some studies show a physiological relationship between stress and time to pregnancy, and one study notes that "Interventions to reduce cortisol prior to commencing IVF could improve treatment outcomes."[4]

"You need a healthy body and a healthy mind," says Dr. Amy Beckley, creator of the at-home progesterone test Proov. "Our cortisol steals from our reproductive system, so if you're too stressed, your body says, 'We do not believe you can carry a child to term,' and turns the needed progesterone into cortisol, a stress hormone." She hates when doctors say, "Just don't think about it." She says, "You have to take actions to manage your stress."

But can we really moderate our stress levels?

I spoke to Tamar Ben-Shaanan, a microbiologist and immunologist studying mice with tumors. In a study published in *Nature,* Ben-Shaanan and her colleagues found that "activating the reward center" in the mouse's brain reduced the tumor, and concluded that "a patient's psychological state can impact anti-tumor immunity and cancer progression."[5] Some recurrent loss specialists concluded that this would be a good line of treatment for people who fail IVF cycles: "It may be a great first step in a new protocol for IVF patients to focus on creating an environment that would lead to activation of this reward system," they write, encouraging patients to do "activities that create enjoyment" and establish a "positive environment."

Ben-Shaanan, who was not involved in that repeat loss study, told me, "It's not a one-to-one ratio: The way our neurocircuitry reacts to our situations in life can perhaps have an impact. It may be hardwired." In other words: We may *not* have as much control over our stress as we want.

Of course, there's also a lot of research showing stress has no effect on fertility. As I always say: Correlation is not causation. Yes, of course infertility causes stress. How can it not? Everyone telling you to "just relax" should try living a normal, happy life while waiting every second for a much-wanted event that hasn't yet happened and they can't be sure ever will. Of course infertility is stressful. Just *please* don't tell me it causes infertility.

"While infertility causes stress, research shows it's not vice versa," says Dr. Janelle Luk of Generation Next Fertility. "Everyone's stressed out, so it's a silly statement," she says. "It's like saying, 'Don't eat without biting the food.' "

In fact, total fertility rates are often highest in countries that experience the harsh conditions of war, poverty, and famine. In an analysis of fourteen studies of 3,583 infertile women, researchers concluded: "Emotional distress caused by fertility problems or other life events co-occurring with treatment will not compromise the chance of becoming pregnant."[6]

Dr. Luk says, "Going through infertility treatment can be a high-stress event for most women, especially if they have been trying for a while." She notes that while stress can cause menstrual and hormonal changes, "these changes are usually self-correcting and do not have any permanent impact on fertility." So if, for example, you're so stressed that you're not ovulating, that can be fixed. If you're so stressed that you're not sleeping, eating properly, or exercising—well, that can be fixed, too. And fixing those situations will probably help your fertility.

Still, there is one concrete way stress can affect fertility: "Sometimes if you're so stressed out, you might not continue treatment," Dr. Luk says. In fact, in one study, 26 percent of couples ended treatment early because of psychological stress.[7]

Let's face it: Trying is stressful. Infertility is stressful. If you need to take a break to manage your stress, that's okay. And if you need to stop entirely, that's also okay. (See chapter 24 for more about ending treatment.)

In the end, it's important to manage your stress, especially if you decide to stay in treatment. And also, to feel better.

The Problem with "Why Don't You Just Adopt?"

"Maybe all the wealthy parents who can't have kids should adopt the 7+ kids being raised in homeless shelters. Everyone wins . . ."

one commenter of many wrote on one of my *New York Times* "Fertility Diary" columns.

People love to say this to people doing fertility treatment. While I can understand the sentiment, there are so many things wrong with the statement:

1. **Adoption is not cheap or easy.**
Marta is pursing adoption while doing IVF just in case it doesn't work out. But the Florida woman is "flabbergasted" by how hard adoption is. She went through the foster care course but realized the state favors family reunification. Private adoption is no better, with agencies charging tens of thousands of dollars to support the pregnant birth mother with no guarantee for a baby. "Anyone who says 'just adopt,' has no idea what it's like," she says. "It's wild."

2. **People adopt for many reasons.**
While some people choose adoption primarily because they want to help children in need, many choose to adopt after infertility. Consider that more than half the women diagnosed as infertile consider adoption, and women who have used fertility services are ten times more likely to adopt than those who have not, according to the CDC.[8]

3. **Whose responsibility is it to adopt?**
There are more parents wanting to adopt than children available. If there are children needing homes, it's not the infertile couple's responsibility to take care of these kids—it's everyone's!

4. **Why is it okay for *you* to want biological children but not me?**
It's a natural impulse to want to have biological children. You did it—so why can't I . . . even if it might be harder for me? (And if you don't think *anyone* should have children, because of the environment or overpopulation or yada yada yada, well, I guess we have nothing to talk about.)

#TryingNotTrying

You know what really stresses me out? All the stories of people who stopped Trying—who chucked their meds, traveled the world, started the adoption process—and then, lo and behold . . . got pregnant.

"Those are the most annoying stories in the world," says Marc Sherman. "It makes you think that you are part of the problem, that you have to give up on what you want to get what you want." The people who say "just adopt" are the worst, he says, because they don't understand you have to reconfigure your entire journey.

But in the eight and a half years he and his wife, Erin, were Trying, that's *exactly* what happened to them. The first time was after four and a half years, when they were told they'd need IVF. "My wife doesn't even take Advil, and she was completely overwhelmed," he says. They decided IVF was not for them. Thinking, *Let's just get back to life,* they bought a boat, then a Jeep, "went off the deep end," and then . . . found themselves pregnant.

Flash forward a few years: After not getting pregnant again, the Shermans started the adoption process—going as far as to meet with the expecting couple and telling them how much they love being parents—only to find themselves pregnant *again*. (When they called the adoption agency to withdraw the adoption application, the agency told them the birth parents had decided to keep their baby *after they saw how much the Shermans loved being parents.*)

Marc says they kept hearing stories of these "accidental conceptions" from people who had stopped trying and realized that many of their journeys were similar—and now they want to help people mimic that "letting go" state.

To help them conceive?

Maybe—that's not really the point of their company, Organic Conceptions, which offers seven-hour online courses as well as training for medical professionals to help them care for their patients. They want to help couples take back control of their fertility journey, to help them figure out where they are and "optimize their emotional health to determine the best path forward," he says.

When you start Googling "getting pregnant naturally" or "do I need IVF?" or "does stress cause infertility?" you'll find that there's no shortage of people and programs offering to align your emotional and inner self, remove stress, and maybe, just maybe, help you conceive (no promises).

"In addition to collaborating with our healthcare providers and undergoing necessary testing, it's also crucial that we engage fully in our own healing," says Julia Indichova, founder of the Fertile Heart program and author of *Inconceivable: A Woman's Triumph over Despair and Statistics*, which chronicles her own journey to combat secondary infertility (a term that refers to a woman who's already had children and struggles to conceive again). She's worked with thousands of women over the years, using mind-body tools, movement sequences, diet, supplements, and more. "The aim of the practice is to identify what it is that is blocking conception and a full-term pregnancy on a physical, emotional, and spiritual level for women and couples who are on a path to parenting. Most important, it's about recognizing what is stopping them from birthing the family they long for," she says.

I didn't use either of their programs, but I *did* go to a Reiki healer—twice!!—while doing IVF. She told me that I was "blocked" in my uterine area and that I had "negative energy toward motherhood." *Duh, have you ever met my family?*

What I needed to do, she said, was meditate on what it meant to be a mother to connect the feeling of motherhood with positive energy. I couldn't help but feel angry: *So I had a bad childhood and now I'm being punished for it by not being able to be a mother?*

"Never, never, never, never blame yourself. You'd be giving yourself too much credit," Indichova says, noting that her work is about "radical compassion. Self-blame could never fit into that model."

Dear Reader, I did what that Reiki healer said: I tried to envision becoming pregnant, infusing my belly with warmth, connecting to powerful mother figures—I even made all my mom friends write me letters about why I'd be a good mom! I did it all. And still, I did not get pregnant. And when I did, with treatment, I did not *stay* pregnant. Turns out, I wasn't going to be one of those success stories of natural conception, before, during, or after treatment.

Maybe those emotional programs don't work for people with serious medical issues. Maybe they wouldn't work for someone with no tubes, undetectable AMH, repeat loss, low sperm count, or other medical issues.

On the other hand, doctors are awfully quick to dispense the "unexplained infertility" diagnosis. It's not like *they* always know what they're doing, either. If that's your situation, maybe you want to try one of these alternative programs. I've heard too many "oops!" stories to discount them.

"Incorporating psychological interventions into routine practice at [fertility] clinics is beneficial," that study on stress and infertility concluded. "It is clear that psychological interventions for women with infertility have the potential to decrease anxiety and depression and may well lead to significantly higher pregnancy rates."

Find Your People

Psychological interventions "may well" help you get pregnant—or they may not. This whole line of thinking may make you as stressed AF.

That's how it felt to journalist Katy Lindemann, who has been through four IVF cycles, seven canceled ones, and two hysteroscopies—and still no baby. "It's fine to say 'relax' for your mental health; but saying that negative thinking is stopping you from getting pregnant or your mental state is having something to do with outcomes is really pernicious." And it's fine if your "well-intentioned but desperately unhelpful" friends say it, because they don't know any better, but it's "downright cruel" when fertility clinics promote it. "If treatment fails, you've only got yourself to blame," Lindemann says.

During Lindemann's treatment, she was disheartened by all the "rah-rah" messaging she saw on fertility boards and groups. She wrote a Medium post called "Infertility and the Tyranny of Positivity."[9]

What's wrong with so much positivity?

Nothing, she says, unless "it's the only way: If you're not Pollyanna Positivity, then you're wrong or it's bad," she says. "It also glosses over the reality of what it's like, because that's not how it is for most people: You're feeling like shit, you're angry and frustrated. It glosses over the reality of all the messy stuff. And it puts the blame on you for not being positive enough."

Lindemann surveyed five hundred women for her blog uberbarrens .club, where people said things like, "I want to read others' experiences that aren't all positive," and "I want to see what it's really like." She says many people have a real desire to hear the truth, not throw a blanket over the reality.

Look, when I started, all the positivity didn't bother me. But as time went on and I kept failing to get pregnant, I longed for a place to shout out my frustration. The trick is to find what works for you, Lindemann says. "Whatever helps you to get through."

You know what they say: Different fertility strokes for different fertility folks.

"Find your people—find the people that gel with you," Lindemann says. You'll probably have to forgive your friends—and that annoying coworker. "People mean well. No one means to be insensitive, or to get it wrong," Lindemann says, because people *want* to support you. And it's our job to help them get it right. "You need to say, 'This is what I need, and this is what I don't need,'" she says. "People aren't psychic."

So find your online friends, your offline friends, and your family, and get ready to start treatment.

Section II

LET'S GET PHYSICAL
(AND TECHNICAL)

Chapter 6

So Many Doctors, So Little Time: How to Find the Right Clinic

I'm in the rooms with the women and there is such a shroud of secrecy and shame. I mean, there's back entrances, there are people who will come get you from your car with an umbrella. The idea of being found out, like going to a fertility doctor? Oh my god, the jig is up.

—Gabrielle Union[1]

I'm embarrassed to admit that the first time I sought out an OB, I simply picked the one closest to my house. Oh, the OB had other qualifications aside from location: She was a woman. And her name sounded really Jewish—this wasn't as much a qualification as a bonus: I thought having a warm, *yiddishe* mama would be a good way to nurture my pregnancy.

Boy, was I wrong. Yes, she was Jewish, but she was not warm. Yes, she was nearby, but she was not a very good doctor. (She should've taken one look at my age and my early miscarriage and sent me straight to a fertility clinic.)

So when the time came to find a reproductive endocrinologist, you can bet I *tried* to do my research.

But what was I supposed to look for? "Female doctor near me" was clearly the wrong criteria. And who was I supposed to ask? People I knew were not talking about infertility, miscarriage, or how long they tried before they conceived their wonderful bundle of joy.

Online was no better, with doctors and clinic names being thrown about on discussion boards like they were Amazon product reviews. With fertility, it seemed people either loved or hated their clinic— with nothing in between.

"I think word of mouth is an incredibly valuable way to find a doctor," says Dr. Jennifer Hirshfeld-Cytron of Fertility Centers of Illinois.

Being the good, persistent journalist that I am, I sought out anyone I could find who might have had a doctor to recommend. I figured my investigations were coming to a close when one clinic's name kept popping up. I decided to make an appointment.

"In *how* many weeks?" I asked the receptionist when she finally answered the phone. I'd thought she said the next available new-patient appointment was in eight weeks, but that couldn't have been right.

It was.

For most people, finding a reproductive endocrinologist isn't like finding a college, where you visit different universities, meet with students and teachers, ask questions, and then pick one based on complex algorithms such as Best Party School and who will give you financial aid. It's not even like shopping around for a doctor in another field, where you might interview a few, hear their diagnosis, ask pointed questions, and decide if you want to commit to an expensive treatment with them. It often takes months to get an appointment with a specific RE, and those initial appointments can be expensive (my first one was $800), not to mention inconvenient (why, *yes*, I can take three hours out of my busy day to trek across town to see you . . .). Many people do not shop around for their first doctor, and their first doctor is the first one they go to.

CAVEAT: If your insurance covers multiple consultations and you're not in a super hurry, you can interview at a few different clinics. (You can learn more about insurance in chapter 7 and what to ask doctors you're interviewing in chapter 8.)

The vast majority of people do what I did: They ask their friends, or friends' friends—having no clue exactly what to ask them—and a couple of months later they find themselves face-to-face with a perfect stranger quizzing them about their menstrual cycles, thinking, *How did I get here?*

You don't want to be thinking that. Actually, I won't *let* you think that.

You want to be an educated consumer, so you have to do your research *before* your consultation. Because it may be less of a consultation than a plan to start treatment.

Four Out of Five Patients Recommend Their Doctor

When Jake and Deborah Anderson-Bialis were having fertility troubles in their twenties, the San Francisco tech couple found that talking to their young, carefree friends was no help, and neither was talking to strangers. "We just felt like we had nothing in common with the people we talked to about where they got treated," says Jake. "We had a different budget, a different timeline, and ultimately, we were hearing from people who had different issues and a different sensibility." After visiting three different clinics in three different states, "money flying out the door," they felt like "patients on a conveyor belt," referring to the factory-like, one-size-fits-all treatment they received. "We were unable to form an opinion as patients."

They decided they needed to help people like themselves— actually, people *unlike* themselves in every way: all types of people experiencing infertility, but from a different part of the country, or at a different age, or with a different diagnosis. Jake and Deb started gathering reviews from patients all over the country.

They founded FertilityIQ, an education site for patients that also rates doctors and clinics. (Patients can rate doctors on everything from their bedside manner to their communication style, from whether you see them at appointments to their response time.)

Jake says people are overwhelmed, thinking, *I have a lot of data, but how do I sift through it? What's relevant? What applies to me and what doesn't?*

When I plug my zip code into FertilityIQ, I still come up with dozens and dozens of doctors. How could I just pick one?

"Fertility doctors are very different. Not everyone is going to practice medicine the same way," he says, which might sound obvious, but come to think of it, that's exactly the opposite of what I thought when I was trying to find a clinic—*How different could they be?*

He says big cities are similar because most have between two and ten clinics of different types, like two large private clinics, two academic centers, and a bunch of individual practitioners. Here are some ways to classify clinics:

- **Academic vs. Private:** Academic centers are not motivated by profit, but the doctors there might also be committed to research, so you might see less of them. At a private clinic, you might see your doc more, but you should keep in mind that it's a business.
- **Big vs. Small:** Take a look at a clinic's website and see how many doctors they employ. Big clinics *do* have more doctors, more embryologists, more patients, more cycles, so they have more expertise.

"At a clinic of our size—a high-volume clinic—where we see three thousand cases a year, we are open the whole week and don't need to time treatments on an arbitrary schedule," says Dr. Owen Davis of Weill Cornell Medicine about a cycle appointment. (Some clinics might schedule their retrievals and transfers for a weekday.) "There's virtually no clinical situation we haven't seen," says Dr. Davis, who calls Cornell a "tertiary" practice, where many patients come after they've failed at other clinics. Larger centers "generally have more experience," he says. Also, they have a bigger team of doctors, who meet weekly with the lab people and sometimes psychologists to discuss cases. "We're operating as a team, not in a vacuum," he says.

Still, he concedes that bigger is not necessarily better.

"An intimate program can be nice from an emotional standpoint: One can potentially see one's own doctor every day, there's a quieter waiting room, and it could be a good thing from a quality of life standpoint," and, he allows, "if they have a good lab, you can be very well served." (We'll talk more about labs in chapter 8.)

A smaller clinic can also be more flexible, says Dr. Luk from Generation Next Fertility, which has two primary doctors. "We don't have to follow one standard, 'this is how we do things here,'" she says about following one medical protocol. "You're not treated like a number."

- **Star Clinics vs. Small Clinics:** Some small clinics might also be what I'll call "star" clinics—where the practice is set up around one main player. This doc might be a specialist among specialists, focusing on a certain type of patient. Star clinics may not have a whole team like the big centers, but they have a concentration of patients with your diagnosis. Because of their high volume, they may be as busy as the big places. But if the doctor is out or leaves, the practice may not survive.

- **Location, Location, Location:** For some people, location can make all the difference—especially since you'll be there half a dozen times per cycle. "The traveling made it a very grueling process," says patient Jennifer Lowright, who commuted an hour and a half from the suburbs to Chicago for her appointments—not to mention parking and waiting for the doctor. She didn't think she had the option of

Do You Need a Female Fertility Doctor?

I went through IVF and I think that it really did make me a more empathetic doctor. Patients will say to me, "Doctor, I'm so glad you're doing this ultrasound," because a man can be rough with it (not on purpose) or they'll say, "It's hard to talk to the guy about what's going on with my bleeding." It takes a really, really special man to be able to do this.

—*Dr. Lora Shahine, Pacific NW Fertility*

I'd like to think that being a woman can be an advantage. I think the most important thing is that a patient has a good rapport with an RE who they trust, who listens to their concerns, and who provides the highest-quality care consistent with her needs. I'm sure some women prefer a woman and others prefer a man, and I don't think being a parent should matter.

—*Dr. Jessica Brown, NYU Langone*

I don't believe in the idea of only seeking a female RE, because male physicians are just as capable of offering supportive and nurturing care. Many male REs have been through the struggle of infertility themselves so they can connect with both men *and* woman during an emotionally difficult time. On the flip side, there are some aspects of what we do that are likely more understood by a woman, for example, fertility preservation and the inherent want to "stop" the clock. Male or female, the most important aspect of finding the right doctor is ensuring you have a partner that shares common goals in care and communication in this, the most important journey of your life.

—*Dr. Anate Brauer, Shady Grove Fertility*

changing clinics—as she put it, "That's where my 'babies' were," meaning her embryos. But after two failed transfers, she decided to take a break. A year later, she visited another local center—and fell in love with her doctor, who had gone through infertility herself.

Not everyone is located in a big city with a variety of choices. "I didn't really shop around," says Vicki, who lives in Seattle, where there are just five clinics—only two of which took her insurance. "My OB/GYN recommended one of them," she says.

Some cities have even fewer clinics. Hawaii has four, Oregon has two (both in Portland), North Dakota has one (in Fargo), and Wyoming has none. (In that situation, you can either go to the clinic in closest flying distance or, since you're already traveling, you can go to the best clinic.) California, by the way, has over seventy clinics, and Texas and New York both have more than forty.

Bedside Manner: Does It Matter?

Whether you're looking at a website or asking your friends, you might want to ask specific questions about the doctor. What is she like? Does he take time to explain things to you? Will you be able to see her or get in touch with her when you need to? Does he *really* care about your case?

But you also have to know yourself.

"I needed someone who would listen to me and answer all the questions I have. I needed someone I could be comfortable with, who clicks, personality-wise, and has time for me," says Lowright. "I'm not going to settle: I've fired a lot of doctors and I've moved on when I wasn't happy."

I once saw my last fertility doc, Dr. Jeffrey Braverman, cry about another patient who had failed. I saw *tears* in his eyes. These are all the things that go into "bedside manner." (More about Dr. Braverman in chapter 22.)

"It's our job to prepare the patient, and I think it's incredibly important they feel that we are taking care of them," says Dr. Cytron. "The patient is driving the boat and we are the crew," she says. She compares it to a cardiologist: If he tells you to do a stent, you'll do a stent. "We don't direct people—with fertility, people want to be informed about the treatment, the protocol, the advantages, the costs, the side effects." Besides, she says, since many clinics offer similar standards of care, "it's on us clinics to get to know our patients as people." Otherwise, you can find a place that does.

Some people don't care about bedside manner. "Where I'm from, the bigger asshole the doctor is, the better," a friend of mine from Europe said. "I just want him to get me pregnant."

FertilityIQ's Jake Anderson-Bialis says he sees "zero correlation between a doctor's bedside manner and the quality of care they practice." He also says that these days, you don't have to choose between bedside manner and quality. You can have both.

A 2019 Pregnantish survey, "Why I Left My Fertility Doctor," of more than a thousand women (average age: thirty-three) found that the top reasons patients leave a fertility doctor isn't because of success or lack of it (baby), but how they connect with their RE and the clinic. "Many concerns with treatment are related to how infertility doctors and treatment teams manage the emotional components of infertility treatment, not merely how successful the treatment is."[2] Pregnantish plans to provide patient feedback to clinics to help improve the patient/provider relationship, so that the clinics have higher retention rates and the patients' voices are heard.

Maybe in the olden days, it was okay for a doctor to be . . . well, a jerk. But these days, they know they're getting online reviews.

Interestingly, in asking the basic question, "Do you recommend this doctor?" FertilityIQ discovered that, yes, women tend to recommend doctors who get them pregnant, but short of that, doctors who treated their patients more like humans than numbers would often still get a recommendation *even if* the patient ultimately failed to conceive.

During my years of infertility, there were doctors who did not get me a baby (most of them, actually), but I loved them for their attention, kindness, and for making me feel like a person even though I wasn't a mom.

One of the main reasons to find a doctor you like is that you might be with her for a while. Anderson-Bialis notes that the average patient needs two to three cycles to get pregnant, and one of the biggest problems in the field is patients stopping treatment too soon. According to a JAMA study, 65 percent of women get pregnant after six cycles (!!).[3] "For some couples," the study says, "the emotional stress of repeat treatments may be undesirable. However, we think the potential for success with further cycles should be discussed with couples." For fertility treatment to work, especially after one round of treatment fails, Anderson-Bialis says, "People need to continue treatment. If they leave the doctor, there's a very good chance they don't try again at that clinic, or *any* clinic, for that matter."

I Shoulda Been a Statistician

Success. That should be the best way to measure—and find—a doctor. The one who is most likely to get you pregnant, right?

The Society for Assisted Reproductive Technology (SART), established to maintain the standards for the field, provides success rates on their website of reporting clinics (some 90 percent of clinics across the United States)[4] Just plug in your zip, and voilà! You can compare the success rates of each clinic, sorted by category, such as age or diagnosis.

"Just pick the one with the highest success rates!" says Solomon, who studied statistics during his MBA (file under "Things He Didn't Mention on Our First Date").

Not so fast, Anderson-Bialis says. Some clinics take harder cases,

Humor: What Are You Looking for in a Clinic?

1. When I go to a doctor, I want to
   a. know he's the best by his swagger and refusal to answer questions.
   b. understand her time is so precious by how often we're interrupted.
   c. feel like he's my best friend forever.

2. I'm looking for a doctor who
   a. is young.
   b. is a woman.
   c. is human.

3. My doctor's office can be
   a. on the other side of town—who needs to work anyway?
   b. a state-of-the-art facility paved with the gold of all its clients.
   c. an eternal wait, as long as they serve coffee.

4. I expect the nursing staff to
   a. smile when I come in.
   b. look at me when I talk.
   c. not bite my head off.

5. Things I'd like in the waiting room:
   a. coffee and tea
   b. Wi-Fi
   c. chairs

6. My preferred mode of communication is
   a. furtive phone calls at work with no callback number.
   b. long-winded and unclear medication instructions left on my voice mail.
   c. three emails from different nurses all contradicting one another.

so their success rates will naturally be lower, while others turn away patients with poor prognoses so they can keep their numbers high.

SART agrees: "The data presented in this report should not be used for comparing clinics," reads the pop-up window on their website. "Clinics may have differences in patient selection, treatment approaches, and cycle reporting practices which may inflate or lower pregnancy rates relative to another clinic. Please discuss this with your doctor."

So what are the reporting numbers good for? "Quality assurance," says Dr. Kevin Doody, a former president of SART. "We use our data not only for public reporting, but making sure patients get the best possible care," he said, adding that it is meant to keep clinics honest. Dr. Doody also notes that you can compare an individual clinic's statistics with the national averages to see if they fall within range. You can also use the SART stats to tell how big and busy a clinic is. SART doesn't count patients; they count cycles. But if you look at how many cycles a clinic does per year, you can get a sense of the size of their practice. You can also get a sense of what they specialize in.

So would you rather go to a clinic that only takes the most promising patients, or a clinic that takes everyone?

"You have to be frank with patients," Cornell's Dr. Davis says. "You have to be honest where you've had success—it's reasonable to share that." You can also look at a clinic's own website to see the number of doctors employed there, their specialties, and the clinic's philosophy. (*We are super-busy, with long waiting hours and terrible bedside manner, but we'll try to get you pregnant anyway . . .*" says no website ever.)

I personally love to judge books by their covers. I don't want a scary-looking doctor up in my biz, unless perhaps a friend forewarned me, "He's a bit weird-looking, but he's got a wonderful personality *and* success rate!" I always go to the clinic's website to see photos. Yeah, I know, we're not dating here, even if the search for a doc sometimes feels the same.

Tips on Finding a Fertility Doc

1. **ASK** your gynecologist and primary care doctor: Medical professionals are often in the know.
2. **SEE** which doctors are covered by your insurance: Some insurers only cover certain clinics, and that will probably narrow down your choices.
3. **TALK** to anyone you think took a long time to get pregnant or might have had fertility issues. Call her and ask about her doctor's bedside manner and level of information giving (or mansplaining), how often they saw the doctor, the office communications, and the doctor's ability to think outside the box.
4. **CHECK OUT** SART's list of clinics to find one in your area. If time is an issue, look for the ones that are easiest for you to get to. If you're a statistician or married to one, analyze their numbers.
5. **VISIT** sites like FertilityIQ.com, which rates and reviews many doctors, assessing everything from their bedside manner to their office wait times.
6. **JOIN** fertility forums on Facebook, like Matt and Doree's Egg-cellent Adventure or IVF for Women Over 40.
7. **CALL** doctor's offices. See how long it might take to get a new patient appointment.
8. **PREPARE** for your visit. Bring all the tests you've had done (see chapter 2), plus a list of your questions for the doctor.

How Much Information Is TMI?

Talking to people, finding recommendations, and sifting through all the information available online—even *with* helpful sites like FertilityIQ and Healthgrades—it's overwhelming. It is. How much are we, as patients, really supposed to know and research?

"You gotta do your homework," Anderson-Bialis says. "It's easy to abdicate responsibility, to feel that it's someone else's job to explain it to you." He admits he was more like me at first, hoping it was the doctors' job to lead the way. "I've had a change of view," he says. He learned from his wife and company co-founder, Deb, who had more history with the healthcare system and whose family often sought second opinions, that it's up to the patient to be informed. "You have to be a tough, discerning customer," he says.

Dr. Davis adds: "Anyone practicing in any area of medicine should appreciate the possibility of patients wanting to get another opinion."

I'm new to infertility/this city/this diagnosis, someone invariably posts in one of the Facebook infertility group or subgroups I belong to. *Which doctor do you recommend?*

In the end, I don't think there's one doctor or clinic for everyone. (Thank God, because that doc would be even busier than she is today!) For my friend at the end of her rope who has been to four clinics and tried every protocol, I'll recommend the most experimental clinic. And for the woman who's been trying for a year but never had a basic workup done, I'll suggest a small practice run by a cautious RE who I know won't force her into invasive treatment too soon.

As you do your research, one or two doctors' names will keep coming up—and you'll see if they're in network and/or in your neighborhood (or maybe even near your workplace). You'll ask your friends questions, read the doctors' reviews, make an informed decision—and then make an appointment.

And then you'll wait.

Chapter 7

Money, Money, Money

If you do run into struggles, don't give up. IVF, egg freezing, surrogates, adoption—it can all sound overwhelming *and* expensive. But there are ways to find the funds,
from financing to loans. So don't panic. There are *always*
options.

—*Real Housewives of Atlanta*'s Kenya Moore[1]

"Promise me this is not about the money," Solomon begged when I
told him I wanted to start IVF at a different clinic than the one we
were at for IUIs. I'd heard about this new fertility clinic from friends,
who said that it specialized in a lower-medication treatment. Yeah, I
loved the idea of putting fewer hormones in my body—but I'd be
lying if I didn't say it *was* about the money: At this new clinic, it was
$5,000 for one round of IVF, versus $18,000 at my current clinic.

Whoever says, "Money is no object" is someone for whom . . .
money is no object. That, unfortunately, was not us. I'd left the rat

race to pursue freelance journalism, and living in New York City on one perma-salary and my freelance salary didn't leave us with an extra $20,000 lying around.

And that twenty grand would cover only *one* try. I was hoping that would be enough, but I was beginning to suspect it might take longer. Especially since patients usually go through an average of two to three cycles, and may need up to six.

"Maybe we should budget for three IVF cycles *just in case*," my ever-realistic husband had said before we started. At the new clinic, three rounds would cost $15,000, versus $60,000 at my current one. Sixty Gs was *not* in our price range.

How Much Is That Baby in the Window?

Does having a baby really come down to money? It's so unfair—no, outrageous!—that having a baby could be determined by something as prosaic as cold hard cash. (Oh, no worries, they take credit, too.)

"Money is one of the most undiscussed topics of infertility," says Anna Almendrala, a freelance health reporter and formerly the host of *IVFML*, a *Huffington Post* podcast that focused on fertility treatment. "Everybody needs to be more transparent about the money they're using to fund these fertility odysseys," she says. Her first fertility treatment go-round—three IUIs, two IVF transfers, two miscarriages—gave them one daughter. "People are confused—how are people like us paying for it?"

By "people like us," she means people overeducated enough to *know* about IVF but not rich enough to *pay* for it.

It's a common trope that fertility treatment is for older women who waited too long to have children, but one study showed that more than 40 percent of cycles were undergone by women younger than thirty-five.

But the money topic is always there. I once mentioned in my weekly *New York Times* column that, after being told I was miscarrying *but the baby was still inside me,* I went to a spa—and got blasted in the comments section for my "extravagant" ways. (*Poor Amy is going to a fancy spa,* wrote one person.) I neglected to mention in the column that this "spa" was actually Spa Castle, a cheesy structure with indoor and outdoor Jacuzzis populated by rambunctious kids and couples making out. BTW, it cost about $35 ($25 with a Groupon).

Still, because of its sticker price, it's easy to believe that fertility treatment is only for the wealthy: An IUI with medication can cost $2,000 to $4,000,[2] and the national average for one IVF cycle is about $20,000. (FYI: Whatever you think IVF is going to cost, add a third more to that to account for unexpected add-ons, like a laparoscopy or other last-minute surgery.)

Some people hear about these prices and throw up their hands. "I'd had two miscarriages, and, well, fertility treatment just wasn't an option for us," says Natasha, who, now forty-nine, might pursue adoption.

A survey of 858 men and women conducted by CoFertility, a website "answering all your fertility questions," found that 86 percent of respondents would forgo fertility treatment *recommended by their doctor* due to costs.[3]

But fertility treatment need not only be for celebrities and other lucky people who think $100,000 is chump change.

First, you may not have too long a road ahead of you. Perhaps they'll unblock a tube and *voilà!*—you'll get preggers. Maybe your first medicated IUI will work and you can use this chapter to wrap your baby's diapers. Or maybe a long-lost uncle will die and leave you an inheritance.

That's kind of how Almendrala paid for it. "My husband is wealthy," she said unapologetically. I asked her how they approached his parents for money, thinking how difficult it was for us to approach *our* parents for money. Was it hard for Almendrala and her husband, too? Almendrala said no: "He inherited money from a deceased grandparent." I admired her candor.

After six years of failed IVF, singer/songwriter/storyteller Sam

Creative Ways to Fund Fertility

For those of us who don't have inheritances, there are ways to mitigate the costs of fertility treatment.

1. **GET** great insurance. Get a unionized job, like a teacher, police officer, or garbage collector. Sign with a tech company that offers a fertility package. Become a barista at Starbucks. Or change your insurance at work.

2. **MOVE** to a state with mandated insurance coverage of infertility, such as New Jersey or Massachusetts. Or find a company that buys their insurance from that state.

3. **TRAVEL** abroad for IVF. Spain, Greece, Mexico, and Prague offer lower rates—and are nice vacation spots, too!

4. **START** a GoFundMe campaign. Plenty of people are doing this, so you'll need a campaign slogan that goes beyond "I want to have a baby."

5. **HIT UP** your parents and in-laws for money, especially if they're saving it for you to use for a house or another milestone.

6. **TAKE OUT** a specialized fertility loan or sign up with a fertility cycle management company that can offer cycles for a flat monthly fee like Future Family ("one place for all your IVF and egg freezing needs").

7. **WIN** a cycle in a contest or get a grant from a religious organization.

8. **TRY** the shared cycle programs offered for egg freezing, IVF, and donor eggs.

9. **TALK** to HR. Progeny, which handles fertility benefits for companies, says that 65 percent of employers offer benefits because of employee requests.[4]

Shaber and her husband had to stop. That Thanksgiving they told her family and her cousin offered to pay for a surrogate, "no strings attached." Shaber almost said no because she wasn't sure she could "start the circus again." But she immediately reconsidered the generous offer. "I mean, I'm not crazy." Their son was born via surrogate, and she's using her stage skills to host a podcast "of uninhibited interviews" called IVFU.

Navigating Insurance

During my last pregnancy, I was prescribed a daily blood thinner injection. My insurance denied coverage. I appealed. No answer. I went online to check out the cost: $90 . . . per shot. With more than two hundred days of pregnancy left, that would come out to, oh, another $18,000. *WTF.*

I'm not a fan of insurance, but I'll say this: It's better to have insurance than to not. In the US, some 60 percent of women have *no* fertility coverage, and just 20 percent have *full* coverage, according to FertilityIQ.

I was somewhere in between.

"If you have health insurance through your or your partner's employer, talk to the benefits person and find out exactly what is covered from your health insurance," says Barbara Collura, president and CEO of RESOLVE: The National Infertility Association, who noted that the exclusions of your full health benefits plan document are "typically over one hundred pages in teeny-tiny font."

If you have an insurance plan through your state's exchange, you might have coverage if your state has mandated fertility coverage.[5]

According to a CoFertility survey,[6] more than a third of respondents (37 percent) estimated spending three to nine hours on the phone with their insurance provider each month—fighting for approvals, appealing denials, pricing out medications, and trying to make sense of their coverage; 15 percent estimated spending more than *ten* hours each month.

Questions for Your Insurance Company

1. Do I have fertility benefits? Does my partner?
2. Do I have in-network or out-of-network benefits?
3. If I have out-of-network benefits, do I have to pay upfront and then get reimbursed? How long does that take?
4. Are my consultations covered, and if so, what is my co-pay or coinsurance? How many new doctor consultations can I have?
5. What is the maximum benefit—and is it a sum of money or a number of cycles?
   a. If I have a financial cap (i.e., $10,000 maximum for life), does that include the cost of medication? Do treatments covered by previous insurers (or self-paid) count?
   b. Do you reimburse for medication?
6. Are there certain treatments I need to do first before beginning IVF? Can my doctor call in with an exception?
7. Do I need approval for each and every cycle, and how long does approval typically take?
8. If I don't have IVF coverage, which parts of the treatment are covered (i.e., sonograms and monitoring)?
9. Is genetic testing covered? Is egg or embryo freezing covered?
10. Do you have a dedicated person I can call every time?

Next, go to your clinic of choice, give them your insurance card, and let them explain their benefits to you. Obviously, it's hard to figure out costs before you know what treatment you're going to need. That's why I say call your insurance to find out your general coverage and which clinics offer it in your area first, then meet with your doctor to hear about a treatment plan, then sit down with the clinic's billing department to see how much of your treatment is covered, how much of your meds are covered, and what kind of out-of-pocket costs you can expect to shell out.

But make sure to have your clinic call your insurance as well.

Bethany didn't, and she simply paid out of pocket for her first round of egg freezing—"I didn't think I had any coverage," she says. After she switched clinics to do another round, they asked for her insurance card and got certain parts of the procedure covered. "It was in the hundreds of dollars—but that's still *something*."

Some clinics will list coverage on their website, although not always exact costs. CCRM Colorado's website states:

> Below is our list of contracted insurance carriers. We will bill your primary insurance carrier only if you have IVF insurance coverage and/or infertility insurance coverage and we participate with your insurance carrier and plan. Please note that we are out-of-network with all HMO plans, and that we will only bill your primary insurance carrier. We can bill your services under your partner's policy only if you are an active member on their policy and it is your primary insurance.[7]

Sounds crystal clear, right? Nope. When it comes to finances and insurance, I cannot promise you clarity.

"It's a trap. It's almost purposefully confusing," admits one clinic's insurance coordinator, frustrated on behalf of their patients. "You don't know what's going to happen, it's not predictable: You can speak to one person who will give you one answer, but then you'll often get a different answer from another person. It can make or break your cycle," she says.

Here's a tip I learned from an insurance company consultant: Most companies have a time limit per cost assessment—a cap on how much time they can spend with a customer. So the bigger pain in the butt you can be, the better it may work out in your favor, because they may decide it's not worth it to fight you. (Yes, I'm talking to you, Amazon customer service!) Make yourself known to your insurance provider: They may decide to help you after all.

Humor: Your Insurance Coverage Rider

Congratulations! You have insurance coverage for infertility.[123456]

1. . . . provided you are between ages 25 and 25.5.
2. "Infertility" is defined as trying for more than five years . . .
3. . . . documented with photos, videos, and sworn testimonials.
4. Costs may not exceed $150.47 per year.
5. Coverage includes unlimited Band-Aids, alcohol wipes, and syringe disposal boxes till your third kid.
6. Good luck getting us on the phone.

Beg, Borrow, and . . . Win?

If you're lucky enough to have fertility coverage because of where you live or work, good on ya, mate! Skip to the next chapter. But for the rest of us, who have to scrimp and save enough to afford treatment, a good place to start is with friends and family.

Our insurance covered unlimited IUIs (yay!), which didn't even produce a single positive (boo!). Our insurance also covered meds (yay!), but not IVF (boo!).

We decided we would ask our parents to each cover one cycle (between my dad and his wife, my mom, and Solomon's parents, that would mean three cycles). They wanted more grandkids, right? My husband's parents and my mom handed over a check without asking their usual litany of questions. My father was a bit harder to convince.

Actually, he had a suggestion I found outrageous at the time, but it wasn't a bad idea: Why didn't I apply for an IVF grant? (He actually used the Hebrew word *gemach,* which means "act of kindness" and refers to grants offered in the religious community.) Because I was over forty, with two miscarriages under my belt, I probably wouldn't qualify for any studies or grants. I'd perhaps qualify for a loan, but since I'd prided myself on not having any student debt, I wasn't about to start taking out loans for my unborn child. (My dad came through in the end.)

Many clinics offer qualifying candidates (read: young, first-time IVFers) discounted or sponsored cycles. CoFertility has a "Find a Grant" tool, and RESOLVE has a list of scholarships, loans, and grants, like those from Baby Quest Foundation. Specific communities, such as your church or synagogue, might offer help, too.

Emotionally Speaking: Script for Hitting Up the Rents

Hi, Mom and Dad,

You know how much you love children and are excited for grandchildren? No, we're not pregnant.

And that's actually what we wanted to talk to you about. We haven't been able to get pregnant. We're not exactly sure why.

Yes, I know your best friend's niece went on vacation to Tahiti and got pregnant, but we've been on three vacations already and were pretty relaxed and didn't get pregnant.

We really, really want to start a family, and we think we would be great parents—and you'd be great grandparents. (Well, not great-grandparents—you're way too young for that—but really good grandparents.)

But we're gonna need help. We're making appointments with fertility doctors now. We're not sure what kind of treatment we'll need or how long it will take, but we'd love your support. Yes, thanks for your emotional support! We were also wondering if you could give us financial support?

Thank you. No, this doesn't mean you will get to name the baby.

You may also qualify for a clinical study, which you can find on websites like ClinicalTrials.gov, CenterWatch, and FindMeCure—and you'll be helping mankind, too. Once in a while, companies hold a free cycle sweepstakes, like the one featured in *Vegas Baby,* a documentary about families competing in an IVF contest and the ethics and results of such a contest.

"I know a lot of people were not happy with me because I participated in the 'Have a Baby' contest," says Jennifer "Jay" Palumbo, an infertility advocator who blogs at The 2 Week Wait and who was featured in the documentary. "I was someone who ran out of money to get pregnant. I don't own a house now because we went through treatment. My first IVF was partially covered by insurance, my second was a free clinical trial, and my third wiped out our entire savings." While some may think these contests are crass—would a doctor raffle off diabetes medication?—desperate times call for desperate measures.

"We were in a very bad place: our whole savings account was empty, it was just . . . bad," Palumbo says. From that last cycle, which her family helped pay for, she and her husband had their first child. Then, three years later, she hit the "fertility lottery" by getting pregnant naturally with her second son. She jokes that her elder son is a "timeshare" baby, since her parents, her sister, and her savings account all paid for that last cycle. She has no regrets about the lottery. "People don't have the resources to pay for fertility treatment."

Should You Hire an IVF Consultant?

If I could paint a picture of my three years of infertility, it would show me on the phone yelling at some poor insurance representative. But this doesn't necessarily have to be your experience: Some companies and private IVF coaches will navigate insurance for you.

"Two huge pain points for women and couples who face infertility treatment is the really obvious one, the finances—but it's not just the sheer magnitude of the bills," says Claire Tomkins, CEO of Future Family ("Flexible financing plans and dedicated support for IVF and egg freezing"). She founded the company after her own stressful IVF experience. "It's also stressful to do the clinic management piece, what it's actually going to cost: They'll ask for a credit card and you'll be charged with some random amount." For a flat monthly fee ranging from $150 to $350 for some sixty months, Future Family will handle all your insurance communications, doctors' appointments, and even add fertility consulting to the package.

"People who have insurance don't know the extent of it, and people who don't have it think it's going to be out of pocket, and that doesn't have to be the case, either," says Tasha Blasi, a fertility coach and patient advocate who not only helps clients navigate their cycles, but helps people find thousands of dollars. She has a whole lesson on navigating insurance when you have it, and more important, how to find discounts when you don't have it.

Many people hire consultants to help them through the emotional aspects of the process. "The fertility journey is so overwhelming in so many aspects: So many things are thrown at you and you don't know where to start," says Rebekah Rosler, a licensed clinical social worker who started a Facebook group in 2016 called "Warriors" after her IVF journey, and who offers private consulting. "Having a cheerleader, a friend, an advocate on your side is empowering to have someone educate you and support you, someone who has been there before."

But beware of someone who makes unrealistic promises, like a 100 percent success rate. Hiring someone—be it a therapist, a nurse to give you shots, or a coach—"can only get you so far," Rosler says. "There are no absolutes in this journey."

Hustle & Flow

Some people consider moving out of state—or country—for subsidized fertility treatment. In fact, that's what we did: After our three cycles (so generously sponsored by our parents), we went to Israel, where IVF is free for citizens up to forty-five years old.

But "free" is an interesting word, because it doesn't include ancillary costs: Although we sublet our NYC apartment to pay for living abroad, we didn't take travel costs into account, nor did we know the jobs we had lined up would fall through. And, of course, we had no clue how long we'd be there (eight months) and how there'd be costs for getting resettled once we were back in the US (finding work again, etc.). We *might* have been better off moving to New Jersey. "I do wonder about the cost of living increase and the cost of moving . . . it wouldn't outweigh the IF [infertility] savings?" one Reddit commenter wrote in a thread about moving states for IVF. Others pointed out some caveats to watch out for if you're moving for coverage:

- Some insurance caps for fertility coverage include *previous insurance coverage*—so, for example, if you were on Aetna and spent your $20,000 coverage maximum, then move to Blue Cross, which offers $10,000 toward infertility, Blue Cross might exclude you for having reached your coverage maximum, even though a different company paid for it.
- Some large companies with branches around the US get their insurance from a particular state, which may or may not have fertility coverage. Remember: You don't necessarily have to move. Instead, you can choose to work for a company that has insurance based in a state that mandates insurance coverage for infertility.
- You also have to factor in cost of living. "I moved from Ohio to Massachusetts," says a woman who hadn't done IVF but had her surgeries and consultations covered. "The big downside is that the cost of living and housing might

cancel out the fertility savings." Another one added: "Boston is super expensive and honestly, the money you save could get eaten up by rent if you live in the city."

- Self-insured health plans are generally exempt from state law, and so are plans covering companies smaller than fifty people, so they likely won't offer infertility coverage even if you relocate to a state where it's mandated.
- Some insurances have waiting periods (you must be Trying for six months) or force you to do IUI before IVF.

In short, before you make a move for IVF coverage, make sure you're going to actually receive it! Talk to people at your prospective company, the HR department, the insurance company. Figure out cost of living, moving expenses, and what you'd be giving up by relocating. Nearby family and friends? Your therapist? Your security? For me, living abroad was difficult because I was cut off from my friends and family. At a certain point, I just wanted to go home, *baby or no baby*.

Instead of moving cities, some people find jobs that offer fertility coverage: Tech companies and some finance companies bend over backward to offer good egg freezing and fertility benefits. Government jobs and academia might have coverage, too. One guy started working at Starbucks for their fertility coverage, which is offered to even part-time employees who work a certain amount of hours. He was able to get the testicular sperm extraction he needed due to Starbucks's health benefits.

But the same cost caveats apply: Make sure a new job—even with fertility coverage—is worth more than your old one. (For more on IVF abroad, see chapter 23.)

Advertise Your Troubles

Some people find help on social media.

Husbands Anthony and Kirk, who blog as "Two Beards and a Baby," knew they wanted to have a baby via a surrogate and donor eggs, so their first question was, "How much is this going to cost?" They were getting some monetary assistance from Men Having Babies, a nonprofit providing guidance, advocacy, and financial assistance for current and future gay surrogacy parents, but they needed more. "There were costs we were not prepared for," Kirk says, so they turned to crowdfunding.

In retrospect, they were naive in their first crowdfunding attempt: They set an all-or-nothing goal of $75,000—meaning if they didn't get it all, they'd get none of it. They raised $20,000 from a wide circle of family and friends, but couldn't keep any of it! "It was ridiculous," Kirk says.

Their next campaign was much more modest: They set a goal of $10,000—and raised $12,000. "Where was that other $8,000?" Kirk says, although he kind of knew. Their first campaign had gone wide, getting a lot of visibility and publicity—but that came with its own set of problems.

"It was a really vulnerable experience, trying to start a family," he says, noting that people weren't exactly mean but there was a lot of what he calls "side-eye." "People would say, 'Oh, that's interesting.' And people who wouldn't outright say to us that they thought it was wrong distanced themselves from us." Others still assume they're trying to adopt, "which is weird."

I know just what he means. Out of the five hundred comments on one of my *New York Times* columns, there were probably only a dozen or so mean ones. But the mean ones can really wear a person down. Especially if she's on hormones, experiencing disappointment and loss, and, well, *still* not having a baby.

The need to have a thick skin is something to take into consideration when going public with fertility struggles, especially if you decide to start fund-raising.

The second time around, Kirk and Anthony only shared their campaign with very close friends and family, even if it meant raising less money. "We were not going to share with the public again—that was just too hard."

Socioeconomic Factors Affecting Treatment and IVF

Let's get real: All these machinations are usually accessible to those in the know, to those of us at a certain socioeconomic level, who have white privilege, who have enough time to create a social media campaign, who have the luxury of deciding between a job at Google and a job at Facebook, or who have the wherewithal to pick up shop and head to Boston or the Dominican Republic.

"IVF was intimidating to me," says Regina Townsend, a librarian who chronicled her eight-year journey to have a baby on The Broken Brown Egg, a website she founded to increase awareness around African American infertility and reproductive health. "You're a minority within a minority," she says of being black and infertile. Her journey was complex for many reasons—PCOS, her husband's male factor infertility, and just plain ignorance about her health and reproductive system.

One of her first gynecologists laughed when Regina suggested she might have PCOS: "[My doctor] was in the south side of Chicago, in a lower- to low-middle-class area—she was used to seeing people who *didn't* want to get pregnant. Having someone like me—she may not have known where to start."

One of Townsend's biggest hurdles was finances: "We would try something for six months and then take a break: I lost my job or he lost his job or we didn't have insurance, then our clinic wouldn't take our insurance," she says. Then there were talks with a family member who was considering having them adopt her baby, but ultimately decided against it. "That took another beat. In the grand scheme of things, it was a long time and there were a lot of things in the middle."

By "a lot of things in the middle," she means, of course, life. Both she and her husband are traditional caretakers for their families. "We try to help out with everyone. We're the babysitters, we take everyone's kids to the museum, we're trying to take care of everyone else while seeing everyone else's family grow," she says. "This whole journey of trying to become parents is exhausting."

Also, national statistics are not on her side: It may take African American women *a year* longer than white women to seek infertility treatment,[8] and when they do, treatment can be 14 percent less successful than for Caucasian patients,[9] due to factors like being slightly older, having a higher BMI, and likely having a more diminished ovarian reserve.[10] African American patients also have less access to care than the general population, according to the ASRM ethics committee's report "Disparities in Access to Effective Treatment for Infertility in the United States," which found that "persons of middle to lower socioeconomic status and persons of African American or Hispanic ethnicity are underrepresented in the population of infertility patients."[11]

African American patients being treated for infertility experience fewer pregnancies, higher pregnancy loss, and fewer live births from embryo transfers, despite producing more eggs and more quality embryos than Caucasian patients.[12]

In general, African Americans and other minorities tend to get a "low-value" healthcare experience,[13] not to mention issues related to systemic racism such as access to healthy food, health information, and health services. Other minorities also experience differences in treatment: Asian ethnicity is also an "independent predictor of poor outcome," research has shown.[14]

Until recently, IVF literature didn't even feature people of color. Now, it seems like every clinic website features a rainbow of ethnicities—but many waiting rooms do not.

"Representation matters! A lot of clinics and agencies have gotten the marketing services promoting a visual representation of people of color," Regina says, but what matters is "financial diversity," making sure the payment plans and financing options are available to people of different incomes. "When people go to these sites, they think, 'This is something I can't afford,' and they back away and postpone a dream because it's out of reach."

The Townsends were finally successful and had their son. Although they have more frozen embryos and would ideally like to have more children, "we're trying to make sure we're in a good position to do that," Regina says, referring to both her financial state and her mental state, since she experienced postpartum depression. "Infertility is such a flurry of emotions and stressors; it's really hard to get to where you have to."

Should You Make Fertility Decisions Based on Finances?

In an ideal world, no, no, no, and . . . no!

But the world is not ideal.

After my second (failed) IVF cycle, Solomon informed me that his company had switched insurance plans. We would now get $10,000 in infertility coverage. (Only meds were covered on our previous plan.) I had a new decision to make: Should I use the extra insurance and return to our first (higher-priced) clinic? Or should I stick with the current one and get an extra cycle?

I couldn't fathom switching, dealing with another insurance company, another clinic, another billing department. A more expensive IVF cycle. So I stayed.

Money will likely be a factor for most people.

One friend told me she had to juggle credit cards till she had maxed out each. "Every time I went, I had to remember which credit card to use."

"Most people can't put it on credit," says Anna Almendrala, the *IVFML* host. "I think the more that people are transparent about how they pay for it, the more we'll be able to know as a society the immense burden it is to have children."

That's why so many infertility advocates promote recognizing infertility as a medical diagnosis. "It just drives me insane that infertility isn't covered by insurance," says Palumbo, who works with RESOLVE in addition to running her blog, The 2 Week Wait. "It's not just women who are older who waited to have kids—it's both men and women who have specific medical reasons for not having children, like blocked tubes or low sperm count."

"This really, really is a medical issue," Palumbo says. "People still don't get it. The World Health Organization recognizes infertility is a medical disease and yet most of the United States doesn't. I can't understand it."

Although people like Palumbo and RESOLVE's Barbara Collura are fighting one state legislature at a time to include fertility coverage in insurance plans (and just succeeded in New York!), it's unlikely the whole of America will see free or affordable infertility coverage any time soon. In the meantime, it's up to you to fight for your own care.

Chapter 8

Are You There, Doc? It's Me, Your Patient: What to Expect on Your First Visit

> For those of you who don't know what's been going on in my life lately, I have been going through fertility treatments after 15 months of trying to conceive. In these past 6 months, so many thoughts have gone through my head. "Is it my workouts? Am I working out too much?" "Is it what I'm eating? Am I eating too little or the wrong macros?" "Am I too stressed?" I could go on . . . the answer to those questions is a big nope.
>
> —fitness influencer Anna Victoria[1]

I had mixed feelings about being at a fertility clinic.

On the one hand, I couldn't believe this was me, like, *I* had to go to a *fertility clinic*? (What, me infertile?) I vaguely knew some women had problems getting pregnant, especially when they were older, but not for one moment did I think I would be one of them. I suppose it's like any disease or condition: You have a vague knowledge of, say, diabetes or Crohn's, and may even know someone who *knows* someone who has it, and then, suddenly, *you* are that someone. Now you have to get up to speed on everything, and *fast*.

On the other hand, I was looking forward to hearing what the doctor might have to say. Maybe he'd say something easy and simple, like:

- "You just have to have sex earlier in the month!"
- "Take *these* two vitamins and call me next month."
- "Go on vacation and get rip-roaringly drunk!" (Annoying AF when relatives, friends, and perfect strangers tell you this, but maybe if it was *medically recommended* . . . ?)
- "According to your blood test today . . . you're pregnant!"

Nah, that's not what happened. They did tell us to take a different prenatal vitamin for my MTHFR folic acid deficiency, but it wasn't the magic solution I'd hoped for.

What Do Docs Need from You?

Hopefully, you'll arrive at your first doctor's appointment somewhat prepared. As mentioned in chapter 2, you might already have your recent hormone tests (AMH and/or FSH) as well as a semen analysis from your partner, if you have one. You and your partner might have also done prenatal carrier testing to ensure you're not both carriers of a genetic disorder. (Certain ethnicities and races carry greater risk for certain diseases—like European Jews and Tay-Sachs disease—as do certain families. "But anyone can have one of these disorders," says the American College of Obstetricians and Gynecologists. "They are not restricted to these groups.") Before treatment, you and your partner/donor will likely do genetic carrier screening.

In addition to giving your doctor a thorough family history, you'll want to give them your own fertility history, which might be something simple as one year of Trying, regular periods, never been pregnant, he's never gotten anyone pregnant. It also might be more complicated, including a missing period, a failed pregnancy, a D&C, or a past fibroid surgery.

Include *everything*.

Setting Up Your Fertility Document

Document all your efforts and failures, when they occurred, and a medical history, if relevant. Here's mine:

Amy Klein

Sept. 2011: Natural pregnancy, miscarriage #1, 5–6 weeks

Dec. 2011: Natural pregnancy, miscarriage #2, 9–10 weeks

Feb. 2012: D&E surgery

March 2012: Genetically normal embryo found

April–Aug. 2012: 4 IUIs (natural and with Clomid, no pregnancies)

July 2013: Laparoscopy found one tube blocked

Sept. 2013: Mini IVF, four eggs retrieved, three fertilized, one day-3 embryo transferred

Oct. 2013: Miscarriage #3, 7 weeks

Nov. 2013: D&C, results indeterminate (female contamination)

Dec. 2013: Mini IVF, two eggs, none fertilized

Feb.–June 2013: Three transfers w/ Lovenox and baby aspirin

Oct. 2013–Jan. 2014: High dose (600 Follistim), 14 eggs, 5 pgs tested, all abnormal

March 2014: Donor #1 egg transfer—pregnant!

April 2014: Miscarriage #4, blighted ovum

April 2014: D&C, balanced translocation

July 2014: Immunological meds: Lovenox, Neupogen, steroids

Oct. 2014: Donor #2 transfer

Nov. 2014: Pregnant with singleton

Dec. 2014–Jan. 2015: Intralipid, steroids, Lovenox

July 2015: Baby Girl

Some doctors and clinics will go through this history pro forma, like a tired old detective who has seen one too many burglaries go unsolved.

Sandra was turning thirty-five and had been trying for a year when she went to her first appointment. "I just wanted to find out what was going on," she says. The doctor explained her treatment options, but "she didn't seem too keen on thematically wanting to find out what the problem was," Sandra says, noting that she forced the doc to do a uterine examination to see if there were any blockages. (There weren't.)

Other doctors will be more thorough in their investigation, like an energetic young detective, eager to prove her worth on the force. Depending on your history, those docs might send you in for more diagnostic tests, including either a hysteroscopy or laparoscopy to check that your uterus, fallopian tubes, and ovaries are fully functioning.

"I can't believe it was my fourth doctor who asked if my mother had endometriosis," says Ursula, referring to the condition that affects fertility and that hadn't been diagnosed by her three previous doctors over two years of treatment. When she finally had a laparoscopy—and was found to have endometriosis—it made her lack of a baby make sense.

You'll also need up-to-date STD testing, a mammogram, and a PAP smear from the past year and up-to-date immunizations. Best to get all your vaccinations, too, since you may not be able to while you're pregnant.

Speak Up, Woman!

"So the first thing a patient should ask her doctor is, 'What do *you* think is going on?'" says Dr. Brian A. Levine, the founding partner and practice director of CCRM New York.

I like the way he places the onus on the doctor.

So often we women feel shy, insecure—or worse, ashamed and fearful—when it comes to asking for what we need, especially with something as sensitive as our reproductive ability. A study called "The Girl Who Cried Pain: A Bias Against Women in the Treatment of Pain" found that "in general, women report more severe levels of pain, more frequent incidences of pain, and pain of longer duration than men, but are nonetheless treated for pain less aggressively." If you're poor, or a minority, that care bias is likely to increase.

"Black women—speak up!" says Regina Townsend of The Broken Brown Egg, who says that starting her blog has "given me a voice and a little bit of my power back in a situation that made me feel powerless."

I know, I know: We never want to be *that* woman: the one who asks the teacher too many questions in grade school, who asks the guy for too much in a relationship, and hopefully, in the future, that mom who is dogging everyone about her child.

But this is our health, our money, and our care, and we should be able to be inquisitive and assertive (I say "assertive" and not the sexist "aggressive," which, to me, is akin to using weighted words like "bossy" and "hysterical").

"I started off meek and mild," Townsend says, "but after a year, I knew I had to start asking questions."

Yes, you should ask questions, no matter the pushback.

"I'm so traumatized," one woman says of her experience with her first doctor at a top clinic, calling him "brilliant" but socially awkward. "He wouldn't explain anything—not the blood work, not your options, unless you begged him to."

But you shouldn't have to beg. "There's an unfair alignment: I have a lot of information because this is what I do every day," says Dr. Levine. "There is no silly question—I truly believe that."

I had lots of questions at the beginning, like, *Why the F didn't anyone tell me how hard it was to get pregnant?* and *If they did tell me, why didn't I listen?* But the main question, really, says Dr. Levine, is: "What is my diagnosis?"

Hocus-Pocus Diagnosis

When I went in for my first official evaluation, I'd already had two failed pregnancies. Many women going in for their first appointment are just perplexed, and want an answer to one question: *WHY AM I NOT PREGNANT??*

You'd think a diagnosis would be a simple thing. You've been trying to get pregnant, having unprotected sex during your peak ovulation time—and nothing's happened for the past six months to a year. What could be the problem? Here are some statistics:

1. 15 to 20 percent of couples have been diagnosed with male factor infertility

2. 50 percent have been diagnosed with female factor infertility

3. 20 percent have been diagnosed with a combination of the two

4. 30 percent have been diagnosed with "unexplained infertility"[2]

Ha ha, that's 120 percent! No, but seriously, it's either him, you, or both of you.

We'll talk about #1 in chapter 13, but if your partner's semen seems normal, they're going to look at you. According to the CDC, more than 12 percent of American women ages fifteen to forty-four have impaired fertility, which is about the same number who report that they've used fertility services. So you're not alone.

Here are some possible problems:

- **Hormonal:** They'll take a look at your hormone assessment (AMH/FSH, testosterone, LH, estrogen) and see if you are within a normal range. Is that "normal" for your age? Take me: I had a great FSH for my age (5, thank you!), but didn't find out till much later that while my AMH (.6) was normal for my age, it sucked for fertility.

  Your doctor might call this diminished ovarian reserve

(DOR) or premature ovarian insufficiency/failure (POI/ POF). Frustratingly, there's no standard terminology in the industry.

Your hormone levels might determine your "protocol" (i.e., your medical plan).

If your hormone levels are good—not just good for your age, but good good—the doctor may order further testing to see if there are any physical issues.

- **Physical:** You might have an actual physical reason you haven't been getting pregnant, a condition or disease not diagnosed by your gynecologist (bless her heart). You could have PCOS, endometriosis, cysts, fibroids, blocked tubes, or scar tissue, making conception difficult. Your doctor might order testing like a hysterosalpingogram (HSG) to see if your tubes are blocked, and based on the results may recommend some outpatient procedures to eliminate or correct the condition(s).

- **Infectious:** "The uterus and the prostate are notorious for harboring bacteria," says Dr. Attila Toth,[3] an infectious disease infertility doctor who performs "comprehensive microbiological evaluations" on male and female genital canals (but not IVF). "If you clean your uterus and clean your sperm, you will have a healthy baby."

- **Immunological:** Some thorough doctors might run a basic immunological panel to check if you have any clotting issues or autoimmune markers, but most will wait till you have some failures (or forever, in my case) to run a comprehensive investigation. If you have an autoimmune disease, head straight there. (See chapter 22 for more information.)

- **Weight/Lifestyle Issues:** Your doctor may want you to gain weight if you're very underweight or lose it if you're very overweight before starting treatment, especially if your weight is affecting your ovulation/menstruation cycle. (Some clinics have a BMI limit.)

Obesity and Infertility

Being obese can cause problems with fertility, including dys-regulation of the menstrual cycle, no menstrual cycle, no ovula-tion, altered endometrial receptivity, lower pregnancy rates, and possibly miscarriage, according to "Obesity and Reproduction," an ASRM committee opinion.[4] It may also have an impact on egg quality; research has found that obese women using donor eggs had the same pregnancy rate as non-obese women, suggesting egg quality is a primary factor in infertility in obese women. Obese men may also have sperm problems.

The question is, what to do about it?

Get your ovulation working, see if you have PCOS,[5] and talk to your doctor.

The ASRM committee found that "There is no strong evidence that preconception weight loss in women improves IVF-related pregnancy outcome, and the data is less clear in men." Still, they recommend weight loss to decrease BMI to below 35 before con-ception, in an effort to reduce pregnancy complications and mor-bidity from anesthesia-related surgical procedures, such as egg retrieval.

"Weight loss, however, takes time, and the potential benefit of weight loss should be weighed against the risk of declining ovarian reserve," writes Samuel J. Chantilis in an article titled "Tipping the Scales for Reproduction."[6] Since weight loss doesn't improve IVF outcomes and serious weight loss can take a long time (while your eggs decline), it's best to just start IVF, even if your BMI isn't in the range the ASRM recommends. Stud-ies have shown that egg retrieval is relatively safe with "minor complications" for obese women (those with a BMI over 40).[7] Some clinics do have a BMI limit, so if you're shopping around, be sure to ask!

If they can't find anything wrong with you or your partner, you might get diagnosis #4, my favorite: "unexplained infertility." And you might, like me, be thinking, *I could've told you that!*

As usual, there is no real agreement in the industry on what "unexplained" means.

"Our inability to find the causes of couples' infertility does not mean that there is no cause for the disorder," wrote the editor in chief of the *Journal of Reproduction and Infertility.*[8] Doctors should conduct "extensive research," including "ovarian and testicular dysfunctions, sperm and oocyte quality, fallopian transport defects, endometrial receptivity, implantation failures, and endometriosis."

In other words, sometimes "unexplained" means "Just Not Trying Hard Enough to Find an Answer."

Keep in mind that this is a relatively new industry: It's been less than fifty years since the first IVF baby was born. So as confident as your doctors sound, as certain as they might be on a course of action, there is so much they don't know. Even in the few years since I was in treatment, things have changed at a breakneck pace. And when it comes to diagnosis, maybe you don't need an *answer* as much as you need a course of treatment.

Diagnosis, Prognosis

Please don't panic! You might be like, *WTF? How am I supposed to understand everything the doctor is talking about? Do I need an advanced degree in medicine, biology, reproduction, and infertility??*

Don't worry, it's still okay to ask questions. Here are some good ones Dr. Levine suggests:

- **What is your experience with patients like me?**
  If you have *some* sort of diagnosis, you want to know how experienced this doctor is in, say, male factor infertility, or women with diminished ovarian reserve. I had showed up

at my reputable clinic with two miscarriages, but I didn't know to ask them about their experience with recurrent loss.

- **What treatment do I need?**
  Ask what's next: Does the doc need more tests? Surgeries? Does the doctor want you to start with IUI? And for how long? Or should you jump immediately to IVF? Or maybe you should just go home and keep trying on your own. (Fat chance.)

- **Can you help me?**
  Sure, you may have some problems with your eggs or your uterus, but what can *she* do for *you*? This is a good way to ascertain the doctor's level of confidence in her diagnosis and treatment plan. Also, tell her if there are steps you are *not* willing to take, like if you're not able to go on birth control, are allergic to anesthesia, can't afford IVF, or won't have intercourse with your partner (hmm, maybe *that's* the problem?).

  Since she was diagnosed with "unexplained infertility," Sandra told the doctor she wanted to keep trying on her own: "The minute I said I wanted to hold off on treatment, she closed her book." There was nothing more the fertility doc could do.

- **Tell me about your lab success rates.**
  One of the most important things to know when doing IVF and egg freezing is the clinic laboratory's quality and success rates—how the eggs do, if they fertilize and become good embryos ready for transfer. Dr. Levine says doctors should be able to provide you with these rates.

- **What are my chances of success at this clinic?**
  "What I will counsel a patient is that statistics are a guideline—it's a good place to start," Dr. Levine says. It may help point you down the right path. Say the doc tells

you an IUI would give you a 10 percent chance of getting pregnant per cycle, but IVF would give you a 40 percent chance—you might decide to skip the IUI completely. Also, if you're an economist or statistician (or married to one), you might be able to add your finances on another axis and compare expense with percentage of success to see what's the most cost-effective.[9]

"It's important to explain to patients that each event is an independent event—on a per-cycle basis," Dr. Levine says. Solomon tells me this is called the "cumulative probability," which in IVF often increases after multiple cycles. For example, according to an Australian study, women have a 33 percent chance of having a baby as a result of their first cycle, but this chance increases to 54 to 77 percent by the eighth cycle.[10]

Anna Maria Barry-Jester, a woman who works with statistics for a living, reporting on public health, food, and culture for the website FiveThirtyEight, says about IVF: "These are general statistics. There can be a lot of variation in what the individual might expect to experience, depending on their circumstances." She says you can't think about the general trends: "You lie somewhere in there. You can never know if you're going to be the outlier or the average."

When I was single and dating, I was an outlier: At thirty-nine, I moved to New York City, where there are 38 percent more female college grads than male college grads—and a tenth of those men are gay.[11] Plus, I was looking for a Jewish man on the Upper West Side—a neighborhood replete with single Jewish women. You could say my odds were close to zero. And lo and behold, I met Solomon. For better or worse, right?

I was so hoping to be an outlier in fertility, too. Or to quote my favorite children's book, *The Phantom Tollbooth*, "So many things are possible just as long as you don't know they're impossible."

Cheat Sheet: First Visit Qs

1. What do you think is wrong with me?
2. Do we need any further testing?
3. Are there things we can do before starting treatment?
4. What is your plan of action?
5. What are my chances of success?
6. How many cycles of treatment will I need?
7. Who will be in touch with me?
8. How can I get in touch with you directly?
9. What happens on the weekend?
10. Do you like me? I mean, really like me?

One Last Thing Before You Go

Remember my not-so-warm-and-cuddly OB? At our first appointment, she was *lovely.* She was charming, she was attentive, she looked at me like I was the Most Interesting Patient in the World. I later realized this was because she was selling herself. I'm not saying your Dr. Jekyll will turn into Ms. Hyde, but that first appointment is when you have her attention. Here are a few more questions you can ask the doctor, nurse, or receptionist:

- **How will we communicate?** Ask for the best way to be in touch, and if you can have their email and/or their cell phone (*only for emergencies, I promise!*).
- **How often will I see you during treatment?** Most docs won't do the monitoring—especially for IUIs. (Monitoring is when they assess how your eggs and hormones are progressing, usually via blood tests and ultrasounds, and is done a few times during your cycle.) Try to find out

how often you can expect to see your own doctor or *a* doctor.

- **Am I a good candidate for your clinic?** If your numbers are not great, the doctor might tell you if they won't treat you.
- **What are monitoring hours?** Is it first come, first served? Meaning, is there a line snaking out the door at six A.M. because all the C-suite ladies have to get to their corner offices? Or is there an actual appointment for monitoring on the books?
- **Who is the billing coordinator?** Oh, you'll probably meet her, but make her your very best friend in the world. She holds your life in her hands.
- **What's the outlet situation?** You may think I'm crazy, but I was tethered to that one wall in the corner right near the door just to charge my phone. (PS: Ask if there's a no-cell-phone policy in the office.)
- **Do we have a good rapport?** Maybe you don't need to say this aloud, but you should still ask yourself this question. Do you feel excited about treatment, or at least confident in your doctor's plan to get you pregnant?

"In the end, it's all about patients feeling aligned with their doctors—where they feel comfortable with the outcome the doctor wants from them," Dr. Levine says. "Patients need to understand that it is a partnership." He always tells patients, "This might be the most stressful experience you have in healthcare."

If you don't feel good about your first appointment, the doctor, or the clinic *and you have another option time- and money-wise*, it might be worth considering plan B. "Be honest with your doctor," Dr. Levine says. It's okay to say, "I feel like we don't have a good therapeutic relationship." You can find another doctor at the clinic or find another clinic entirely. Dr. Levine says, "At the end of the day, patients need to be honest—they don't need to suffer."

What Doctors and Fertility Clinics Can Do Better

1. Hire Nice Receptionists
We know you're slammed with patients, but guess what? We're going through infertility. Would it kill you to smile? To pretend you care?

2. Get Good Reading Material for the Waiting Room
I really don't want to read last year's *Time* magazine that looks like it's been in the sperm collection room. Also, coffee, tea, and snacks would really help the morning wait. (Let *me* manage my caffeine and sugar intake.)

3. Schedule Morning Monitoring
What are you, the cable company? I have better things to do than wake up at six A.M. to push to the front of the line for blood work or have to wait an hour in line. Mid-morning and lunch monitoring would be nice, too.

4. Know Our Files
Doc, thanks for telling me to do another retrieval and forgetting I have two embies on ice. Can you be familiar with my file before talking with me?

5. Put a Dedicated Nurse on Our Case
Speaking of calling or emailing me, it would be so great if there was a dedicated person assigned to my case, not a rotating bunch of clinicians and nurses.

6. Billing, Be Exact
Why am I getting a hidden-cost bill four months after my baby was born? Please give me a detailed list of all the costs I should expect. Better yet, put them on your website!

7. Follow Up After a Failure
I know I'm at my most moody and hormonal when my period comes and I'm not pregnant. But if you called now and gave me comfort and guidance for next steps, it would make this shitty

time feel a bit more hopeful. (And by follow up, I do *not* mean send me to billing to start another cycle.)

8. **Validate Parking**

There's nothing that would make me like to come back for another visit more than a sticker on my parking ticket that says "free!" At least *something* is.

Chapter 9

_____

The Turkey Baster: The IUI First Try

> No romantic dinner, long-stemmed roses, smooth wine, or flickering candlelight preceded this event. Instead it was a date with a cold sterile room, bright overhead lights, and awkward stirrups. It didn't matter. Nothing could dampen our spirits because we knew that science and humans had given their best efforts, and now the re- sults ultimately lay in God's hands.
>
> —Kate Gosselin, *Multiple Bles8ings*[1]

I was glad to finally be at the fertility clinic.

After my two natural pregnancies failed, we'd been Trying on our own, and all of that planning, charting, temp-taking, and stick- peeing was taking its toll on us. Now the doctor could be the archi- tect of our fertility and give us the kick-start we needed.

There's a reason doctors talk about time to conception. That's a fancy way of saying "how long it will take you to get pregnant and have a baby." Solomon and I had already clocked in eight months, and while I'd never been one to obsess about my biological clock (if I had, maybe I wouldn't have been in this predicament), I could feel it ticking. I wanted to be a mom already.

I wanted to try an IUI.

Monitor Me, Please

I always think of intrauterine insemination (IUI), also known as artificial insemination, like a turkey baster procedure, a DIY impregnation kit. It's way less invasive than IVF because with IUI, all they're doing is getting the sperm inside you at the exact right time (ovulation) and then hoping the sperm fertilizes your eggs and the embryos make their way to your uterus. (During IVF they have to extract eggs from your body, fertilize them in a lab, and put the resulting embryos back inside you a few days later.)

As mentioned, you *can* do an insemination at home (ostensibly *not* with a kitchen utensil), but then you'd be missing out on one of the things I would soon look forward to: monitoring, i.e., how your doctor assesses your cycle. It's usually done using a blood test to measure your hormones and an ultrasound to examine your uterus.

At the start, they'll want to make sure you're ready to begin a cycle, that you have no cysts or other conditions, and that your hormones are where they need to be. When you're closer to ovulation, they want to assess the state of your uterine lining and when you will ovulate—or more precisely, when to *make* you ovulate.

That's why I appreciated the monitoring: Let *them* figure out what was going on and when. Let them bring the sperm—our sperm—to the party. At least I wouldn't have to wonder anymore about when to have sex. Oh, don't get me wrong, I still wanted to! It was just . . . thinking about what my eggs were doing and where his sperm were going while we were doing it was getting me down.

Let science figure out how my egg was growing and when it was ready to meet its mate. Then, they'd take Solomon's sperm, "wash it" (separate the sperm from the semen in a centrifuge machine), and shoot me up.

Superovulation!

When I got my period at age twelve, my mom explained to me what to expect from menstruation (blood, tears, and embarrassing moments that could be solved by carrying a change of clothes), and biology class further explained the technicality of the uterine lining shedding when the sperm did *not* find an egg (the message always seemed to be how to NOT get pregnant).

Yet it was only when I did my first IUI that I understood how the mechanics of reproduction actually works during the cycle. ("IUI: Taking the Magic Out of Reproduction, One Cycle at a Time.")

Inside your ovaries are follicles—"like a water balloon with an egg inside," is how Dr. Isaac Sasson, a Shady Grove Fertility RE in Pennsylvania, puts it. Each of your follicles contains an oocyte, or an immature egg. At the start of your cycle, the follicles should be in a "resting" state. Throughout the cycle, your estrogen rises and the follicle grows.

"When the follicles are 20 to 24 millimeters in size, and peak estrogen is around 200, the body has an LH [luteinizing hormone] surge," he says, "causing ovulation 36 hours later, when the eggs complete the first stage of meiosis," a special type of cell division.

That's when the party starts.

"Ovulation is the craziest part of reproduction," Dr. Sasson says, because the ovary and the fallopian tube aren't actually connected to each other. The released egg bounces around the woman's belly ("peritoneal cavity") until the fallopian tubes "vacuum it up," and there it sits, waiting for the sperm. (We women, always waiting for the man: for him to call, for him to pay the bill, for him to propose, for his sperm to impregnate our eggs.)

But wait! There's something called superovulation, the hero swooping in from fertility clinics everywhere. It's when you add meds to your cycle to trick your brain into releasing a couple more eggs (or, if you don't ovulate at all, which happens to some women, it helps your ovary release one egg).

"The goal is *one* healthy baby," Dr. Sasson says, echoing doctors everywhere, because having multiples is risky to the babies' health, as they are likely to be premature. But with an IUI, "you can't prevent multiples. I have more multiples from Clomid than IVF," Dr. Sasson says, referring to the drug used most often with IUIs. (With IVF you can transfer just one embryo.) If Dr. Sasson sees three follicles growing, he may cancel the cycle to prevent high-order multiples. "It's a conversation," he says.

Some gynecologists or doctors give women the meds without monitoring them. That's how you end up with crazy reality show sextuplets, and why some parents have to "selectively reduce"—i.e., abort some of the fetuses so the others will survive. (Kate Gosselin, of *Kate Plus 8,* was under the care of a fertility doctor, who performed an IUI with four follicles.)

When the follicles are mature (18 to 22 millimeters in size), you'll do a "trigger shot," to stimulate ovulation 36 hours later. If you're doing an unmedicated IUI (you may choose to do this if you react badly to medication), you then have to play a guessing game with ovulation. In general, Dr. Sasson encourages at least using a trigger shot to "control" the timing of ovulation. Then you can either have timed intercourse or an IUI.

Shoot Me Now!

"Put on this gown and the doctor will be in soon," the nurse told me. Even though it was spring, it was cold in the office, so I left my lucky socks on, as well as my shirt and bra. Over time I would realize I should wear a skirt or dress for easy access. I tied the hospital gown behind my back and waited for the doctor to return. *Should I have gotten a bikini wax?* I thought. *Nah, if I don't do it for my husband, the doctor can live with it.*

When the doctor entered, he seemed distracted. It was only later that I realized why: For him, IUIs were minor procedures. Easy-peasy, like an In-N-Out Burger drive-through. Sometimes the doctor wasn't even there to monitor me.

Still, no matter who was conducting the ultrasound, I always liked watching them measure my follicles for their fifteen minutes of fame. *Who knows?* I thought. Maybe one of these two minuscule egg sacs would become my baby.

Although the medical establishment prefers singletons, I was still hoping for twins.

I understood there were health risks to multiples: it's hard on the mom's body and the babies are often born prematurely, which could cause long-term health risks. But I couldn't help but want to be one and done, i.e., have one pregnancy with two kids. I was almost forty-two: After ten months of pregnancy, and a year of recovering from having a baby, I would be almost forty-four! I couldn't count on having a second baby . . . even if I got pregnant *that very cycle.*

"Okay, get dressed," the doctor said. "I'll be back soon."

Back then, I was shy about undressing in front of him—a veritable stranger who was suddenly so intimate with me. One day, a year in the future, I would not be shy anymore. I would laugh that the doctor would leave the room while I changed, that he'd call me "Ms. Klein"—all things to keep distance between us even though he was closer to me and my vagina than my husband. But for now, I was shy.

The doctor came back into the room and told me it was time to trigger.

I'd never really had a problem with injections. I didn't exactly love someone poking me with a needle, but I sucked it up for most of my

Myths About IUI

1. **You should always try an IUI before IVF.**

Not true—depends on your age (only under thirty-eight) and other factors.

2. **IUIs are better than timed sex.**

The actual method of insemination is less relevant for couples with normal sperm.

3. **If you have a blocked tube, you can't do IUI.**

Your other tube may be fine! (I only had one open tube.)

4. **If your tubes are open, everything's okay.**

Even if they're open, they might still be unhealthy.

5. **If you had an ectopic pregnancy (where an embryo implants outside the uterus), you can do another IUI.**

Actually, with an IUI you're at increased risk of another ectopic pregnancy, even if the damaged tube was removed.

6. **If Clomid doesn't work, you should try shots like Follistim with IUI.**

There's not much added benefit to using a stronger gonadotropin medication like Follistim in IUI, and it increases your risk of multiples.

7. **Sperm count doesn't matter.**

If the sperm have a normal semen count, chances of pregnancy are the same, no matter *how much sperm there is*, but if sperm count is "on the low end of the spectrum," IUI pregnancy rates fall, according to a Shady Grove study.[2]

life in the hopes of getting a purple lollipop from the pediatrician. But then I started fertility treatment and discovered that:

- Solomon faints at the sight of a needle.
- I was going to have to inject myself.
- Some people hire nurses to administer shots.

The first few times I needed a trigger shot, I made Solomon stand there with me, even though he had to turn his back as I injected myself. Afterward, I'd give him the empty *covered* needle so he could dispose of it in one of those cute red sharps boxes (which would pile up until I remembered to take them to a pharmacy or doctor).

One important thing about the trigger shot: It's the only medication that needs to be administered exactly on time. The trigger shot is actually hCG (human chorionic gonadotropin), which does the same trick as your LH surge, inducing the egg's final maturation. (It's also the same hormone your body releases when you're pregnant, which is why you can't take a pregnancy test till it leaves your body.) And 24 to 36 hours after the shot . . . ovulation!

Less than 36 hours after I injected myself, Solomon headed to the clinic's collection room (PS: It's a porn room: tough life), then handed his semen over to be washed, a procedure that separates chemicals and sperm from the semen and is thought to improve fertility.

Then I was up! Clean sperm coming my way. I promise, it didn't hurt. They injected the semen beyond my cervix, closer to the egg, another reason to do an IUI over plain old regular sex.

IUI by the Numbers

Here are the live birth rates after one IUI.[3]

AGE OF WOMAN	LIVE BIRTH RATE
20 to 30	13%
31 to 35	10%
36 to 38	9%
39 to 40	7%
over 40	3%

And as I lay there, tilted up in the chair (*way* better than contort-ing myself at home), I was happy that the sperm were getting where they needed to be ('cuz you know how men love asking for direc-tions).

Reconsidering the IUI

In women under thirty-eight years old, including women with ovula-tion disorders, secondary infertility, normal ovarian reserve, or a partner with low sperm count, "IUI should be considered as an op-tion," one study found.[4] It can help give them the push that's needed. It's much less invasive than IVF, not to mention much less expensive, so psychologically and financially, it may be an easier start.

"In other cases, IVF should be discussed as the first-line treat-ment," the same study found. Ask your doctor if IUI is worth it for you. "In a couple with a normal semen analysis, I'm going to skip the IUI," says Dr. Sasson, noting that he'd still opt for the superovulation medication and monitoring, but tell the couple to have sex at home the night of the shot and then again a day later. "Ejaculated sperm live longer than washed sperm."

A recent trial of a fertility treatment called FASTT (short for "fast track and standard treatment") showed that the most effective treat-ment for women under forty was three cycles of medicated IUI, then moving straight on to IVF.[5] And another small study, known as FORT-T (the "Forty and Over Treatment Trial"), found that for women who went straight to IVF without doing IUIs, the time to pregnancy was faster, there were fewer treatment cycles, and almost 85 percent of the pregnancies came from IVF.[6] Dr. Sasson may send older patients straight to IVF. "I don't want you to miss your oppor-tunity. Age is what predicts egg quality," he says.

Guidelines suggest no more than four IUIs; after that, it's unlikely to be effective.[7] Also, although IUIs may be cheaper than IVF, their emotional toll cannot be measured. As one study concluded, "IUI can be characterized by half the price but twice the time."[8]

Emotionally Speaking: Going the Unmedicated Route

When I started fertility treatment, I was insistent that I wanted to do it "naturally." I did not want to put hormones in my body. I did not want to mess with my menstrual cycle. And so I started IUI without the hormone-stimulating medication. (Dr. Sasson calls this "pointless.") And then, when I started meds for IUI, I wanted as little as possible. It didn't stop there: I started IVF on as minimal a dose as possible (see chapter 20 for more on "mini IVF") before moving on to maximum IVF.

The problem with all that? As I tried my incremental phases, my egg quality was deteriorating. I should have started at the *highest* dose of meds, then started *decreasing* if it didn't work. (Some women actually respond better to lower doses of medication.)

I have many friends who *really* don't respond well to medication. Like, their systems shut down. They might have to go the unmedicated route. But if you don't have that problem, the question you have to ask yourself is this: *Do I want to do it my way, or do I want to have a baby?*

I'd Like to Thank IUI For . . .

I *had* to do three IUIs before I could move on to IVF because my insurance mandated it. Insurance can be crazy—mandating IUI for same-sex couples, or a genetic disease carrier who doesn't *want* to try naturally for fear of passing on a disease like cystic fibrosis, or even women over forty who don't have the time to waste.

Although I did not get pregnant during my four IUIs (the last, actually, was converted to timed sex because I was going camping and couldn't make the doctor's appointment), I *did* learn to navigate dealing with my insurance, find the best nurses at the clinic, and balance my schedule with treatment hours. (I guess that's like saying I got really good at navigating Tinder without finding a partner.)

It's easy to look back on IUI treatments and call them "easy" or "not invasive" or "cheap," but truthfully, when I was doing them, they were none of those things. Each and every time, I was filled with hope, buoyed with the ineffable optimism that *this* would be my month, my baby, our year, our life.

That's why I want to tell you about the two-week wait.

Chapter 10

The Two-Week Wait

For everyone going through infertility and conception hell, please know it was not a straight line to either of my pregnancies. Sending you extra love.

—Anne Hathaway

I was terrible at dating. Oh, I was great on the date itself, all light-hearted and amusing—*you're so funny and I'm so fun and we're having the greatest time in the world and I have not a care in the world!* was the attitude I was hoping to convey, with a few well-placed touches to his arm.

But the minute the date was over, the voices in my head would start up: *Will he call? Will we go out again? Will he be the man who changes my life? Or will he be abducted by aliens like the five hundred men before him who said they'd "be in touch" and never graced me with their presence again?* The thrum of this thinking pulsated throughout my day, while driving to work, sitting in meetings, hanging out with my friends. I'd pretend to be there, with them, giving my undivided attention, but I was aching to check my phone to see if he'd texted or (gulp) answered my follow-up text: *Hd a gr8 time.*

I wasn't an anxious person. It was *dating* that made me that way. It was *waiting* that made me that way.

That waiting, though, was *nothing* compared to the Two-Week Wait.

While You Were Waiting

Anyone who has been Trying knows about the Two-Week Wait (or 2WW), that maddening time after ovulation until your expected period (which you're hoping won't come!). I like to think that the acronym actually stands for "Two Weeks of Worrying."

If you're trying naturally, you're probably (hopefully!) thinking about when to have sex, how much sex to have, and if that sex got the job done. And you probably (hopefully!) know when your period is supposed to arrive, are keenly hoping it won't, and are disappointed when it does because, well, you're not preggers.

After fertility treatment, the 2WW can be especially agonizing, because medicine has taken the guessing game out of the equation: If you've been through daily monitoring, then you know *if* and *when* you're ovulating. You know when the optimal go-time is. You don't have to wonder, *Did I not ovulate? Did I miss my fertile window? Did I not read the ovulation stick right?* (You definitely need a PhD to read it.)

When you have an IUI, you don't have to wonder, *Did he finish?* (I'm always too embarrassed to ask.) You don't have to obsess, *Did the sperm make it into my vagina? Are they headed to the uterus?* Nope, you don't have to, because it's already been placed there by a doctor with a speculum.

During your 2WW after an IUI, you're just hoping the sperm has made it into an egg (or two eggs, if you've taken fertility drugs), and that they're happily coursing through the fallopian tubes together in wedded bliss as an embryo.

And if you're doing IVF (which we'll talk about in the next chapter), you don't have to wonder, *Did the sperm make it to the egg? Did the sperm penetrate the egg? Did the embryo make it into the womb?* No, in the IVF 2WW (and that's the most acronym usage you'll see in this book), you *know* there's an embryo in there, and all you have left to wonder is, *Am I pregnant?*

The Emotional Roller Coaster

If I couldn't manage the relatively low stakes of dating—which, after all, came with a free meal or drink—how was I gonna get through the loaded two-week wait of conception?

I'll tell you a little secret: I couldn't.

Now that I've revealed my dating neuroses, that shouldn't come as a surprise. But it *was* a surprise to me how nerve-wracking each waiting period was. At the beginning, I had a handle on keeping the wondering to a minimum, while getting on with my life—especially since I had a life outside of fertility then.

But once I started treatment, from that very first doctor's appointment, I was admitting, YES, I WANT TO BE PREGNANT! I WILL PAY YOU TO GET ME PREGNANT! I WILL WAIT ON AB-SURDLY LONG LINES AND SIT IN INCREDIBLY UNCOMFORT-ABLE WAITING ROOMS IN THE HOPES THAT YOU GET ME PREGNANT.

And so, pretending to be chill about it all during my two-week wait—*Why, sure, I'm just so relaxed! And if it will happen, it will happen! And if not, there's always next month!*—well, that kind of thinking, just like my joie de dating vivre, went *pfft*, down the drain.

When you're spending time and money and so much emotional energy to conceive, and you've become hyperaware of how your body works (or how it's *supposed* to work), it's tough to be nonchalant.

Your two-week waits can go from exhilarating to excruciating, depending on how long you've been at it.

How do people get through it?

"I was fine in the first week, but in the second week I would lose my mind," says Palumbo, the infertility/women's rights activist and author of The 2 Week Wait, a blog about that and the entire fertility

---

Scientifically Speaking:
Is Laughter Good Medicine?

They say that laughter is the best medicine, but what *kind* of laughter?

In a 2011 study at an IVF unit in Israel, half the patients had a visit from a medical clown, a specially trained jester who tends to the psychosocial needs of the patient.[1] According to the study, the clowns entertained women who had just had an embryo transfer using jokes, tricks, and magic for 12 to 15 minutes. The women clowning around were 2.67 times more likely to get pregnant than the ones who weren't.

"Laughter may have an effect on the embryo-uterine interplay," the researchers posited, either through hormonal pathways or stress reduction, increasing uterine receptivity.

So do you need to laugh during your two-week wait?

While I'm all for laughter—give me Tiffany Haddish in *anything*— I'm not sure this small study translates: It was about a medical clown—an actual *person* coming to a woman's room, interacting with her, and entertaining her. If a clown came to my hospital room here in the USA, I might run out screaming.

Still, there's no harm in filling your life with comedy: If you can find something or someone that actually makes you LOL, it can't hurt.

process. As a mom of two boys—her first conceived at thirty-eight after four years of IVF, her second unassisted—Palumbo, in retrospect, finds her blog's name amusing. "For many people, the two weeks feel really permanent, and it really stuck with me," she says. For her, the two-week wait is actually symbolic of every part of fertility treatment. "I felt like I was terminally stuck in waiting—you're waiting for two weeks when you're cycling, appointments are two weeks apart from each other, then after you're pregnant, it's two weeks between appointments. That two-week wait kept coming up." During the two-week wait, Palumbo tried to distract herself with things she enjoyed, like getting pedicures and binge watching *The Golden Girls, RuPaul's Drag Race,* and other shows where there was no chance of pregnancy or infertility talk, or even an errant diaper commercial.

Symptom Spotting

For those of us who are not so great at compartmentalizing, there's not much to do during the two-week wait except . . . wait.

And relentlessly monitor your symptoms.

Back in the beginning, before I started treatment, we had a holiday party. Solomon and I had gotten married in September, been pregnant for a short time in October, gone on a honeymoon in November, and, well, I was expecting my period around the holidays in December. I hadn't been charting or monitoring or anything—I don't think I even knew what basal body temperature was!—so I had no idea exactly when or if I ovulated. But at that party, I was *wondering.*

I set up for the party, thinking, *Should I be lifting things?* I put on my makeup, noticing, *Wow, my cheeks seem really flushed.* "Oh, hi!" I greeted all my single friends, thinking, *Is this the last time I'll have a kid-free holiday party?* (It was—but only because in the infertile years to come, I wouldn't feel like having parties.) As I flitted around the room, refilling the appetizer trays and chucking the empty wine cups,

I had a smile plastered on my face, but a thumping in my heart. *Pa-pa-pa-regnant?* I actually snuck out during the party to purchase a pregnancy test. And I was!

This, my friend, was a disaster. Not just because I lost that pregnancy, but because after that experience I was *sure* I could predict when I felt pregnant.

Symptom spotting is one of the worst parts about the two-week wait.

"The more time goes on, the more I realize that I don't actually have 'two-week waits.' I have a one-week wait, and then a week of all the PMS symptoms that a girl can handle: cramps, backache, break-outs, nightmares, moody, weepy, migraines and retaining water," Palumbo wrote on her blog while she was doing IVF.

The most irritating thing about looking for proof of pregnancy is how similar the symptoms of pregnancy are to those of PMS—especially if you're on progesterone (side effects: fatigue, loss of appetite, "foggy thinking").[2] During my waits, I loved to examine those pink bubble charts online comparing PMS symptoms to pregnancy: sudden increased appetite could mean you had PMS, and nausea or vomiting could mean you were pregnant. Breast tenderness, stomach cramping, fatigue, and mood swings? Could be either one. Bitchiness? Well, Solomon might say that was just me being me and could go either way.

I thought I was an expert at predicting pregnancy: *Is that cramp the embryo implanting?* (No, it was me having to go to the bathroom.) *Aren't those crazy dreams about babies a sign?* (No, just my usual psyche working out my desires.) *Oh, I skipped eating that Snickers bar, maybe it's the baby making me healthy.* (It was all the vitamins I was taking.) *I feel so tired, is this how it's going to be for the next ten months?* (Perhaps it was the decrease in caffeine.) *Is that implantation bleeding?* (No, it's my period starting.)

"PMS symptoms and pregnancy symptoms are the same," says Palumbo when she finally found out she was pregnant. "I *HATE* saying this as I think it prolongs the torture for many of you in the two-week wait, but sadly, it's true. Whichever entity came up with that really needs to be bitch-slapped."

I do think some people can distinguish the difference between pregnancy and PMS, but the symptoms are *not* universal. I think the only way you can symptom spot is if you really, really know your own body and its PMS symptoms.

What does your body feel like in the days leading up to your period? Are you nauseous or eating everything? Does your stomach bloat like a boat and your boobs fill up like water balloons? Do you collapse at eight P.M. or get crazy insomnia the way I do?

The more time I spent Trying, the better I became at discerning between feeling pregnant and feeling premenstrual. At one point I even thought I could *smell* the hCG. (Just like dogs!)

I found that a *lack* of symptoms was most indicative. The suspension of my PMS—no bloating, no mood swings, no insomnia—meant no period. All those other pregnancy symptoms? Nausea, sensitivity to smells, fatigue? Those came much later.

During my last two-week wait, I was no longer symptom spotting. I'd been doing this for so long that I'd gotten good at ignoring that long running dialogue in my head: *Do I feel a cramp? Is that a brown spot on my panties? Is the smell of my husband making me ill?* (No, darling, never!) It had just become background noise. I didn't know I was pregnant until the doctor told me.

People love to say, "Don't think about it," or "Try not to worry about it." But I'm guessing those people have never yearned to be pregnant or spent many, many years Trying. In many ways, searching for proof of pregnancy is about searching for control during a time when you have very little, and that's totally normal. Don't beat yourself up about it. Although in the end I stopped symptom spotting, I also stopped trying to control my thoughts and feelings. I was always going to think about it, and I just had to learn to accept that about myself.

To Test or Not to Test

If you're symptom spotting, you're probably going to want to take some pregnancy tests.

"Try to avoid temptation," a woman's magazine article advised, when it comes to "the all-encompassing urge" to take a home pregnancy test (or POAS as many refer to Peeing On A Stick).[3]

Yes, there are downsides to testing at home:

a) Waiting for the second line to appear can be the most excruciating 2 to 5 minutes of your life.

b) If you test too early, you may see a false negative, giving you unnecessary grief.

c) You can get a false positive if you've taken an hCG trigger during IUI or IVF: It's the same hormone the pregnancy test measures. Which can also give you grief.

Yet what doctors, Internet articles, and women with willpower who advise not to test don't understand is that there are many reasons to take a home pregnancy test.

a) You like getting your own pee on your hand.

b) Pregnancy tests can give you an answer much sooner than your follow-up appointment.

c) You'd rather deal with the information on your own than learn about it from a phone call.

I was the type of kid who would fail the marshmallow test, and I've grown into an adult with even less willpower: I was going to test. Boy, was I going to test *and* double test daily. So instead of spending $25 on one pregnancy test, I bought them in bulk on Amazon (twenty-five for $10 bucks).

I didn't know then that there is a difference between the tests. Home pregnancy tests measure hCG, the hormone made by cells formed in the placenta, which nourishes the fertilized egg after it has attached itself to the uterine wall.[4] So, what you need to know when testing at home is the minimum milliliters of hCG a test can detect. Some are more sensitive than others and can detect early. The expensive ones can detect as little as 6 milliliters of hCG in the bloodstream, promising a result some six days before your expected cycle. The cheaper ones can detect 10 to 25 milliliters. (Anything over 5 milliliters is technically pregnant.)

But here's the thing—you're not going to know exactly what the test means until you go to your doctor. Which is why most docs don't recommend at-home testing. But they're not the ones agonizing over the two-week wait, analyzing every hiccup and pimple. (God, if I could just put the doctor in my head for one day, he wouldn't last a minute without testing!)

So, if you're going to test, the question is when?

- If you haven't gotten an hCG trigger shot, you can begin testing 7 to 10 days after your IUI, because implantation (when the embryo nestles into your uterine lining) usually occurs 6 to 12 days after ovulation/IUI.[5] If it's negative, keep testing! You may not have a test that detects low levels of hCG. If it's positive, keep testing to make sure the line is getting stronger.
- If you *have* gotten an hCG shot, some women "test it out." They start testing soon after their IUI/IVF transfer until they see a "not pregnant" test, meaning the artificial hormone is out of their body. This can take up to a week postshot.

You know how they say that people stuck in the desert will hallucinate an oasis where there is none? A woman Trying will always see a second faint line—even when her husband refuses to support this vision. Luckily, there are Facebook groups devoted entirely to analyzing pee stick lines.

Even when I managed to refrain from testing for most of the two-week wait, I'd cave at the last minute. I came to hate getting a phone call from a nurse—a stranger who had the power to change my life. That hopeful feeling when the phone rings? The cheery-sounding nurse? *Maybe she sounds so happy because she has good news for me,* I'd think in those last two minutes of bliss. No, she was just being polite. Because then she'd say: "I'm afraid you're not pregnant."

I tested because I wanted to know first. (Control freak, much?) And because I could handle the disappointment more easily on my own. (Some people have a negative at-home test and then the blood test proves them wrong!)

So now that I've revealed the true nature of my insanity, you might decide to be the Un-Me and not test at home. Good for you! Head on over to the clinic to get the accurate blood test (see chapter 12).

What If You're Negative

It's okay to be negative. By this I mean two things: It's okay to have negative thoughts, to be sure this isn't going to work. And it's also okay to have a negative pregnancy test.

You don't know anything for sure until you test at the doctor.

If you're not pregnant, I'm so, so sorry for your loss. And it *is* a loss—of hope, of potential, of possibility, of time, of effort. It's devastating to see that single line on your home test, or hear the nurse give you the news over the phone (or, if you're smart, read it in an email so you don't have to be mean and slam the phone down on her like she's a random telemarketer).

Here's what truly bites: A negative pregnancy coincides with an actual period. Watching the blood flow out of my body was the definition of adding insult to injury. Not only did I have to suffer the mood swings of PMS and the pain (and inconvenience) of my cycle—which felt one hundred times worse *after* medication!!—but on top of that, I had to deal with the dejection of my barrenness. I hate that old biblical word; it feels so . . . so final! But after a treatment failure, it felt like the right word, conveying the sheer emptiness in my womb and in my heart.

Whether you choose to continue with another IUI or move on to IVF, you will definitely have to endure another two-week wait.

How the hell are you going to go through that again?

"Don't judge yourself," Palumbo says. "Be forgiving of yourself to get through it: Two weeks is temporary. This is not going to be the rest of your life. Even if you decide to stop treatment, use donor eggs, adopt, this is not going to be the rest of your life. You *will* have a resolution: It might not be the resolution you expected, but you'll have a resolution," she says. "For me it felt like the pain would last forever—but nothing does."

Chapter 11

Next Up, IVF: What to Expect During Your First Cycle

These are the needles that it took to make Moses. . . . These came with pain, tears, and it began joy. And so I wanted to share this because all of these went into my body so that I could become a mom.

—Tamron Hall[1]

After four failed IUIs, I was relieved to begin IVF. I felt like it would take chance completely out of the equation. (Although I was soon to learn that chance—or luck, fate, God, whatever you want to call it—is always part of the equation.)

IVF is cheating, a "short-circuit of the system," says Dr. William B. Schoolcraft, founder and medical director of the Colorado Center for Reproductive Medicine (CCRM), a network of eleven fertility centers across North America.

If you've gotten this far, you probably know how conception

works: The ovary releases an egg, that one egg has to get "captured" by the fallopian tube (as Dr. Schoolcraft says), the sperm have to get there and fertilize the egg, and that fertilized egg has to make a five-day journey to the uterus.

"That's a lot of things that have to go right—with only one egg. And if one thing fails, it doesn't work," Dr. Schoolcraft says, noting that IVF bypasses half the steps of natural conception and IUI—namely, the eggs being fertilized and making their way to the uterus—and "IVF delivers the embryo directly to the uterus."

That's what I loved about it. I felt like I had more control of the process.

Of course, not everyone is as excited to start IVF as I was. Some people are really bummed about it.

Aside from the sheer practical problems—the money, the time suck, the waiting, did I mention the money?—doing IVF means another dream you have to relinquish: conceiving your baby naturally. (Some people prefer the term "unassisted." I prefer "free.") Although those IUIs weren't exactly natural, because you still had to go to a doctor's office to jump-start the sperm, at least the baby-making was happening *inside your body.* Conception—the sperm meeting the egg—was happening on its own.

I won't try to talk you out of your bummed-out-ness. This is an "all feelings are legitimate" zone, a safe space for rants about IVF, pregnant friends, rude family, and terrible triggers (like the seemingly innocuous story "Infertile Snails Have Recovered along the Norwegian Coast,"[2] which made me cry: *Even the snails are recovering from their infertility?*).

All I can say is yes, it does suck.

But consider what Dr. Schoolcraft says: "We give you medicine to carry a dozen eggs instead of one. . . . With natural conception you'd have to ovulate twelve times to get that amount of eggs."

When you think about it that way, it's amazing we don't all do IVF.

Are There Health Risks to IVF?

Here are the questions to ask your doctor:

· **What are the risks of IVF medication?**

Ask about the side effects of *every* medication you'll be taking, and tell them about any other meds you're on. Ask about the long-term risks of medication: Is there a limit to how much you can take and how close together you can take it?

· **What are risks for the procedure?**

Ask about complications that can arise from the egg retrieval procedure and if there are any long-term risks, too.

· **Are infertile women/men at risk for other conditions?**

Ask your doctor if you're at risk for other conditions and diseases because you're infertile, and if the medications increase those risks. Many of the studies saying "IVF causes XYZ" actually correlate infertility with XYZ, meaning that people with infertility have a higher risk of XYZ.

· **What are the health risks for IVF pregnancy?**

Are there risks during pregnancy (like preeclampsia, preterm birth, and C-section)?

· **What are the risks for children born from IVF?**

Ask your doctor about the risks for children born from IVF, and from other add-on procedures like genetic testing of embryos. What are the incidents of birth defects, disease, and development?

Be sure to ask about the actual risk, rather than the relative risk, which one study of how doctors communicate the health risks of IVF found to be deceiving.[3] For example, although the relative risk of a child having schizophrenia is 300 percent higher if the child is born to a sixty-year-old father versus a twenty-five-year-old father, the absolute risk only increases from 1 percent to 3 percent chance.[4]

Also discuss with your doctor who the subjects of the study are and if you are similar enough to the study group that the risks apply to you. Sometimes, things are out of our hands. "Most importantly, we explain to them that there are things we just do not know," that study found.

Resistance to IVF

When I was growing up, there was a science-fiction-y, futuristic aura (cue the *Twilight Zone do-do-do-do* music) attached to the mention of a test-tube baby, to the fact that we can create babies outside the womb like pods in *Invasion of the Body Snatchers*.

So I was shocked when I belatedly realized that babies conceived via IVF were, in fact, what they called test-tube babies. It seemed *so normal*.

In vitro literally means "in a glass," but has come to be defined as "outside the body." (PS: The egg is fertilized in a petri dish, not a test tube.) Let's not forget that the first test-tube baby, Louise Brown, was only born in 1978. Since then, more than eight million babies have been born using IVF.[5] Back then, it was considered freakish, premature, and was "accompanied by a loud opposition from the press and members of the public," according to *In-Vitro Fertilization: The Pioneers' History,* a book that fascinatingly recounts the origins of the science behind IVF all the way back to a rabbit egg transplant in 1891.[6]

I bring this up because if you, or busybodies around you, have reservations about IVF or any of the technology associated with it, you should understand that certain fears always seem to accompany new science and technology. Routine operations like heart or liver transplants were once considered verboten, and it seems that nearly every improvement to reproductive technology provokes panic.

If, in the future, an entire pregnancy can be gestated outside the womb (like I saw attempted on *Grey's Anatomy*), IVF will be considered downright old-fashioned! Then, if we IVF moms wanted to feel superior to women "having" babies in artificial wombs, we could say, *Well, my baby was in human utero for nine months.*

My point is that IVF might seem strange at first, but you'll get used to the idea.

For those of us who are a bit further down the line, we've gotten way beyond discomfort over the procedure—and well, we'd give our right ovary to be at the beginning of our first cycle.

Because the first cycle is, in many ways, *magical.*

Attrition Rate in IVF

Some say that in traditional IVF, at every step of the process, you can expect your results to decrease by up to one-third. Start with:

- How many follicles you have at the start of your cycle
- How many follicles you have before retrieval
- How many eggs were retrieved
- How many retrieved eggs were mature
- How many eggs fertilized
- How many embryos made it to day 3
- How many embryos made it to day 5
- How many embryos you can genetically test
- How many embryos turned out to be genetically normal

When Doc Knows Best

Your first cycle is magical because it's a mystery. Why, it's a magical mystery tour! (In a good way.) No matter how high/low your hormone levels are, no matter what you've done prior to this—timed sex, stimulation meds, IUIs—no one really knows exactly how you will do in your first IVF cycle.

Right now, you're a blank canvas ready for the masterpiece of conception.

Your doctor does not really know how your body will respond to medication (although if you've done medicated IUI, he may have a clue and can adjust your IVF medication accordingly), how many eggs your body will produce, how many of those he will be able to extract, how many of *those* will be good (mature) eggs, and which of those eggs will fertilize and turn into embryos ready for transfer.

When I started IVF, I didn't know much. Yeah, sure, I knew the basics—egg + sperm=embryo, yada, yada, yada—but I was still on the "Doc Knows Best" plan. And Dr. Chang really did seem to know a lot—more important, he was generous and patient about explaining it to me. (No wonder he was always running late.)

Here's why I felt like the process was magical: I was getting a front-row seat to my own fertility. During the transvaginal ultrasound exam—yes, they stick a cold, gooey wand inside you—I saw my follicles being measured. And there were six of them. Six!! Because we were doing mini IVF (using less medication to create fewer eggs, which I'll discuss in chapter 20), six seemed like an embarrassment of riches. Solomon and I only wanted two kids: *What am I going to do with all these babies?* I thought. Yes, back then I thought my follicles would all become children.

At the beginning of the process, you have to sign off on what you're going to do with surplus embryos: discard them, donate them to science, or donate them to another couple. I magnanimously chose the latter. *Well, Catherine is trying on her own and Maya has always been so generous with inviting me over to her house,* I thought, mentally bequeathing my embryos to the two other women in the clinic. I felt fertile, wealthy, and benevolent.

And that feeling continued throughout my wondrous first cycle. I loved seeing my follicles on the screen, watching Dr. Chang insert the catheter into me and pinch out my eggs during the retrieval. (I had a local anesthetic, where I remained awake but felt little, especially with the Valium.) He retrieved four. I was a bit disappointed, but he said, "That's great!"

So maybe I wouldn't be gifting embryos anytime soon, but four embryos was more than the boy-girl duo I'd planned.

Even more wondrous than the retrieval was the transfer: Three days later, as I lay in the dark room, with my bladder full, as required for a transfer, I felt like I was viewing my own personal Discovery Channel on the big screen. Dr. Chang guided the three-day embryo back into my womb. This, this . . . speck of dust, this droplet of water! . . . could be our first child. Oh, but first he had to verify with the embryologist in the lab that the embryo had actually made it off the catheter (like glitter, embryos can stick to everything). "You're in!" he said.

As I was wheeled to the post-retrieval room and settled in my pink scrubs into the soft recliner in a peaceful Valium haze, I dreamily thought of Dr. Chang and the embryo transfer. (It was *transferred,* not *implanted.* Transfer is the process, and implantation is when the embryo embeds itself into my uterine lining, which, I hoped, would occur in the next week or so.) I was a little in love with him and a lot in love with science.

Now all I had to do was wait.

Wait, What Are We Doing Here, Exactly?

Yes, for that first, magical cycle, I was on the "Doc Knows Best" program. But as the cycles accumulated with no babies, I felt like I switched to the "Learn as You Go" program, then the "Let's Get Smarter Than the Doctor" program. Meaning: There were failures. There were mistakes. There were disappointments. And I want to help you skip some of those.

If you're not on the "Doc Knows Best" program and are following the "Verify, Then Trust" program instead, the first thing you'll want to know is what your protocol is—that is, what is the plan for your medical treatment? How much medication will you be taking, which days will you be taking it, and when can you plan for a retrieval?

As you probably know by now, things here don't go exactly according to plan, but it would be nice to have a *general* strategy.

"There's only one protocol," says Dr. Schoolcraft, referring to the

This Is Your Lifestyle During IVF

When it comes to lifestyle choices during your cycle, "There is no real definitive guide to what should be done during IVF," says Dr. Eric J. Forman, medical and laboratory director of Columbia University Fertility Center. His advice:

Alcohol: Probably okay in moderation (i.e., one glass of wine) during stimulation, but Dr. Forman recommends abstaining from alcohol after embryo transfer and during pregnancy.

Exercise: Safe in moderation, but as the ovaries enlarge, exercise should be reduced as there is an increased (though still very small) risk of torsion—twisting of the ovaries. Dr. Forman advises against increasing core body temperature with very rigorous exercise or activities like hot yoga.

Sex: Safe until you get closer to egg retrieval, when your ovaries are enlarged (see "torsion").

Water: Traditionally, Dr. Forman says, he tells patients to avoid baths, hot tubs, or otherwise fully submerging themselves in water for one week after an invasive procedure like egg retrieval and until pregnancy is confirmed after a transfer.

Bed rest: There's no evidence that bed rest helps with anything. In fact, Dr. Forman says, evidence suggests it's safe to get up immediately post-embryo transfer and resume a more or less normal activity level.

fact that there's only one basic goal: to stimulate egg production. Of course, it's not so simple. Different combinations of drugs are appropriate at different times and for different people, and which combination your doctor uses takes into account many factors, including your hormone level, your age, your height and weight, and your previous reaction to fertility medication. "The way you execute the protocol is important, the dose is important, the timing is important," Dr. Schoolcraft says, noting that the embryology lab is the most important part.

Here are the basic meds:

1. **Gonadotropins** override your natural endocrine system and get your ovaries to produce more eggs—but not too many!—and grow those eggs "evenly," at the same rate, so they'll be ready for retrieval at the same time.

2. An **antagonist** (no, not an evil enemy) will be given to make sure you don't ovulate on your own.

3. A **trigger** will make you ovulate.

Some women agonize over which medicines they are taking and at what dosages, and if they were doing a "long" or "short" protocol (meaning how long you are being stimulated).[7] I was never one of those people who got involved in my medical protocol—I trusted my doctor to choose the right medications and dosages. You'll have to decide which approach feels right to you.

You can ask your doctor what drugs she is prescribing and why, but, Dr. Schoolcraft says, "It's not the protocol, it's when to stop it," meaning the timing may be more important than the type of medicine.

Also, remember, if this is your first cycle, you're a blank slate, right?

I suggest that rather than focusing on the whys, you should focus on the hows.

How are you going to get through every step of the cycle?

Here are some prep questions:

- Who will administer your shots? (Not my husband!)
- How should they be stored?
- Can they be reused? (And what about that little bit that's left over?)
- Do the shots have to be administered at a certain time— and what happens if you miss that time?

Scientifically Speaking:
IVF By the Numbers[8]

- For women younger than 35, the percentage of live births per egg retrieval is 54.4 percent.
- For women ages 35 to 37, the percentage of live births per egg retrieval is 42 percent.
- For women ages 38 to 40, the percentage of live births per egg retrieval is 26.6 percent.
- For women ages 41 to 42, the percentage of live births per egg retrieval is 13.3 percent.
- For women ages 43 and up, the percentage of live births per egg retrieval is 3.9 percent.

Prepping for Retrieval

Before some women start IVF, they are given oral contraceptives, estrogen, or sometimes testosterone, which is called "priming" the ovaries, to improve ovarian response or create more symmetrical growth of the follicles, according to CCRM.

Then, you'll start going to the clinic on day 2 or 3 of your cycle to get your hormone level assessed and your follicles checked out. That's when your doctor will decide how much medication to give you and when you need to return.

Then you'll start your shots. Ice everything! Poking holes in your stomach and/or butt is easier when you can't feel anything. And, yes, alternate sides. You'll look like a pincushion, but the only worse thing than taking shots every day is taking them in the same spot. And drink lots of water.

You'll probably have to go in every other day for ultrasounds and monitoring, and your doctor will adjust your meds accordingly. The monitoring is usually done early in the day so the doctor can give you instructions by a certain hour. However, that means you're stuck sitting by the phone like a high school senior waiting to get asked to prom. (Good luck if you don't have cell service in your office, or if you're in the subway or if you, like, have a *life*.) Make sure they also email you *everything*!

"Sixteen, eleven, twelve," the ultrasound technician called out like they were lotto numbers. In truth, she was measuring my follicles on the screen to monitor how they were growing and when they were ready to be "triggered."

After eight to ten nights of injections, the follicles will reach a mature size and your doctor will proceed to egg retrieval. Retrieval happens 35 to 36 hours after your trigger shot. The trigger shot is the only med where the exact time you take it really matters, because ovulating early and missing your retrieval is one of the worst things that can happen. (The doctor cannot retrieve your eggs if your ovaries release them early.)

You won't miss your retrieval. I hope.

It is now, right before retrieval, when they have a pretty good idea of how many eggs they'll try to retrieve, when you'll have to answer more questions:

1. **Will you be getting local or general anesthesia?**

   Some clinics make that decision based on the number of eggs being retrieved—if it's only a few, they may go local.

2. **Are you using fresh or frozen sperm?**

   You may be using frozen sperm if you're going it alone, if you're in a same-sex partnership, or if your partner is unavailable. If your sperm supply is limited because you purchased it or it had to be extracted via surgery, you will need to discuss how much is to be defrosted.

3. **Are you freezing your eggs?**

   If so, congratulations! This is where the process ends.

4. **What type of fertilization will you be doing?**

For normal fertilization, an embryologist places some 50,000 to 100,000 sperm in a petri dish with one egg and hopes for the best. An added process is intracytoplasmic sperm injection (ICSI), in which the embryologist micro-injects only *one* sperm into the shell of the egg. When you don't have a lot of sperm—whether that's due to male factor infertility or because you purchased it—ICSI is preferable because it uses less sperm. (Some studies show ICSI is not helpful for regular couples, i.e., those without male factor infertility.[9])

For your first cycle, doctors will probably not do ICSI, but you can sign up to have "emergency ICSI" within a few hours if fertilization fails. If you are testing your embryos (see #8), you need to have ICSI.

5. **Are you going to do a fresh transfer?**

After the retrieval, the eggs are fertilized with sperm. You can do a **fresh embryo transfer** in the same cycle, or you can freeze all the embryos to transfer at a later cycle, which is known as a **frozen transfer**. (If you do a fresh transfer, you can freeze the remaining embryos for a later frozen transfer.)

Some doctors believe a "freeze all" strategy is better, freezing all the embryos created from your retrieval and not doing a transfer that month. They think this gives your body time to recover from the stimulation meds and retrieval so you'll be healthier for transfer during your next cycle.

Others believe that it's better to start with a fresh transfer to avoid subjecting your embryos to cryo-preservation. According to a recent study, for women with fewer eggs (less than 15), it's best to start with a

fresh transfer.[10] (The remaining embryos will be
frozen.)

Some clinics have a strategy set for all patients, and
others take a "wait and see" approach to how your embryos develop.

6. **If you're doing a fresh transfer, will it be a day-3 or
day-5 transfer?**

These days, most clinics prefer day-5 transfers, believing
that the longer an embryo survives, the stronger it is.
For your first cycle, they will probably aim for a day-5
embryo. Some old-school clinics, believing the less time
the embryo is outside the womb, the better, still do day-3
transfers, especially for older women or for women
whose embryos may not survive five days.

Studies show that blastocysts (day-5 embryos) have a
50.5 percent chance of implantation, and cleavage-stage
(day-3) embryos have only a 30 percent chance.[11] Of
course, statistics vary between clinics and labs.

7. **How many embryos will you transfer?**

In the past, twins and triplets were a common result of
fertility treatment, but today, with better laboratories and
technology, doctors are aiming to reduce the risk of multiples because they present health risks to the mother *and*
the children. Multiples are more likely to be born premature, which increases the risk of health problems.

"In continuing efforts to promote singleton gestation
and reduce the number of multiple pregnancies," the
ASRM recommends transferring as few embryos as
necessary for one, healthy baby.[12] In women younger
than thirty-five, that's usually one embryo. The guidelines change depending on your age, if you've given
birth, and the quality of your embryos. (Women forty-

one and over may have three or four untested embryos
transferred.)

8. **Will you be genetically testing your embryos?**
   Since many people don't do embryo testing in their first
   cycle, we'll discuss it in depth in chapter 20. If you do test
   your embryos, you will not be doing a fresh transfer, as
   they have to be biopsied, then frozen, at least until your
   next cycle. Also, if you do test your embryos, most docs
   will only transfer one.

After Your Retrieval

Back when I did IVF, there were very few Facebook secret/private
groups (I still don't know the difference) devoted to every stage of
IVF, from two-week-waiters to positive-pregnancy-testers to repeat-
pregnancy-lossers to donor-egg-moms. So I did not *know* I was supposed to be anxiously waiting for the phone call to hear how my
eggs/embryos progressed. I was blissfully ignorant during my first
cycle in a way I wouldn't be for the next three years.

After your retrieval (day 0), you'll find out how many eggs were
actually retrieved, how many were mature (have a "visible polar
body"[13]) and, the next day, you will probably get a phone call disclosing how many eggs fertilized.

The calls may come again on day 3 or day 5. By day 5 or 6 the clinic
will grade your embryos, something like "5AB, 6BC." Most clinics
rate your embryo's speed of development and its morphology, the
shape or appearance of cells in the embryo. (One note: Don't compare
grades between clinics, because they each have their own system.)

And then you get the call: My nurse always, no matter what the
results were, sounded unbearably upbeat. I mean, millennial-uptalk
upbeat.

"Hello? Is this Amy?" she'd say. (It probably wasn't even the same person every time, but they all had the same affect.) "We wanted to let you know? That you'll have a transfer tomorrow? And we'll freeze the rest of your embryos??"

"Okay?" I said, subconsciously mimicking her.

If everything is okay, you'll have your transfer. And if it isn't, *call your doctor!* If you are overstimulated—i.e., produce too many eggs—you will be in danger of ovarian hyperstimulation syndrome (OHSS), a condition characterized by enlargement of the ovaries, fluid retention, and weight gain, which can be serious and painful.[14] (I never did have any health side effects from a retrieval, but if you have OHSS, or react adversely to the drugs, transfers may have to be postponed until another cycle.)

Let me tell you something about transfers: They're easy, especially compared to everything you've been through with the retrieval, the medications, the side effects, and the timing.

Hopefully, you'll be successful on your very first try. (If not, head over to chapter 20.)

Secrets of the Embryo Lab

"Embryo Man," as he's known on Twitter, has been working in an embryology lab for over three years and spent a decade before that in various research positions. He started his blog, Remembryo .com, to look at evidence-based research for IVF.

Q: How can a lab or embryologist make a difference?

A: The embryologist is the caretaker for the embryo, and without the necessary skills to handle the gametes/embryos, the success for the patient could suffer. Good labs have good quality controls. Besides checking incubator temperatures, gas levels, etc., we need to be confident that the embryologists are doing their job appropriately. Statistics can be tracked (like fertilization rates) and proficiency testing can be performed (to ensure skills are good).

Q: Does embryo grading really matter?

A: Embryologists are the judges who decide which embryo looks best. For each stage of an embryo's growth (cleavage, morula, blastula) there are different criteria that are used to assess quality. These qualities can be correlated with the embryo's potential to create a pregnancy. *But* there are other factors that determine success, besides grading, including endometrium and maternal age. Higher-graded embryos have a better chance than lower-graded embryos but even poor-graded embryos make babies.

Q: What do people not understand about embryologists?

A: My experience in a high-volume clinic is that *we have very little time.* It might surprise people to learn how long things can take, and when you have a bunch of those things piled on top of each other, you don't have much time for anything else!

I hear all the time, "But you only need one sperm!" Yes, I only need one sperm, but the problem is *finding that one sperm.* Literally impossible at times. It can be tough. But it's pretty awesome when you do find it and it fertilizes!

Chapter 12

So, You're Pregnant! What to Expect Before You're Home Free

The best part about being open is when you really don't have anything to hide, it's just liberating and free. . . . The thing at hand that felt so heavy to carry doesn't feel so heavy anymore. It's not a burden.

—dancer Julianne Hough[1]

I strode into the doctor's office with a secret weapon in my hand. I walked behind the desk to the phlebotomist (the word sounds so much better than "the technician drawing my blood") and unsheathed my plastic sword: "I'm pregnant!" I chanted, proudly waving around the home test with the pink lines. She took a dubious step backward, no doubt worrying about getting splattered with urine.

"Don't worry, I washed it," I assured her.

She gave me a tepid half smile, not *nearly* as pleased as me. Didn't she hear me? *I'm PREGNANT.* I wanted to shout it from the rooftops, blare it on my blog, run screaming through the quiet, white clinic.

Instead, I sat there patiently as she wrapped my arm in a tight tourniquet and stabbed me with a needle. *This will all be over soon,* I thought. *No more blood tests, no more doctor visits, no more dumb fertility acronyms (NMDFA), no more planning my day around doctor's appointments, because I'M PREGNANT! I'm done! I'm outta here!*

Not So Fast

And I was also . . . naive.

I'd been so obsessed with getting pregnant, with seeing those beautiful lines on my at-home pee stick, with envisioning my protruding belly and fat cankles (be careful what you wish for) that I had no clue about what came next: *staying* pregnant. Before I could celebrate, the clinic would want to calculate whether I was going to go on to have a healthy pregnancy or whether this was a false start.

That's why, when I was waving around my positive test with panache, the gang at the clinic was taking it all with a grain of salt. It might have been my very first IVF, my first retrieval, and my first fresh day-3 embryo transfer, but they'd been to this rodeo before. Here I was thinking I'd hit a home run, while they knew I'd barely gotten to first base. (If there's anything worse than IVF acronyms, it's probably sports metaphors.) Let's just say it was only the beginning.

"Hi, Amy?" the nurse said later that day. I wondered if she was calling to tell me when my first ultrasound appointment was or if I'd forgotten my credit card at the office (again).

"I just want to let you know your beta is ninety-eight."

"My what is what?"

"Your beta hCG?" she said. "The hormone measuring your initial pregnancy level. Come back in two days to measure it again?"

I hung up and went about planning the rest of my life (okay, surfing Facebook). I had no clue what she was talking about, had no clue that some women wait by the phone for that first test, knowing that their initial number can possibly predict the future of the pregnancy, as can successive numbers.

I was so green that I went hiking the day of my third or fourth hCG test—I can't even say which because I wasn't paying attention. When someone from the fertility clinic called, I had to tell everyone else in the crowded car to quiet down. (We were so new on our journey that we were still hanging out with raucous, happy singles.) "I just wanted to let you know your hCG is three thousand something something?" she said, not even giving me the benefit of a round number.

"Great!" I said, trying to stop from laughing at the antics in the car.

"Well . . ." she said, this time not ending her sentence with a question mark.

"Well what?" I said a bit too loudly because everyone suddenly shushed themselves.

"Well, it's not exactly great. . . . We want you to come back in two days for another blood test," she said. "The numbers aren't exactly where we want them to be."

"The numbers?" Was I supposed to be paying attention to them? Was there a place they were supposed to be? And if so, how come nobody told me? What were those numbers, anyway, and what the hell did they have to do with my perfect pregnancy?

A Little Bit Pregnant

I'm not an idiot. (Well, I guess you can judge for yourself.) I knew that a pregnancy test measures your hCG hormone level and predicts whether you're pregnant based on that. But I thought there were only two outcomes: yes or no. I did not know there was a "maybe," a might be, a possibility, an in-between place. I was led to believe there's no such thing as a little bit pregnant. But actually, I was soon to learn, there is. This is just another injustice we IVF warriors must deal with. (Side note: When you get pregnant naturally, you take your at-home test, which tells you only if you're pregnant or not pregnant. Then you go to the doctor a month or so later for an ultrasound to confirm it. But with fertility treatment, they want to monitor your hormone levels from the start to see if you need extra support and if your pregnancy will be viable.)

Is there a magic number for what is called your "beta," your first hCG blood test? Well, yes and no. The higher the number, the stronger the pregnancy. And if it's really high, it could be multiples.

Technically, anything over 5 mIU/mL hCG is pregnant. But as I learned from the time I got an 8 (come *on*, embryo, not even a 10?!), anything lower than 25 is likely a chemical pregnancy (i.e., it does not progress to a pregnancy, which we will discuss in chapter 21).

The problem with comparing betas for viability is that clinics do the tests on different days, the numbers vary for day-3 and day-5 embryos, and they also may vary for fresh or frozen transfers.

"A single quantitative hCG measurement cannot reliably distinguish a viable intrauterine pregnancy," Dr. Robert Barbieri editorialized in *OBG Management*.[2] So one test isn't enough; you're going to need what they call serial hCG measurements.

There are many different "doubling times" in regards to how your hCG should increase in the beginning of the pregnancy. Some docs and website calculators say your hCG should rise 66 percent every two days in the beginning, but slower-rising hCG can still result in a healthy pregnancy, especially with medical support.[3]

I hate to give exact numbers because I have heard so many stories of successful pregnancies with low-starting numbers or slow-rising hCGs.

Consider this post on a mom board[4] (it will help you get used to how women write on these things):

1st hCG level was 995 on 12/21, 2nd was 1388 on 12/23, and third level is now 2800 on 12/28. This is approximately a 5-day doubling period. Is there any hope for this pregnancy? For some reason my doc is not concerned because levels are increasing. I have had no cramping or spotting. Any encouraging stories?

There were plenty: One woman's didn't double every 48 hours for the first few weeks and then skyrocketed—and she had twins! Another's took five days to double, but resulted in a healthy baby. (Unfortunately, the original poster wrote later that that pregnancy did fail, but she eventually went on to have a baby.)

"A minor disadvantage of serial hCG measurements is that patients may become anxious and fearful as they await the result of life-altering test results," Dr. Barbieri writes. (Um . . . *may* become???)

Falling or plateauing hCGs usually indicate a failing pregnancy.[5]

Once I started playing the hCG game, it was hard not to get obsessed. You can find different hCG doubling calculators on the Internet, and if you plug in two numbers, it can tell you their doubling times. As your pregnancy progresses, the doubling time takes longer. However, there is still so much that is unknown: "The minimal hCG rise in early pregnancies that correlates with good reproductive outcome has yet to be determined," according to a recent study.[6]

Come to think of it, my last pregnancy beta was 55. It seemed terrifically low for 8 days post-transfer of a day-5 embryo, but my doctor told me he only needed it to be above 50. So, instead of doing obsessive calculus yourself, talk to your doctor. She will probably know predictive values, what she likes to see as an initial value, and how much she likes to see it double and when.

A word of warning: In early pregnancy, you might see blood. Don't panic—it could be what they call "implantation bleeding"—brownish blood from your beautiful embryo burrowing into the uterine lining. It also can be the loss of one of the embryos (like when my twin pregnancy turned out to be a singleton). It could also be an SCH (subchorionic hematoma) from blood collecting between the gestational membranes and uterus during the first and second trimester.[7]

I have a non-IVF friend (yes, I have a couple of those!) who was bleeding for about a month, thinking it was a very long period. Finally, she went to the doctor and found out she was sixteen weeks pregnant. (We don't hate her, because she had been Trying for two years.)

Beyond Blood

Your clinic may do three or four hCG blood tests in the first few weeks. When your hCG reaches the low thousands,[8] your doctor will probably take a transvaginal ultrasound to see the gestational sac, the cavity of fluid surrounding the embryo. Some clinics wait until week 6 or 7 to see the fetus and hear a heartbeat. (At this point, you probably know the pregnancy-counting scam: the minute you miss your period, you're considered four weeks pregnant. Even though we doing fertility treatment know *the exact date of conception,* they're still counting it from your last-known menstrual period [LMP].)

So to recap: Around the day you're expecting your period, you do your beta blood test, repeat it two or three days later and maybe a couple more times until you have to wait for a 6- or 7-week ultrasound.

Here's one reason why you shouldn't live or die by your hCG: During one pregnancy, I had wonderful rising numbers, starting out of the gate at over 100 (twins, maybe?) and rising so nicely that everyone told me not to worry. And I didn't: My cheeks *were* flushed, my pulse was fast, I felt happy and high on hormones. My body *felt* pregnant. But I went for the ultrasound and I had an empty gestational sac. So bully for rising hCG.

On the other hand, my 55 doubled appropriately but I felt *nothing*. Well, except a mounting panic, probably based on all my previous failures.

"Do you want to come the day before Thanksgiving or the day after for your ultrasound?" Dr. Jeffrey Braverman, my final IVF doctor, asked me.

"The day after," I said, thinking the pregnancy wouldn't be viable. *Let me enjoy my last supper,* I thought. Even though I couldn't drink the specialty pumpkin mimosas and could barely swallow my aunt's famous scalloped potatoes, never mind the juicy turkey.

Somehow, I made it to the day after Thanksgiving, certain it would be my worst. When the doctor finally waved that magic wand over my jiggly belly and we heard the shocking *ba-bump-ba-bump-ba-bump-tat-tat-tat* sound of the heartbeat, I was flooded with what I can only say was *relief,* rather than joy.

IVF Complex Equations

- If Amy had an initial hCG reading of 55 and 3 days later had an hCG of 135, what is the rate of increase of her hCG?
- How much does your hCG need to go up if it's at 125 and your next test is in two days?
- What is 1.5 percent of 542, and does that mean it's twins?
- Why did you become an English major and not a scientist like your mother wanted you to be?
- Do you think your brain will explode if you keep doing hCG math all day long?

Case Dismissed!

Can you believe that Regular Pregnant Women—i.e., people who have never seen a basal body temperature thermometer or the inside of a fertility clinic—generally don't go to the OB till they're eight to twelve weeks pregnant?

It feels strange going to the fertility clinic when you're pregnant. You want to shout your news from the rooftop, but you also want to be sensitive to your silent, suffering sisters.

I hope it happens for you soon, I prayed for the other women in the waiting room.

Most clinics will dismiss you by the end of your first trimester. Ask your clinic for OB recommendations if you need to see a high-risk doctor.

Do You Need a High-Risk OB?

It often feels precarious to be pregnant after fertility treatment—especially after multiple tries. But it doesn't mean you will have a high-risk pregnancy.

A high-risk pregnancy is one that threatens the health of the mother and/or the baby. It can result from a condition that developed before pregnancy (or was discovered during fertility treatment), such as a clotting issue or an immunological disorder; or from your surgical history (including a previous pregnancy); or from diseases or chronic health conditions like diabetes, high blood pressure, and HIV.[9] But a pregnancy can also develop into one that's considered high-risk, such as if there's an RH incompatibility (when the mother and fetus have different blood types) or an abnormal placenta position. Multiple pregnancies usually need a high-risk OB.

It used to be that "old mothers"—over thirty-five—were automatically considered high-risk due to the risk of preeclampsia. But these days, I've seen forty-one-year-olds released to regular non-high-risk clinics. If you have no prior losses or other complications (like bleeding during early pregnancy), this may be you no matter your age.

A high-risk clinic will monitor you more often and more closely. I was going every two weeks until week 30, when I went every week. And I was happy to have the constant attention. After all my time at the fertility clinic, I was used to it.

If you feel you need your pregnancy to be monitored frequently, you can seek out a high-risk OB.

Upon dismissal, you may feel elated, but you also may feel irrationally panicky, wanting to throw yourself at your doctor's feet and say, "Don't leave me!" But you won't. Because you're sane. And you're pregnant—so you don't want to be throwing yourself around anymore.

Instead, take a good look around the office, at the white walls, the hopeful women, the busy receptionists who always seem to be on the phone (but never seemed to answer when *you* called). And bid them adieu with all the joy of Marie Kondo cleaning her closets.

Choose Your Own Adventure

If you're going to do another cycle, continue to chapter 20.
If you're pregnant, continue to the epilogue.

Chapter 13

It's Not You, It's Him: Male Factor Infertility

> I remember sitting up in the middle of the night thinking, *Jen would be a great mother and I don't want to get in the way of that so I'll let 'em tinker with my balls for a few hours.* And tinker, they did. I limped out of outpatient surgery a few hours later ... and for eight days I walked around New York City like a cowboy in snow. People were like, "What happened?" I was like, "Unnecessary ball surgery."
>
> —storyteller Mike Birbiglia, "The New One"

Am I a *terrible* person?

When our first IVF doc came back with the results of our diagnostic tests and didn't find anything wrong with Solomon, I was disappointed.

A tiny part of me (or bigger) wanted the problem to be with my husband.

The doctor didn't know exactly why I couldn't carry a pregnancy.

My FSH was fine (and no one thought to test my AMH till many docs later). Was it my MTHFR gene variant, which meant my body couldn't process folic acid? Or was it my slight clotting tendency? They didn't know, but all I could hear was *YOU, YOU, YOU,* with an Uncle Sam finger pointing hostilely at . . . well, me. Me, me, me.

I was too old.

I was too broken.

I was not able to carry a pregnancy to term.

So yes, of course, despite Solomon's speedy and voluminous sperm, I had been hoping, *Maybe it could be him.* I thought it would be easier to have someone else to pin it on.

Little did I know that male factor infertility is no picnic, either.

What's Your Problem, Dude?

After a year of unprotected sex, 8 to 15 percent of couples do not get pregnant. Some estimate that male factor infertility—when the reason you're not getting pregnant is due to the sperm—accounts for 20 percent of infertility, and another 30 to 40 percent is due to a combination of male and female problems.[1]

It should come as no surprise that men are a factor in infertility. Even though we women go through the lioness's share of testing, invasive diagnostic procedures, repeated monitoring, time-consuming appointments, and, hopefully, pregnancy and birth, "Men are *one half* the genetic contribution to making a baby," Dr. Marie Davidson, a psychologist at the Fertility Centers of Illinois, likes to remind the couples she counsels. "Many men will come to a fertility practice and feel like they don't even count—that's crazy," she says. "I've also met many couples where there is a joint fertility issue. Sperm is never off the hook, no matter what the semen analysis reveals."

And neither is the man, who should be getting the third degree about his reproductive history, too, including if he ever got anyone pregnant, had any childhood illnesses like the mumps, or has had any STDs, surgeries, or hernias, as well as his current medications and allergies and past or present exposures to toxins.

Before proceeding with *any* treatment, every clinic should do a semen analysis, evaluating the health and viability of the sperm. (Did you know that semen and sperm are not the same thing? Semen is the fluid men ejaculate, and it contains sperm, the male reproductive cells.)

"Ideally sperm should be collected at the laboratory," says the ASRM committee opinion on the evaluation of the infertile male.[2] "If collected at home, the specimen should be kept at room or body temperature during transport and examined in the laboratory within 1 hour of collection," the committee opinion recommends.

The lab sperm test will check the semen volume, sperm concentration (the number of sperm in the semen), sperm motility (how they move), and sperm morphology (their shape). If any of these numbers are abnormal, a second test is recommended, and then a referral to a urologist or male infertility specialist.

If a couple has "unexplained infertility," or infertility even after the woman has been treated for her issue (tubes unblocked, endometriosis scraped, period regulated), it also may be time to look at the man. If you're undergoing IVF and your embryos keep arresting at day 3— i.e., fertilizing but not making it to blastocysts at day 5 or 6, it may be time to reevaluate the sperm.[3]

Many urologists believe that male factor infertility is *way* underdiagnosed—and likely responsible for up to half (!) of all infertility cases, according to Dr. Paul Turek, a urologist specializing in male factor infertility and sexual health. "Even if everything looks normal, and they're not conceiving, I assume it's male until I can prove it's not."

In fact, "sperm DNA damage is a useful biomarker for male infertility diagnosis and prediction of assisted reproduction outcomes," one study found, noting its association with reduced fertilization rates, embryo quality, and pregnancy rates, and higher rates of spontaneous miscarriage and childhood diseases.[4]

Scientifically Speaking: The Male Biological Clock

Women love to read articles about the male biological clock—that age affects men, too—but is it true?

Studies do show that it takes longer for older men to conceive.[5] For men older than forty-five, there was a fivefold increase in the time to pregnancy relative to men younger than twenty-five.

"In the past we thought men's fertility was not affected by age," says Dr. Natan Bar-Chama, director of male reproductive medicine and surgery at Mount Sinai Medical Center. "Now we've learned there is a component to paternal age to try to conceive." A number of studies link older fathers to increases in the risk of autism and schizophrenia in their children.[6]

"But when you look at the numbers, you have to separate the absolute risk and the increased risk," Dr. Bar-Chama notes. "The absolute risk is still really very small."

A 2015 review of ninety studies found that sperm declines as men age.[7] "Male age needs more recognition as a potential contributor to the negative pregnancy outcomes and reduced offspring health associated with delayed first reproduction," the reviewers noted. If clinics would focus on DNA fragmentation and sperm's declining motility (speed), it "may lead to better patient outcomes during fertility treatments of aging couples," they said.

A 2019 study, "Maternal, Infant and Childhood Risks Associated with Advanced Paternal Age: The Need for Comprehensive Counseling for Men,"[8] suggests just that, as children born to fathers over forty-five have increased risk of complications, and have increased psych, neurocognitive disorders, and childhood cancers, "reproductive counseling and sperm banking may be an option in men who are planning to delay fatherhood."

Diagnosing and Treating Male Infertility

Before you start any IUI, ask about the results of the initial sperm test. And not just for the numbers and the percentages, but what they *mean*. What numbers do you need for an IUI and IVF? Is the sperm good? Not just "good enough" for fertility treatment—where reproductive endocrinologists will simply try to bypass the sperm's deficiency rather than correct it—but actually, really good?

Dr. Turek calls semen analysis a "blunt instrument," which often needs a more thorough evaluation than a regular fertility clinic may provide. "There's more to a man's fertility than is revealed by a semen analysis," he says, noting that there's a "preponderance of unnecessary infertility treatment" going on because he believes reproductive endocrinologists love assisted reproduction. "There's a desire to do it because it's expedient," he says.

It makes me sad to hear that fertility doctors may overtreat women's infertility. But it's not all their fault: According to "Limitations and Barriers in Access to Care for Male Factor Infertility," other factors that cause men to be undertreated and women to be overtreated include education level, household income, cultural norms, religious beliefs, geographic location, and "the availability of specialty-trained reproductive urologists."[9] Couples don't know what they don't know.

Should you have sperm tested?

- If there is absolutely nothing wrong with you as a woman— you're young, your uterus and tubes are clean, your hormones are stellar—you might want to get your male partner evaluated by a urologist for a second opinion before IUI/IVF.
- If your partner had a vasectomy, cancer or another illness, or a surgery that would deplete or destroy sperm, you should *start* with a urologist.
- If you have repeat miscarriages, sperm may be a contributing factor.

A urologist will do a full semen and hormonal evaluation, a thorough medical history, a physical exam, and often a genetic exam (although that may be a second line of treatment). Some men have low sperm counts, others have slow sperm, and a few have absolutely no viable sperm. Dr. Turek says that abnormal results could mean:

- An infection
- A hormonal imbalance
- A disease
- A blockage
- DNA fragmentation
- Genetic defects [10]
- A lifestyle issue (diet, weight, drugs)
- A medication issue

Glossary: Male Factor Infertility

DISORDERS

Azoospermia: The absence of spermatozoa in the ejaculate, either from:

- Obstructive azoospermia (OA): Blockage of the reproductive tract.
- Non-obstructive azoospermia (NOA): A failure of sperm production in the testicle.

Cryptozoospermia: So few sperm in the semen that they are identified only after concentration and centrifugation of the sample.
Elevated sperm DNA fragmentation (SDF): A measure of sperm quality that is unrelated to the simple semen analysis. A high-level of DNA damage in sperm cells can lead to infertility and poor IUI and IVF outcomes, as well as miscarriages.[11]

Oligospermia: Low sperm concentration in the semen.

Y chromosome microdeletion (YCM): Genetic disorders caused by missing gene(s) in the Y chromosome, which is present in many men with reduced fertility, but no other symptoms.[12]

PROCEDURES

Testicular mapping: Sperm mapping is a minimally invasive, nonsurgical procedure performed under local anesthesia to find sperm in the testes of men who have no ejaculated sperm due to testis failure.

Microsurgical epididymal sperm aspiration (MESA): A sperm-retrieval technique that uses a small microsurgical skin incision to collect fluid and sperm from the epididymis.

Percutaneous epididymal sperm aspiration (PESA): A sperm-retrieval technique in which epididymal sperm are aspirated using a fine needle directly through the skin of the scrotum.

Testicular sperm extraction (TESE): A sperm-retrieval technique in which testis tissue is taken using small incisions in the testicle.

Microdissection testicular sperm extraction (micro-TESE): A sperm-retrieval technique that is larger and more invasive than TESE and that is used to find small numbers of testicular sperm in men with poor sperm production.

Varicocelectomy: Surgery performed to remove enlarged veins in the scrotum to restore proper blood flow to the testicles and improve sperm production and male fertility.

Vasectomy reversal: A vasectomy cuts or blocks the vas deferens, the tubes that carry sperm from the testes to the epididymis, where they are stored until ejaculation. In a vasectomy reversal, these tubes are microsurgically rejoined.[13]

There are different modalities of treatment for male infertility:

1. **Lifestyle and environmental changes:** Lifestyle changes could be as simple as coital therapy, such as teaching people to have sex during ovulation and to not use spermicide. Other lifestyle treatments include refraining from hot tubbing, smoking weed, and drinking alcohol excessively. If a man has ejaculation issues, counseling or medical therapy may be helpful. Antioxidants might help DNA fragmentation. (Some of the supplements recommended in chapter 3 for egg quality might also help.)

2. **Medicine and hormonal treatment:** Antibiotics may be necessary in the case of infection, and steroids may be given to suppress antisperm antibodies. Hormones can be given to those with conditions such as hyperthyroidism and testosterone excess or deficiency.

3. **Surgical treatment:** Surgery might be necessary if obstructions are being removed, if sperm is being retrieved, or if varicoceles (dilated veins in the scrotum) are present. Dr. Turek says that 40 percent of primarily infertile men will be found to have varicoceles, and in cases of secondary infertility, it's 80 percent, if evaluated properly.

Not all male infertility can be treated or solved. Sometimes a man has no sperm, or a genetic defect that can't be fixed. Sometimes surgeries fail. And sometimes the cause of the infertility is simply unknown.

"Evaluation of male factor infertility should be conducted to uncover life-threatening conditions and correctable problems that present as infertility," Dr. Turek writes in "Practical Approaches to the Diagnosis and Management of Male Infertility,"[14] noting that IVF should not be a first line of treatment, especially since some processes to overcome bad sperm, like ICSI, may actually be harmful to the offspring.[15] About half the time, a cause can be found, he writes. But most "lady doctors," as Dr. Turek colloquially refers to fertility doctors, do not treat the man. "There has been a recent trend to avoid specific male factor, potentially curative, treatment in favor of assisted reproduction. This is unfortunate, as many male factor treatments help infertile couples conceive without assisted reproduction," he writes.

Do you want another reason to investigate the cause of male infertility? There's a correlation with mortality, a study shows.[16] The idea of sperm counts being a biomarker of a man's health has taken root over the past decade, especially after published studies[17] (by Dr. Turek and others) showing that men with low or no sperm counts have higher rates of prostate and testicular cancer years after infertility.[18]

It's important to remember that correlation is not causation. "Men with a diagnosis of infertility are not at a higher risk of death than the general population, although having a diagnosis related to infertility may be linked to a higher risk of death," a Swedish study of more than forty thousand men found.[19]

When Men Are Infertile

An infertility diagnosis is never easy. But I was a fool to wish it on my husband, because well, human decency, but also, according to a study in the *Journal of Sexual Medicine*, couples struggling with male factor infertility "have a lower sexual and personal quality of life" than couples for whom infertility is unexplained or is due to the woman's biology.[20]

And, unsurprisingly, "women feel it's their fault no matter what," psychologist Dr. Davidson says. Even if they don't feel like it's their fault, "they want to protect their husband's feelings," she says. (See "emotional labor," chapter 14.)

"I felt responsible for our inability to conceive, as if my egg had willingly refused to be fertilized," medical sociologist Liberty Walther Barnes writes in her book *Conceiving Masculinity: Male Infertility, Medicine, and Identity.*[21]

Dr. Davidson says male factor infertility can cause conflict within couples due to coping styles. Men might not want to worry or pursue treatment until after a few months of Trying, but women dealing with infertility might want to seek out treatment ASAP because they're worried their egg quality might be deteriorating the longer they wait. "There's a lot of pressure on the male partner, because the woman is saying, 'We can't wait, my eggs are going to expire!'" Dr. Davidson says.

Emotionally Speaking: What He's Thinking

Here's what some men think when told their sperm doesn't work:

- You should have married someone else.
- It must be a mistake.
- That wasn't a good sample.
- It must have been from that football injury.
- I better not tell anyone.
- No, I do NOT want to talk about it.
- I don't want another man's sperm inside my wife.
- Do we really need to have children, anyway?

A male infertility diagnosis is "hitting way below the belt," punned Dr. Turek. "They don't know how to handle it." He finds that men tend to blame themselves, wondering if it was something that happened in childhood, like getting hit with a soccer ball, or some college indiscretion that caused the problem. Because male infertility is much less discussed in the media than female infertility, it could come as a surprise to a man when diagnosed. "It's a biological identity crisis," he says. "Men just aren't prepared for that in life."

Adam certainly wasn't. The thirty-year-old was shocked when he found out he had very little sperm. "I thought my body would work and follow the plan I had for myself and my family," he says. He felt like the initial diagnosis was a "mistake"; he felt debilitated, then incredibly sad. "It feels like I've let everyone down and I feel like an outsider from the rest of the world." The general expectation on men in society, he says, is that sperm are readily available and a man should just be able to produce them whenever. "I know now this isn't always the case, but that didn't help me feel any better. My self-worth has been damaged: I honestly have a general sense of inferiority knowing this," he says.

Medical sociologist Barnes, whose husband had "dead sperm," wonders about the social framing of male infertility: "How do ideas about gender, including women's reproductive responsibility and the fragility of masculinity, become enmeshed in medical knowledge and practice?" she writes.

In a chapter in *Conceiving Masculinity* called "Masculinity and Virility in the Social Milieu," she writes about idioms like "shooting blanks." "Compare the idea of 'shooting blanks' to other colloquial jargon such as 'grow a pair" and 'that takes balls.' These fragments of language illustrate the prevailing cultural belief that healthy testicles producing potent sperm are a symbol of strength, courage, power, manliness and masculinity," she writes.

Adam spent many hours online reading every study. He also underwent three biopsies to extract sperm for IVF with ICSI (recommended for male factor infertility). "The worst part is that everything always looked great—so there was always a reason to try again," he says. "*What if* is a seriously powerful drug." The sperm extraction surgeries were "scary AF, but much easier to recover from than imagined," he says. "That being said, having been through three biopsies, I hate what it's done to me physically. Now I have the scars as reminders of what will never be."

Adam's sperm failed to fertilize his wife Zoe's sixty (!) eggs, re-trieved over numerous IVF cycles. That's when they decided to use a sperm donor—but not just any donor: his brother.

"It's amazing what things you're willing to do and accept being in a situation like this," he says, noting that because he and his brother share genetics, it made using a donor an easier pill to swallow—especially when his wife got pregnant. "I envy those that can live their lives without ever having to consider some of the choices we've been forced to consider." Amen.

When It's Time to Use a Sperm Donor

It's never an easy decision to use a third party for reproduction (see chapter 23). But in some ways, it's harder for a man to go the donor route than a woman, because at least she will carry the baby.

Although Eric Schwartzman was born with an undescended tes-ticle and was always on the lookout for testicular cancer, he was still shocked to learn he had an extremely low sperm count—six months before his wedding. "I was so thrown off guard," he says, "I gave her the option of backing out."

Schwartzman and his wife did IUI and IVF with ICSI, and he felt even more guilty about that: "Here I am, it's my fault we're in this place but then I have to give my wife intramuscular shots and she's up in stirrups, and it's all me. It really takes a toll on your marriage." He agreed to move on to sperm donation for her. "I wanted a child with my wife, and I wanted her to have that experience going through pregnancy and going through childbirth." He started a blog about it, Life as Dad to Donor Insemination (DI) Kids, and then founded a Yahoo group for "non-bio dads via Donor insemi-nation."

"The men usually go through a loss, then an acceptance, then a rationalization for why it's okay for you to use another man's sperm to have your children," Schwartzman says. "It's hard to adjust: Another man's sperm is going to be entering your wife," he says. "It's an intimate act taking place even though there's no sexual act."

Men have differing attitudes to using a sperm donor: Some can't get past another man's sperm in their wives; others feel it's just a "genetic" contribution to having a family; others choose adoption; and some don't have children at all.

That's what happened to Greg, a Twitter user (@gotnosperm) who goes by the name "Balls Don't Work" who was diagnosed with a genetic deletion at thirty-two. "I didn't realize how badly I wanted to have a child until I was told I would not be able to," he says, saying that he and his wife exhausted all their options. "It's really hard to go through it as a couple—it's *our* journey—and I lost sight of that for a long time. It's her loss, too."

Many men, however, decide to proceed with a donor. "It wasn't easy, but you need to look at the end goal and end the pain," Schwartzman explains. Schwartzman found a donor with the same medical and ethnic background as himself. His son and daughter knew from when they were young about their donor-conceived status— something Schwartzman is very vocal about on his blog and in the Yahoo group. "Adoptive parents go through a hell of a lot more than parents choosing donor conception," he says, wishing that people choosing sperm donors would have to go through similar counseling as adoptive parents "to prepare them for what issues are out there," he says. For example, his children are in touch with their half siblings, and his daughter wants to be in touch with the sperm donor. "Most parents don't know the issues out there," he says.

Can Wives Help?

Schwartzman, who is divorced, says his ex always wanted him to just get over it. "For her it was a done deal; we had our children, and she never dwelled on donor conception. She always wanted me to get past it."

Adam's wife was also wishing he could be as thrilled at the pregnancy (with his brother's sperm) as she was. "It's happy with an asterisk," he told her. When his wife tries to make him feel better, telling him it doesn't matter, he says, "Don't diminish my feelings."

News alert: Men have feelings, too. "Part of the problem is there's no outlet for it," Dr. Turek says. "Men won't discuss their infertility while they're playing basketball or talk on the phone for hours, like a woman might." But, as he's observed from male patient discussion groups, men, like women, "are wonderful individual beings with serious feelings." One admitted, "I had trouble crossing the street without crying every day on my way to work."

His advice for getting your guy to talk about it sounds a lot like women's magazine advice for getting them to talk about *anything*—go for a drive or a long bike ride and see if anything comes up. "A lot of guilt, shame, anger comes out," Dr. Turek says. "A lot of it is lack of control over the situation—a Western/provider culture, and you can't provide. They spin out of control."

A Healthy Perspective

There's an aphorism that when a woman trips on the sidewalk, she gets upset at herself, but when a man trips on the sidewalk, he looks at the sidewalk as if it's the sidewalk's fault. Women have a tendency to blame themselves when things go wrong more than men do.

Maybe, then, we women can learn something from men when it comes to infertility. According to Barnes, many men saw their infertility as "just a medical condition" as opposed to a moral failing. Several men told her that infertility "has no more bearing on what masculinity means than any other disorder, injury, or illness."

Perhaps if we all, men and women both, were to realize that it doesn't matter which partner is the "cause" of the infertility, we'd be able to move on more easily to the most important part: how to solve it.

Section III

EMOTIONALLY SPEAKING . . .

Chapter 14

In Sickness and in Health: How to Preserve Your Partnership

> It was maybe then that I felt a first flicker of resentment involving politics and Barack's unshakable commitment to the work. . . . He read all the IVF literature and would talk to me all night about it, but his only actual duty was to show up at the doctor's office and provide some sperm.
>
> —Michelle Obama, *Becoming*[1]

"Why can't you ever wash any*thing*?!!" Solomon shouted and threw the empty container from the fridge across the room at me.

To this day, he claims he was throwing it "near" me, "into" the sink. Prepositions notwithstanding, it was clear he was losing it.

Normally unflappable and practical to a fault, Solomon's the type of guy to say, "Why is she depressed?" about someone. And for the millionth time, I'd have to womansplain that emotions aren't logical and some people can't always "snap out of it." He tended to not want to fight or get upset about much.

But we'd just found out our natural pregnancy—that second one, before we started any treatment—wasn't viable. We'd already heard the baby's heartbeat, we'd already started tossing around names ("something easy to spell at Starbucks," he'd insisted), and then we found out our ten-week baby (boy, we later learned) had somehow stopped growing in my body.

There I was, lying on the couch, immobile, and Solomon was trying to go about his regular business—cleaning the house and planning our trip to his family's party the next weekend.

How was he doing anything? I still had a . . . a thing . . . inside me, and I had to figure out how to get rid of it. Aside from *that* minor detail, I was wondering if we'd ever be able to have a kid.

And who would we be if we were alone together, forever, without children?

Emotionally Speaking: Top 10 Things Couples Fight About in IVF

1. How much money you're spending.
2. Whose fault it is you don't have a baby.
3. What you're telling other people, if you're telling anyone, or just plain lying.
4. Whose sonograms pissed you off on social media.
5. Why you should *not* visit that quack health guy.
6. How come you can't have more sex?
7. When will you just buck up and get over it?
8. What do you mean, you can't go to her baby shower?
9. If his mother really meant that you should "just relax."
10. Can't we talk about something else anymore?

Apparently, a bickering couple focused on mundane things like housework.

"You want me to clean the fridge? Now??" I yelled, shifting forward on the couch for the first time. "Excuse me, I have to first get rid of a dead baby. And how can you even think about going to a party at a time like this?" At the thought of my unpregnant future, I burst into tears.

And on and on we went.

What's Your Coping Style?

It was one of the first times we fought about infertility, but it certainly wasn't the last.

While all medical conditions are stressful, research shows that IVF takes a harder toll because both members of a couple are going through it. "Healthcare professionals should remember that infertility is a stressful life event for both women and men," found the "Study to Assess the Level of Stress Among Women with Primary Infertility."[2]

During fertility treatment, couples tend to have a stereotypically gendered way of fighting. "Men used proportionately greater amounts of distancing, self-controlling and planful problem solving," found one study of more than one thousand men and women.[3] That sounded familiar.

It's like that scene in the classic film *White Men Can't Jump* where Rosie Perez tells a young Woody Harrelson: "See, if I'm thirsty. I don't want a glass of water, I want you to *sympathize*. I want you to say, 'Gloria, I, too, know what it feels like to be thirsty. I, too, have had a dry mouth.' I want you to connect with me through sharing and understanding the concept of dry mouthedness." In response, Harrelson throws a glass of water in her face.

Infertility was giving me and Solomon a crash course in each other's coping styles:

Me: Sit and cry on the couch and process every feeling, thought, and musing that popped into my head, like I had done after a million boyfriend breakups. (Thought I'd be done with *that* after marriage.)

Him: Keep on keeping on.

Me: Rising annoyance at his imperviousness.

Him: Wondering if I'd *ever* get up—and what he'd gotten himself into. (Those were his exact words when I later interviewed him in *The New York Times.* "In the beginning, I had the ugly thought, 'What have I gotten into?'—but that's what separates the man from the boy. And of course I didn't make a mistake marrying you. I'm happy I married you, with or without this.") That begat another whole fight. Had he really considered leaving me then? When it was all his fault for the late proposal? Or *mostly* his fault?

Over the three years of our baby-making experiment, I remember a few doozy fights:

- That time he had a pot brownie (it was legal—we were in California) even though we were still doing treatment and many studies show marijuana use depletes sperm count.[4]
- When I couldn't be happy for a friend who was pregnant and he thought I should be a better person than that (see chapter 17).
- When he told me the hormones, did, in fact, make me look fat. "You want the truth, don't you?" he said, revealing a fundamental misunderstanding in our relationship. *No, no, no, I don't ever want that truth.*

Those are some of the fights we had *aloud.* I'm not counting those nights I lay awake arguing with him in my head (and won!).

During the months/cycles/years of IVF, everyone likes to tell you, "Oh, you'll have a child at the end of this, somehow." But when you're in it, you don't actually *know* that. You don't know when the end will come or what it will be. And that multiplies the stress of the whole process by a gazillion.

One minute, you're on the road to your blissful future with 2.2 kids, and the next, there's an orange flashing detour sign taking you down an unknown long and winding road that may or may not bring you to your desired destination. To boot, the road's adjacent to a cliff, and you're driving at night, in the rain, with wild animals shrieking around you. It's only normal that the driver and passenger will end up, at some point, screaming at each other—or retreat in silence to their own corners.

The crux of our fights was mostly emotional: how we deal differently, how public we were about fertility treatments, how much we allowed it to take over our lives, how we recovered from disappointment and failure, and how we decided to move forward.

"What's the point of fighting over this if there's going to be no 'us' left by the time we have a baby?" Solomon always said. I could see his point—protecting our partnership should have been primary.

There's no one right way to cope, but it can help to know what you're up against. I've talked to many couples dealing with infertility, and I've learned there are a few issues that tend to come up in the process.

Tips: To Be a Supportive Partner, Say . . .

1. Do you want me to come to your appointment with you?
2. Let me take over billing/insurance/the pharmacy.
3. I was doing research on X and found Y.
4. What did you think of what the doctor told us?
5. How are you feeling that X failed?
6. Do you still want to do more treatments?
7. Would you like to switch clinics?
8. I wish there was more I could do.

Managing Expectations

When beginning treatment, you're not thinking, *Hey, this will take three years and $100,000, so let's plan for that.* Nor should you: A recent study of more than 250,000 British women found that nearly 30 percent of patients had IVF success on their first try.[5]

That's why many people take it one day/cycle/retrieval/transfer at a time. If you're doing your first IUI, why even consider IVF? Should you talk about testing embryos if you've never even had a successful egg retrieval? Is there a point to discussing finances and how many cycles you can afford before you even meet with your first doctor?

Yes, a discussion needs to take place at some point.

Because that same study also found that couples who persevered— doing at least six cycles—were the most successful. Now, no one *wants* to be doing this for six cycles or six years, but chances are, it's probably going to take longer than you thought—so it's good to align your expectations.

"It's so hard for people to understand how to contain their anxiety around what might or might not happen," says Lori Gottlieb, author of *Maybe You Should Talk to Someone: A Therapist, Her Therapist, and Our Lives Revealed.*[6] Gottlieb is a psychotherapist specializing in reproductive counseling who helps people deal with their emotions through all stages of their fertility journey. She also helps couples manage their expectations.

When you start Trying, you and your partner are most likely on the same page: You want a kid! But add in medical science, tens of thousands of dollars on maxed-out credit cards, and oodles of needles, and your expectations may change: Will you go to the ends of the earth to have a baby? How about Colorado? How much medicine are you willing to take?

"Each person has a different threshold for how much time, money, and emotional and physical energy they're willing to put into this," Gottlieb says.

"I could never do that to my body," said one woman who heard about the medications I took to carry my pregnancy to term.

How much money would you spend on the process? "Some young couples have enough for a house—this baby *is* our house," a young woman told me.

How do you feel about a donor? "I'd rather adopt than use a donor egg," one woman in a support group said, noting that if she wasn't going to get to pass on her genetics, her husband wasn't going to, either.

"You might be going through your third IVF and the other person might be relieved it didn't work out and you don't want to give up," Gottlieb says. "So how do you talk about it together? How do you make decisions based on that?"

Some people see a counselor or join a support group.

"I still remember walking into a RESOLVE program and seeing one hundred people in a room, all those people going through the same thing I was going through," recalls Barbara Collura, president and CEO of RESOLVE: The National Infertility Association. The organization has three hundred live volunteer-run support groups across the country. "Emotional support is our mission," she says.

Others, like me, don't want to devote *more* time and money to dealing with infertility. What Solomon and I eventually did was map out a plan: how many IVFs we'd try, what we'd do next if it didn't work.

Managing expectations can help a couple stay on the same page—and help with decisions, like which doctor to choose, which treatment to do, and how much time and money you will put in.

In this game, making decisions is just half the battle.

The other half? Who makes them.

Emotional Labor

One of the primary causes of conflict in IVF is division of labor—actually, what's come to be known as "emotional labor." "It's the unpaid, often unnoticed labor that goes into keeping everyone around you comfortable and happy," says Gemma Hartley, author of *Fed Up: Emotional Labor, Women, and the Way Forward*.[7]

One person takes on the role of "carer"—in heteronormative relationships, it's usually the woman, Hartley says, "because they are culturally trained to take on this role. They care about all the details: what's on the calendar, what's for dinner, what needs to be done around the house, where everyone's belongings are—relieving the other partner of the mental load." Not only that, but what's pissed her and half the Internet off is that if the designated carer wants to delegate some of the tasks, she has to ask in "the right way" to ensure it gets done. *Honey, can you use your big, strong muscles to take out the garbage because little ol' me is too scared to go out in the dangerous dark to do it?*

With IVF, emotional labor "gets pushed into overdrive," Hartley says. "There's so much more to manage emotionally, physically, and logistically."

Logistics seems like nine-tenths of treatment: which doctor you'll go to, when and how you'll get there, how you'll pay for it, who will watch your other kids, where you'll get your meds, who will administer them, who's going to receive the results, what you'll do after. Someone has to be in charge of managing that—and that someone is often the woman, especially since it's usually her body under the microscope.

"You're better at it, I'll just go with whatever you decide," Solomon said at the beginning, when I was clucking around like a headless chicken looking for a fertility doctor. I didn't mind then, since I *wanted* to make the decisions . . . it was only when we were in it forever, when the decisions kept piling up, that I began to feel overwhelmed.

In the beginning, Solomon came with me to the initial doctor interviews. For our last and final doctor, when I was debating between two immunologists, he got to make the decision. Since all my choices had been unsuccessful, I hoped he'd have better luck picking.

"The biggest thing I can stress to the partner on the non-carrying side of it is do whatever it is you can to make the other person feel they aren't alone," says Matt Mira, cohost with his wife, Doree Shafrir, of *Matt & Doree's Eggcellent Adventure,* an hour-long podcast following their IVF journey and answering listeners' questions on the topic. "Whether that means going into work a little late if you have to be at an appointment—even if it's just an appointment to count follicles, it's still important to go to those," he says. "You can't inject yourself with everything they're injecting themselves," he says, reminding me of the time I begged Solomon to take some of my hormone pills so he "could feel what I felt." He refused (shocking). "So this is the least you can do," Mira says.

Shafrir says her husband tried to come to all the appointments. "He tries to be a part of it—it's easy for men to say, 'It isn't my thing and I don't have to be there.' I think a lot of men feel powerless in this situation and they don't know how to participate."

Mira says he saw himself as a "stabilizing dorsal fin: I feel like she can swim straight and I help her keep her eyes on whatever thing a fish would swim to. I'm not like, 'This is going to be real easy,' but like, 'Let's just stay going forward.'"(After more than one hundred podcast episodes, a lot of treatment, and a lot of discussions about the treatment, they finally gave birth to a baby boy.)

There's no reason that one person in a partnership should take on everything—especially when this could be a loooong process. Most couples do find a balance: One person handles the finances, the other handles the appointments. One person handles getting the meds, the other takes them.

"I couldn't deal with any of the technical information. I just let Evan talk to the doctor and make the decisions," Soraya says, noting that her husband literally just brought her the paperwork and told her to sign on the dotted line. Sounds good, but I couldn't picture ceding that kind of control.

"It's too upsetting for Frannie, so I asked the doctors to talk to me directly," Ben told me. He and his young wife have been battling a mysterious problem for years and he was trying to protect her, a busy lawyer, from anything that would affect her equilibrium at work. He does the research, the calls, and the appointment-making, and she shows up.

"If there were ever a time for a partner to step up and take on more emotional labor, this is it," Hartley says, noting that when she went through back-to-back miscarriages between her second and third child, it was a turning point in her relationship. "My husband made the painful calls to family, cooked dinners, took charge of our other two children, listened to me when all I wanted to do was talk about it, and sat with me when I didn't want to say anything at all." In times of intense stress or grief or uncertainty, she says, the balance of emotional labor can either make or break a couple. Fortunately, "Instead of becoming isolated from him, it brought us closer together."

Couples Survive

STANDARD ADVICE	REALITY
1. Have clear communication with your partner.	1. Sometimes it pays to go to bed angry.
2. Don't expect to feel the same way about everything.	2. Obviously you're always right.
3. Rely on others for support.	3. Chew all your friends' ears off until they dump you.
4. Take care of yourself (you do you!).	4. If it doesn't include drinking, pigging out, exercising, hot tubs, or sex, how can it be comforting?
5. Keep up your life so it's not just about fertility.	5. Every movie, TV show, or play you see will reference infertility.

Intimacy During Infertility

The thing about infertility is that it hits a couple in their most private realm: their sex life.

A study of some two hundred women titled "Is Infertility a Risk Factor for Female Sexual Dysfunction?" found: "Women with infertility reported a lower sex-life satisfaction . . . in addition to arousal and desire domain scores, indicating worse sexual functioning, compared with women without infertility," and noted that women with infertility were 50 percent more likely to have sexual dysfunction than women without.[8]

But you don't need research to tell *you* that. "Sex will often take a turn from hope and connection to a reminder of failure," therapist Beth Jaeger-Skigen writes in the article "How to Reconnect Sexually During Infertility."[9] "Once fears of failure or inadequacy enter a relationship, it will drive further disconnection."

During IVF, I had so many medical and psychological reasons not to have sex:

- Before a retrieval: too nervous
- After a retrieval: on antibiotics
- After a transfer: waiting for a positive pregnancy test
- After a failure: too depressed
- While pregnant: nervous about the baby

Sometimes treatment can drive couples apart. Especially when it doesn't work.

One study of almost fifty thousand Danish women found that women who don't have a child after fertility treatment are *three times* more likely to divorce or end cohabitation with their partner than those who do.[10] In a study of almost eight thousand couples in Shanghai, researchers found that couples who did not have children were 2.2 times more likely to separate.[11]

That's what happened to Gigi. She'd been with her partner for three years and really wanted a baby, but Karl had had a vasectomy after he had kids with his ex. He had a vasectomy reversal and they did three rounds of IVF, but finally, Karl said he didn't know if he wanted more kids. "He said he didn't want to prevent me from having that experience—he thought I would be a great mom. It was a great act of love on his part," Gigi says.

Three years later, Gigi got pregnant with a new partner and had a son. But if she and Karl had had a kid, she believes they'd still be together. "It was the fertility treatment that ruined us."

Some newer research shows, though, that infertility doesn't cause relationships to end. A recent five-year study of American couples who failed fertility treatment found that 86 percent of the childless couples stayed together.[12] "Marital stability significantly predicted the initial status of infertility stress and infertility stress growth levels," the study noted. In other words, if your partnership is going strong beforehand, it will survive this, too—no matter the outcome.

So are couples going through infertility treatment likely to split up?

Pregnantish founder Syrtash, who has studied relationship trends and went through seven years of treatments with her husband, says that stressful life moments inevitably test a couple's strength and the way they work as partners to address challenges. "There's research to support the claim that infertility and IVF treatments do *not* directly lead a couple to divorce. If a couple breaks up over this, chances are the couple would separate over another life challenge ahead."

A study titled "Fertility Treatment Does Not Increase the Risk of Divorce" concluded: "We also know that despite all the strain that this infertility can bring, going through ART [Assisted Reproductive Technology like IUI and IVF] can actually bring benefit to a couple's relationship, because it forces them to improve communication and coping strategies."[13]

Actually, almost a quarter of men and women surveyed in "Does Infertility Cause Marital Benefit?" said yes![14] The men who used "active-confronting coping"—letting feelings out, asking others for advice—had better marriages. And the men who used "active-avoidance coping"—turning to work to take their mind off things, avoiding being with pregnant women or children, keeping infertility a secret, and having bad communication—were less likely to report getting closer from infertility.

So are Solomon and I closer after infertility—and better off?

Look, I'll never be one of those people who sanctimoniously says, "Everything happens for a reason," or who welcomes a challenge as a "learning experience." And we weren't one of those couples, like Doree and Matt, who say they "never fight" about infertility, nor did either of us do therapy like Gottlieb advises. But we made it through three years of treatment, four miscarriages, one fraught pregnancy, and the birth of our daughter.

And that's probably the best reason to try to keep your partnership healthy: When you have a kid, *however* you have it—as new parents, you're going to really need each other.

Chapter 15

Defending Your Life: How to Have One During Treatment

> I can't imagine being that nosy, like, *When are the kids coming?* Because who knows what somebody's going through, who knows if somebody's struggling?
>
> —Chrissy Teigen

The day we got the call, I remember the wind blowing through my hair.

I wasn't even in a convertible (I'd sold my Beetle convertible when I left L.A.) but that New York fall day, I distinctly remember the wind whistling past my head as I poked it out the window like a happy Labrador as we hit the road.

Solomon and I were headed to a small college town in the Catskills, where we'd sometimes hole up at a cheap motel in the woods, go for hikes by day to watch the waterfalls, and drink local wine and beer in the pubs by night. I probably wouldn't be drinking too much on this trip (read: at all), as we were in the middle of an IVF cycle, but it was still wonderful to have a little break.

I promised myself that for the next two days, I wouldn't talk about IVF, about how many follicles were currently colonizing my ovaries, about what kind of side effects I was feeling from the meds, about how I would spend the days after my transfer so it would result in a better outcome this second time around. No, I wouldn't fret over my past losses, my lost time, the embryos on ice, the family we were itching to start, and the life we were yet to begin.

I was going to enjoy the stunning palette of fall foliage, the unseasonably warm weather, the vast, fresh outdoors, and my relatively new husband. I was going to live in the moment and enjoy our freedom.

And then we got the call.

I had to roll up the window and assume my serious voice just in case it was work. "Hi, this is Amy."

"Hi! This is Kallie," said a woman who I belatedly recognized was calling from my fertility clinic. They probably needed a new credit card or something financial. I was beginning to notice that although they might get behind on my med orders, appointments, or lab results, they were always, always, *always* on top of my money.

"The doctor would like for you to come back tomorrow."

"Tomorrow?" I said so loudly that Solomon clutched the wheel.

"Tomorrow," she repeated. There had been some mix-up with the results of my latest monitoring and they wanted to check my eggs again to see if perhaps they would trigger me (i.e., give me medication that would force me to ovulate) the next day so they could do a retrieval.

"Tomorrow?" I said again.

There would be no break, no hiking, no motel, no Not Thinking About IVF. The only foliage we were going to see was on the way home. Solomon had already turned the car around even before I hung up. We both knew I was headed back to the fertility clinic the next morning.

How the hell was I supposed to live like this?

This Is Your Life on IVF

When you start fertility treatment, you hope that you will be successful quickly. Sure, you might take an hour off work to call around for a consultation. Maybe you'll have to wake up an hour earlier for morning monitoring, or leave a bit earlier from work to stop by the pharmacy on the way home, and once in a while skip the gym because the meds make you feel unwell, but it probably won't affect you that much, you think.

You'd probably be wrong.

What starts out as missing work for one appointment morphs into a whole lot of hours: of getting to and from the clinic, waiting at the clinic, talking on the phone to insurance, desperately searching for meds when the pharmacy is late/closed/swallowed up in a mysterious earthquake, having to take mornings off for retrievals and afternoons off for transfers.

All of a sudden, I was *in* it. This fertility treatment wasn't a temporary way station along the road to pregnancy, but a base camp where I would be setting up shop for a long while. Something I was going to need to plan for, allow for, carve out time for in my very busy life.

When I was looking for a husband, people always told me you have to make room in your life—clean out a nightstand drawer, stop hogging the whole bed, even leave a few gaping holes in your schedule so that when he does show up, there's a placeholder. That you shouldn't miss out on meeting the love of your life because you're too overprogrammed.

Now, I won't tell you to do the same thing to make room for baby (baby will make puh-*lenty* of room for herself when she comes), but at a certain point, you're going to have to make room in your schedule for fertility treatment: at work, at play, and at home, with colleagues, family, and friends.

Shout, Work It Out

Fertility treatment is a full-time job in and of itself.

Although you may be able to go to monitoring at six A.M. and pick up your meds at seven P.M., you're still going to have to take off a day of work for the retrieval—especially if you're going under anesthesia—and likely take off the day of your transfer as well.

" 'How thick is your cervical mucus?' " Tamika recalls the unique discussion she had with her boss at a women's health tech company. "It was weird, everyone there knew I was trying to conceive—I don't think I've ever had any of those discussions with my girlfriends. . . . It was still a little scary to share that I was trying to conceive, but we talk about TTC, babies, and parenthood all day long, so I realized that I had a bunch of resources at my fingertips," Tamika says. "It felt a bit odd at first to share it, but at the end of the day, my company is working to make the workplace more supportive of women and families. And if we truly want to do this, we need to be able to talk the talk."

Tamika realizes, though, that her frankness is probably unique to her type of women-led, health-focused company.

Many do not discuss their fertility at work.

In one study, 43 percent of the women surveyed did not disclose to their bosses they were going through treatment.[1] "Women being treated or evaluated for infertility must have a flexible work schedule and be willing and able to go for frequent office visits. This can lead to hours and sometimes days missed at work," the study found, observing that treatment is time-consuming (oh, you have no idea!). "For working women, this necessitates understanding, flexibility, and cooperation at the workplace from co-workers and supervisors, which would require in some instances disclosing one's infertility," the researchers noted, and the study subjects were more likely to do so if the boss was a woman. "This may be because women have a greater comfort level with other women when discussing infertility." (Duh.) Yet whether you disclose that you're undergoing fertility treatment shouldn't be dependent on your boss's gender or family status.

Your Rights in the Workplace

The "finance" industries—tech, consulting, and banking—are the top three providers of fertility health benefits, according to FertilityIQ's Industry Ranking.[2] (Surprisingly, "fashion" came in fourth, although "retail" came in last.) Still, despite the growing number of companies offering coverage for IVF and egg freezing, it's still unclear *what* exactly they are offering to people who have to actually *utilize* those benefits.

In industries where people put in sixty- to eighty-hour workweeks, those same managers, team leaders, and HR departments may not realize that you have to take off a few hours a week to get those eggs frozen, a few afternoons a month to have those embryos transferred, not to mention the time you might need if a pregnancy fails.

Yet it doesn't matter what fertility benefit your company does or doesn't offer and what your manager or HR department knows or doesn't know about infertility. Since the American Medical Association designated infertility as a disease in 2017 (in agreement with the World Health Organization), you might be protected.[3]

The US Supreme Court held in 1998 that reproduction does qualify as a major life activity,[4] according to the Americans with Disabilities Act (ADA) of 1990.[5] Legal experts say that women may be covered under the ADA, the Family Medical Leave Act (FMLA), Title VII (sex discrimination) of the Civil Rights Act, or the Pregnancy Discrimination Act (PDA).[6]

"If you're getting IVF treatment and you need an accommodation in the workplace, that's covered in ADA," says Tom Spiggle of the

Spiggle Law Firm, which is devoted exclusively to helping employees win workplace disputes and fight wrongful termination. "The ADA requires that the employer engage in an interactive process with you in an effort to find accommodations, so that you can continue to perform the essential functions of your job," he says, "as long as that does not affect the essential function of your job." So if you're a firefighter or a cop and you have to be on call 24/7, your job may not be protected. But if you're in an office job, it's a different story. "For most people, it's not going to affect the essential function of your job," Spiggle says. "It's going to be hard for the employer not to give you time off."

Of course, if you approach your employer for some time off for fertility treatment and they simply say "yes, of course!" (which I'd hope every employer would), there's no need for an official "interactive process" meeting. Too bad we don't live in an ideal world—employers are not always eager to hear about a pregnancy, let alone a woman *intending* to become pregnant.

But what if you don't envision asking for some specific time off or extraordinary provisions for infertility? Should you still tell your workplace?

"My recommendation? You should tell your employer, and then if they do try to discriminate later because of that, you have it on record," Spiggle says.

He recommends the same thing to pregnant women: Your employer is "going to know eventually. It's better to tell them earlier rather than later—a manager may hear it from the grapevine and, because of their own prejudices, force you out," he says.

The best way to tell your employer is to send an email to HR and your manager, he says, because then they have a dated record that they received it. He suggests saying simply: "Just so you know, I'm undergoing IVF treatment."

Spiggle adds: "Then they are on notice: If all of a sudden you've been doing great for ten years and then you send the email and you get poor performance reviews, it's an easier burden of proof. If there's no record they knew, it's harder to prove that case."

You can also tell your employer that you might need some time off or you may be in late some mornings—but that's not required. And actually, according to the Equal Employment Opportunity Commission (EEOC), "Under the ADA, an employer's ability to make disability-related inquiries or require medical examinations is limited,"[7] meaning they can't pepper you with questions like "What does that mean?" or "When will you need off?"

What if you're working at a small mom-and-pop shop with fewer than fifteen employees? Check your local state and county ordinances for protections.

Sample Email to HR

To: Human Resources
CC: My Wonderful Boss
Subject: Infertility Treatment

Dear _____,
I just wanted to let you know that I am going through fertility treatment.

This may mean I will have to sometimes miss the morning meeting, or leave early once in a while. I will give you advance notice when possible, as procedures are often scheduled at the last minute.

I want to assure you that this will in no way impact my work and dedication to the company. I hope that my treatment will be quick and painless and I appreciate your continued support and discretion.

Best,
Amy

But *Should* You Tell—and If So, Whom?

It's one thing to tell your boss you're going through fertility treatment and might be late to a few morning meetings. It's another thing to announce it to the world.

Maybe you don't tell anyone at first, because hey, it's only one appointment. But after six months of flaking on girls' night out because you don't want to be drinking during treatment, after a year of RSVP-ing no to every bachelorette party, out-of-town wedding, and out-of-the-country fortieth birthday party (why are these celebrations even a thing?!), you might want to be honest with people.

When I initially got pregnant naturally, I told a few friends who I thought could help me find an OB—but then I had to tell all of them when I lost those pregnancies. I realized I was the type of person who did not want other people to know my business.

"Everyone is different," says Katie Lynch, a psychotherapist, fertility advocate, and host of *The Fertile Nest* podcast. "For me it was very important not to go into hiding," she says of her own fertility journey. "For some people that's not their comfort zone, and that's okay. Ask yourself, 'What will be best for me?'" she says, noting that "Do I tell people or not tell?" comes up a lot for her clients with pregnancy.

She tells them to think of the best- and worst-case scenarios. "There are certain people you need to be around you when shit goes down," she says frankly. "If my beta doesn't double, I'm going to need you," she says, referring to the hormone that needs to increase to indicate a healthy pregnancy. When she realized her pregnancy was failing, she was glad she'd included her friends. "I had to have my husband tell people why I was checked out."

But a lot of people are secretive about needing infertility treatment. About 6 in 10 couples (61 percent) try to hide their fertility troubles from family and friends, according to a national survey.[8] And more than half of all couples (54 percent) agreed it was easier

IVF RSVPs for Every Occasion

1. Sorry I can't make it to
   a. the office meeting.
   b. your dog's bark mitzvah.
   c. your wedding in Tahiti.
   d. your life.

2. But I'm currently
   a. lying upside down in my bedroom hoping the sperm will meet my eggs.
   b. trapped in the waiting room stalking my celebrity fertility doctor.
   c. on hold with my insurance company for the last seven hours.
   d. crying in the men's room because there was no line.

3. I really wish I could be there, but
   a. I'm only working for you so I can keep my health insurance.
   b. my psychic healer says I need to spend all my time envisioning a baby.
   c. my therapist says it's better to pretend to be happy from afar than to be bitter in person.
   d. I don't have any money left.

4. I hope you don't
   a. steal my pot brownies from the office fridge.
   b. expect me to make up the hours I lost (or I'll sue you).
   c. tell me any long-winded stories about people who accidentally got pregnant.
   d. ask me a thousand times how I'm doing (not well).

5. I hope in the future
   a. I'll be missing work because I have morning sickness.
   b. my insurance company not only answers the phone but pays for my treatment.
   c. you won't invite me to anything so I won't have to say no.
   d. the world ends.

just to *tell people they were not planning to have children* rather than admit to their struggle.

Now, I'm all for lying when it helps you out (Solomon is very disturbed by this fact), but let me tell you, when infertility and treatment become such a big part of your life—affecting your schedule, your emotions, your finances, and your relationships—it becomes a really hard thing to hide.

And yet, when you open yourself up, you *really* open yourself up: More than 6 in 10 couples (63 percent) reported in the survey that they were tired of people asking them how the process was going or offering suggestions on how to conceive. Couples were frustrated about all the unsolicited advice they got, like:

- Just relax and stop worrying so much (78 percent)
- Health advice like changing their diet (42 percent)
- Get more exercise (41 percent)
- Get more sleep (38 percent)

After not telling anyone about my struggle for a long time, it became rather public in a big, big way—as in, a weekly online column in the *New York Times* Motherlode blog. And boy, did I open myself up to the trolls. "Should We Be Sympathetic to a 42-Year-Old's Fertility Struggles?" one bitter comedienne wrote on the Babble website. (Um, yes?)

Still, despite the national audience to my infertility, I found a way to be private. I never, ever told anyone any dates of any treatment—not when I was beginning a cycle, not when I was doing a retrieval, and certainly not when I was doing a transfer. I wanted the space to absorb the blows and grieve the pitfalls on my own. I didn't want people asking me, "How many eggs did you get?" or "How many fertilized?" and, worst, "Are you pregnant?"

"When there's something to tell you, I'll tell you," I told my inner circle, which was getting smaller and smaller. But I reserved the right to cry to any of those close friends whenever I wanted—without the third degree about why I was crying and what was next. Interestingly,

I chose my child-free friends. They had no kids crying in the background, no judgments on how I'd waited too long, and no skin in the game: They could care less if I became a parent. They only wanted it for me because I wanted it for myself.

"You don't need to tell everyone your business," Lynch says. Whether you disclose is up to you—and either way, "you can set boundaries in a gentle, loving way that preserves relationships." Actually, Lynch says, it's our *right* to set boundaries.

"Learning these skills is really invaluable for life," she says.

Work-Life Balance

Speaking of life, the phrase of the decade is "work-life balance." If you're going through infertility treatment, you need work-infertility-life balance.

How much of your life are you going to cede to this greedy monster?

Will you forgo your social life because of the weird IVF schedule—and your mood? Are you going to cut out all travel because you can't plan treatment around it? Or will you double down, refusing to budge an inch on anything, because you don't want to let infertility take over your life?

When I began, I *refused* to let infertility take over, but as the process wore on, I started bailing on plans, nixing travel, and generally deleting anything not related to fertility treatment from my life. (Every Memorial Day, I'm filled anew with guilt that I didn't make this one out-of-town wedding because I thought I would be pregnant.)

But my friend Karlee was the opposite. When she did IVF for both her children, she never let it become all-consuming. "You have to keep it separate," she says. She did it by "uber-compartmentalizing."

How?

"Fertility is the biggest thing going on," she says, but not the *only* thing—and you can't let it take over, "because you can drive yourself crazy." She has a point: "It's not like if you put one hundred percent of your energy into it you'll get one hundred percent what you want, so you have to be careful not to dedicate everything you have in you—physical, emotional, mental—to fertility."

Great advice, but harder to put into practice.

"I'm not saying you can never think about it. That's not what I did." She says you just "put it in a drawer" to control your emotional state. Say: *I'm just not going there.*

She saw many of her friends become obsessed, letting it dominate every aspect of their world. (*Moi?*) While they did know more than her about every single treatment option, she trusted her docs enough not to enter the deep dark web of infertility. "But that kept me really positive."

As a full-time media executive, she says she had too much else going on between work and family (and then doing fertility treatment to try for a second child while she already had one kid). Besides, she couldn't devote herself full-time to fertility. "I needed my job to help fund my fertility—that kept my eyes on the prize."

Therapist Katie Lynch believes you need to seriously make room for treatment in your life. "We are asking our bodies to do immense work—both physically and emotionally." She remembers when she was working on a statewide trauma response team: "During critical incidents in our community, I help people understand that when their bodies experience a trauma they need to get down to the basics: How do you take care of yourself, your physical body?" she says, asking if they're eating properly, getting enough rest, etc. For many, infertility can be a traumatic experience. "Naming infertility as trauma—and the physical, emotional, and psychological symptoms that they are often experiencing—can be very grounding and validating for many clients. Helping them recognize and give themselves permission to get down to basics and tend to their needs is critical."

Lynch says to ask yourself, "What do I need?" Do you need an IVF break?

After a vacation—from IVF and from life—people may feel relaxed or recharged and reconnected. "Don't be afraid to be selfish, to focus on you and what you need, because it's all more tolerable when you feel like you are taking the best care of yourself you can."

Of course, if the clock is ticking and you can't take a break, you may need to downsize at work. "What are the things you *must* do and what are the things you are *supposed* to do?" she asks clients.

"The reality is that every single woman is doing the best they can at any given moment."

All Aboard the IVF Train

I love David Sedaris's four-burner theory, which posits that in the stovetop of our lives, we have four major burners: work, family, friends, and health. You can only have three on at once in order to be successful. And in order to be *very* successful, you can only have two of the four burners on. Say fertility treatment is health—then that means you might only have room for *one* other thing.

As an extrovert, I needed my friends. And also work.

I actually *lost* my job a few weeks before I lost that second pregnancy. I realized that what I had lost was not just an income and a place to go, but the essential work that would distract me from myself, from my plummeting hormones, and from incessant Googling.

A year later, I was working as an editor at a different magazine and doing IVF. I could walk to the clinic in the morning, get the blood results back in the afternoon, and do my work *no matter what the results*. My meds hadn't arrived in time? I could scour the Internet for alternatives while still proofing pages. My hormones were falling? I could still find the photos I needed for my section. I needed to schedule a D&C? I did so the day after the editorial meeting.

My point is, even if you're at a job you don't love, there's a lot to be said for one that you're comfortable with, where you can still phone it in. I'm forever grateful for that job for keeping me sane—and social. Because despite being an extrovert, when I was doing IVF, I had to retreat, limit my circle of friends, and minimize my social calendar.

On the other hand, if you're terribly unhappy at your job and want to start looking for a new one, you don't have to wait till you're pregnant or have a baby to begin your search. If you have it in you to make the change while going through treatment, do it!

As Lynch says, we're all different.

That's the bottom line for balancing IVF with the other things going on in your life: Make it *one* of the two or three burners you have lit, not the only burner.

"For most of us who have been in it for years, it feels like a really long time," Lynch says. "It's actually a sliver of our life, not forever: For this small amount of time, we can give this to ourselves."

Chapter 16

You Gotta Have Faith: How Religion, Prayer, and Community Can Help

People talk about the miracle of birth. No. There's the miracle of conception . . . I did IVF, but nothing happened. So I began to think of adoption, and then I got pregnant. It was definitely a miracle.

—Iman, *Parade*

"What do you want to pray for?" the rabbi asked me.

I shrugged. I had only come to this kabbalist—a mystical rabbi—as a favor to my cousin, one of his followers. Even though I was in my early thirties, I was nowhere near wanting a husband or children, despite my strict Orthodox Jewish upbringing, so I had no idea what to ask for.

"Um, I guess, my brother, well, he's been trying to have children for a while . . ." I offered. My youngest brother, also a rabbi, had married young, but almost four years later still had no kids. He and his wife didn't talk about it, but in a community where people had as many kids as possible for as long as possible, I knew it must have been painful.

The kabbalist told me they should say a specific prayer until a specific Jewish holiday, and on that day, they needed to go to this ancient rabbi's grave in Israel, where they lived at the time. They would have a son, whom they would name after the ancient rabbi.

"The bus was so crowded I thought I was going to be trampled," is how my brother recounts the story to his synagogue congregation in California. Apparently, thousands upon thousands of people went to that specific grave on that specific day. "I literally feared for my life," my brother says. He made it to the grave, unscathed, to say the prayer. "I had prayed before, of course I had prayed, but maybe that was the first time my heart was really open," he says. Some ten months later, my first niece was born. They didn't end up naming her after the ancient rabbi, but they did choose a name that means "And God has answered my prayers."

Faith, Prayer, Healing in Fertility

What is the power of prayer, religion, or faith when it comes to health in general and infertility in particular?

In a study of some two hundred women undergoing embryo transfers, the half that had people praying for them ("intercessory prayer") had much higher pregnancy rates than those that didn't.[1] Of course that study could be correlative—people who belong to prayer groups might have a stronger support system, a stronger community, or a stronger sense of self than those not connected to prayer groups.

On the other hand, a Harvard study on random intercessory prayer in cardiac patients found no difference between the people prayed for or not prayed for.[2] The patients themselves did not pray, nor did they know if they were being prayed for. It's as if the scientists were trying to see if prayer could be used like medicine, regardless of the patient's knowledge.

So . . . I'm not here to scientifically prove to you the power of prayer, God, faith, or religion. (I tell this to my nonbeliever husband all the time.) But perhaps this study says it better: "We must keep in mind that religion is based on faith and not on proof. This implies that, if God exists, he is indifferent to humanity or has chosen to obscure his presence. Either way, he would be unlikely to cooperate in scientific studies that seek to test his existence."[3]

While it's true that prayer has been found to have the same beneficial effects of meditation,[4] lowering blood pressure, reducing stress, alleviating depression and anxiety, and that some studies[5] have found that religious people in general are healthier, both physically and mentally—that doesn't mean you atheists should jump out of your foxholes and into the confession booth.

But if you *are* a person of faith, someone who believes in a specific God or religion, or in a higher power, if you belong to a religious community or attend worship on a semiregular basis, you might find some particular challenges in dealing with infertility.

You might also discover some particular ways in which this belief system and community provides you strength.

What Religions Say About Fertility Treatment

"And God said to them, 'Be fruitful and multiply and fill the earth,'" Genesis states in the first book of the Bible, and reiterated again after the flood: "And God blessed Noah and his sons, and He said to them: 'Be fruitful and multiply, and fill the earth.'"

It's all well and good that God's first biblical commandment is to be fruitful—but what does He want us to do if it doesn't work?

Fertility treatment has only been around for half a century, so obviously there's nothing written about it in the Bible. Still, religion scholars opine on all sorts of modern-day ills, everything from birth control to euthanasia. And even fertility treatment.

For the most part, Jews, Protestants, and Muslims are in favor of infertility treatment, with various nuances among the sects, and ca-

Scientifically Speaking:
Curative Effects of Religion

"A whole person is someone whose being has physical, emotional, and spiritual dimensions," Dr. Harold G. Koenig writes in "Religion, Spirituality, and Medicine: Application to Clinical Practice."[6] "Ignoring any of these aspects of humanity leaves the patient feeling incomplete and may even interfere with healing. For many patients, spirituality is an important part of wholeness, and when addressing psychosocial aspects in medicine, that part of their personhood cannot be ignored."

In fact, those who attend religious services at least once a week (women in particular) appear to have a survival advantage over those attending services less frequently another study of four thousand people (aged 64 to 101) found.[7]

People who never attend services have 1.87 times greater risk of death compared with people who attend once a week, according to the data from the National Health Interview Survey—Multiple Cause of Death.[8] This translates into a seven-year difference in life expectancy at age twenty between those who never attend and those who attend more than once a week.

In a self-reported study of substance abusers, researchers noted that "among recovering individuals, higher levels of religious faith and spirituality were associated with a more optimistic life orientation, greater perceived social support, higher resilience to stress, and lower levels of anxiety."[9]

But it's not just mental. *The Journal of Health Psychology* found that effects of prayer, religiosity, and service attendance meant lower cortisol responses: "Findings suggest that spiritual and/or religious individuals may experience a protective effect against the neuroendocrine consequences of stress."[10]

So if you're suffering from infertility and want to pray, attend services, or engage in other religious practices—go ahead. Science has got your back!

veats on how to follow them, especially when it comes to embryo creation and disposition.

Muslims, for example, allow both IUIs and IVF for married (heterosexual) couples, as long as the treatment uses both the husband's sperm and the wife's eggs and uterus. This means no donor eggs, donor sperm, donor embryos, or even a surrogate. (There are differences between Sunni and Shi'a rulings. In Iran, which has a Shiite majority, third-party reproduction is permitted.)

Male factor infertility is often the culprit in conservative religious communities, says Dr. Richard Grazi, medical director of Genesis, a fertility clinic in Brooklyn, New York, who deals with a lot of devout Muslim and ultra-Orthodox Jewish patients, and author of the book *Overcoming Infertility: A Guide for Jewish Couples*.[11] "The women tend to marry young, so they haven't had time to develop advanced endometriosis, and they don't have sexually transmitted diseases that might have caused tubal damage, so you've eliminated a lot of causes of female infertility [typical in the secular community]," he says. "What you're left with is a relatively high preponderance of male factor infertility."

Judaism, for the most part, is on board with all parts of assisted reproductive technology, from IUIs to IVF. Although they permit fertility assistance, many devout Jewish religious leaders have problems with sperm collection because of the prohibition against wasting seed, Dr. Grazi says, noting that it may even make semen analysis, an otherwise routine initial test, difficult. (Devout Muslims may have problems with this, too.) "Many ultra-Orthodox rabbis say that you need to do all the testing on the woman to make sure it's not her issue, and only then do semen analysis," he says. After, the rabbis may allow sperm collection with a laboratory-grade condom for use during sex that contains no spermicide, to show there is no wasted seed.[12]

Many religious couples use a "fertility supervisor" to monitor procedures in the lab to make sure there are no mix-ups (like the recent case of a New York couple who gave birth to two babies belonging to other parents).[13]

One boon for Jewish conception can be family purity laws, where observant Jews abstain from sex during a woman's period and for the week after, until the woman immerses herself in a *mikveh*, or ritual bath, to cleanse herself spiritually. That means couples are usually having sex during their most fertile time.

At least the Jews and Muslims can *do* IVF. Catholics and Orthodox Christians are forbidden from using any assisted reproductive technology.

"They dissociate the sexual act from the procreative act," the Catechism states.[14] "Under the moral aspect, procreation is deprived of its proper perfection when it is not willed as the fruit of the conjugal act, that is to say, of the specific act of the spouses' union."

The Greek Orthodox rule: "In vitro fertilization technology is a gross interference in the mystery of child-bearing," Archpriest Oleg Stenyayev says.[15] Archpriest Pavel Gumerov says, "We must accept the Lord's will."

Some religious couples only create one embryo at a time through "natural IVF"—working with only one egg at a time instead of stimulating the ovaries—so they won't have to deal with the disposition of extra embryos. Others may try newer technologies, like INVOcell, which incubates an embryo in a device placed in the uterus.[16]

Some women go to "natural fertility centers," like the Saint Paul VI Institute for the Study of Human Reproduction,[17] which says it offers "reproductive health care that fully respects life," meaning no IUI or IVF. Their NaPro (natural procreative) technology combines fertility awareness with diagnosis and treatment of the underlying causes of infertility—such as charting, monitoring cervical mucus, etc., or treating endometriosis or male factor infertility or other conditions that should be first-line treatment before reproductive technology.

Obviously, if you follow a particular religion or religious leader, ask what you can do to treat infertility.

To those who are not religious, many practices may seem strange and weird. "The truth of the matter is that I respect the process," Dr. Grazi says. "Part of practicing good medicine is to be culturally sensitive. People from all cultures, backgrounds and beliefs suffer from infertility and we need to respect those differences during their treatment."

"So, When Will You Start Your Family, Already?"

For a religious person, one of the biggest challenges may be how to exist in a family-centered community.

When I first moved to Los Angeles in my early thirties, I explored the main Jewish drag as a potential place to live. Walking into the synagogue on the Sabbath, I saw that the giant entryway—the size of a basketball court—was filled with strollers.

No way, I thought, since I was years away from . . . anything. So, I moved to the beach to work on my surfing instead.

I can't imagine going to that type of weekly worship while going through IVF.

"When you don't have a family you can feel left out of the whole church experience," says Elizabeth Laing Thompson, a North Carolina minister, speaker, and author of *When God Says "Wait"* and *When God Says "Go."*[18] She and her husband started trying to get pregnant at twenty-five, and during her almost three years of infertility, she found it challenging to be in church.

"The Christian faith community tends to circle around family life—marriage classes, Sunday school kids' classes, youth groups." She remembers at one point, six women in her midsize congregation were pregnant at once—all expecting baby boys due within a three-week period. "I could hardly walk through the church fellowship without brushing up against someone's belly. The whole church was so excited, hovering around all the moms-to-be, making them meals, throwing them showers—and there I was, infertile all by myself."

No one was *purposefully* being unkind, "but that was a painful period when my situation felt particularly isolating."

I sympathize. I remember having to go to a good friend's circumcision ceremony after a miscarriage. When I ate the challah bread—considered a sign of good luck and fertility—it stuck in my throat as I felt tears forming. I had to excuse myself for a cry in the bathroom.

Sure, some people might say to absent yourself from these kinds of torturous events (I give you creative ideas for avoiding baby showers in chapter 17), but it's hard to shut yourself out of religious life, especially when it can provide great comfort.

Thompson says that she found a great deal of support in her faith community: Friends at church prayed for them for years. And so did the college students where she and her husband served as campus ministers.

After nearly three years, her third IUI resulted in pregnancy. When they finally told their ministry students they were pregnant, "we were mobbed by screaming, crying college students, all shouting words I could hardly understand." Finally it was explained to her: A group of girls had been secretly fasting and praying for them for more than a year.

"To this day, I count their secret sacrifice as one of the most precious gifts I have ever received," Thompson says.

How Faith Can Help You

"It can be isolating to want to participate in family-based practices while struggling to have a baby," says Rabbi Idit Solomon, founder of Hasidah, an organization that provides financial assistance to Jewish families seeking infertility treatment, which she started after her own treatment. "Fertility touches one of the most basic parts of our humanity—creating another life is a connection to the Eternal Source of Life," she says. Of course, most people don't usually think about it that way—until you find out you can't have a baby. "All of the sudden, deep and hard-to-articulate questions come up about life's meaning, connection to the future, providence and punishment."

"I believe that the best religion is one that makes us most fully human," she says, and for her that is Judaism, which "keeps people connected to the community, to each other, and for those who are more spiritually inclined, to God." She points out that there are plenty of stories in the Bible about infertility—Sarah, Hannah, Rachel—and while those can be difficult to read, they can help people feel less alone, showing how deep the yearning is to have a child and how painful it is.

Infertility is so isolating. If you attend weekly services and have a community with you—praying for you, supporting you—"it can remove isolation and help people have a sense of wholeness during their fertility journey, wherever it leads," Rabbi Solomon says. Because, in the end, she says, "we are not in control of whether we are going to have a baby or not."

The Thompsons were lucky to have three children, but Elizabeth had to struggle with prayer and faith, questioning God, and feeling let down and disappointed. "Here on the other side of that journey, I still have strong faith," Thompson says. "I have learned that there aren't always easy, pat answers to questions of suffering and loss."

Some women see their struggles as a challenge from God to take on more, religiously. "I am considering putting on the Hijab again because I have a lot of struggles with infertility," Samira Amen-Fawaz said on the short-lived TLC show *All-American Muslim*, as she started fertility treatment. "All these things I feel are a little sign from God saying, 'When are you going to wake up and listen to me?'"

Infertility Prayers

CHRISTIAN

SAINT GERARD'S PRAYER

Good Saint Gerard, powerful intercessor before the throne of God, wonder-worker of our day, we call upon you and seek your aid. You know that this marriage has not as yet been blessed with a child and how much [husband's name] and [wife's name] desire this gift. Please present these fervent pleas to the Creator of life from whom all parenthood proceeds and beseech Him to bless this couple with a child whom they may raise as His child and heir of heaven. Amen.

—From Santa Teresita Hospital[19]

ISLAM

"He Who has created you from a single person (Adam), and (then) He has created from him his wife [*Hawwa* (Eve)], in order that he might enjoy the pleasure of living with her. When he had sexual relations with her, she became pregnant and she carried it about lightly. Then when it became heavy, they both invoked Allah, their Lord (saying): 'If You give us a *Salih* (good in every aspect) child, we shall indeed be among the grateful.'"

—From *The Noble Qur'an*, Al-A'raf, 7:189[20]

JUDAISM

May it be your will God, our Lord and the Lord of our forefathers, that you shall hear my prayers and bless me with full breasts and womb. Remember me for good, and help me become pregnant quickly and grant me an easy pregnancy. That with your mercy, I may give birth to sons and daughters, and shall have enduring offspring. Give me and all those without children the strength and courage to persevere on our journeys. Grant us healing and comfort. Strengthen us and surround us with love and support. As you remembered Sarah, Rebecca, Rachel, and Hannah, and just as you have heard the voices of the righteous men and women when they beseeched you, please listen to my beseeching. Listen with mercy and willfully hear my prayer. Fulfill my wishes for good, and so may it be Your will, and let us say Amen.

—From Yesh Tikva, a Jewish infertility support group, with help from Dr. Moshe Sokolow and Shlomo Zuckier

When Faith Is Not Enough

For some religious people, infertility is enough to push them over the edge.

Katelyn was raised Catholic—from school to camp to church choir, the whole bit—but started "falling away" in college. Still, it was her four years of infertility that really made her examine her faith—or lack of it.

She married at twenty-four and started Trying at twenty-eight, to no avail. "Getting the infertility diagnosis was hard for me, especially as people around me were getting pregnant by accident," the Ohio teacher says. "I was already struggling with religion when we started trying but was still on the fence about what I really believed," she says. "The Catholic Church doesn't support any medical intervention."

Despite the church's ban on any intervention, they started treatment—many, many, medicated IUIs, a miscarriage, and two rounds of IVF, which resulted in one baby at age thirty-two.

People told her they'd pray for her, and when she was pregnant they'd say, "Oh great, we have been praying for you every night and it worked!" She was skeptical. "Right, not the thousands of dollars and science," that gave them the baby. "Don't discount the work we've done to get to this point."

Infertility was "the final nail in the coffin" for her faith. "For me, it's more comforting to think this is happening to *me*, this infertility happened for no reason. My sister got pregnant with an IUD in—and how do people look at me and say that's God's plan—you lose your baby and my sister gets pregnant?"

Katelyn knows that many modern people are "Cafeteria Catholics"—picking and choosing what they want from the religion's tenets, like ignoring the ban on fertility treatment or birth control. But she doesn't want to do that.

"I don't feel comfortable practicing a religion that doesn't feel my baby should exist," she says. "I wouldn't *have* this baby without this intervention."

Are You There, God?

During my years of miscarriages, I also questioned God. Not that we were on close terms anyway. Although I was raised an Orthodox Jew, attending religious yeshiva from age three to nineteen, by the time I was in my thirties, I was more of a bagel-and-lox type of cultural Jew: Sometimes I'd celebrate the Sabbath with family and friends, but I was no longer observant. When I married Solomon, a staunch atheist, I knew I was leaving religion behind for good.

Still, when faced with my repeat miscarriages over the next three years, I couldn't help but wonder if it was God's revenge. Especially because my religious friends and family kept telling me they were praying for me.

I should have been grateful that they wanted to help, but instead I was mad.

Are my prayers not good enough? I thought. *Does God really have the power to give me a baby? And if so, why isn't he doing it? Am I not deserving?* After my fourth miscarriage, this time with a donor egg, I felt abandoned by both medicine *and* God.

By the time I was ready for my last transfer, it was the Jewish High Holidays, the only time of year I still went to synagogue.

"You owe me, God," I murmured into my prayer book, bowing my head and ignoring the official liturgy. My sister was pregnant with her first; my brother, the rabbi, pregnant with his fifth (that kabbalist's blessing sure went a long way!). *You owe me this one baby,* I demanded.

But that's not the way God works, says Rabbi Chaim Poupko, leader of the Orthodox Congregation Ahavath Torah. "I know bad things happen to everybody and who is to say I deserve this less than anyone else?"

Bad things did happen to him. His third daughter, at the age of one, was diagnosed with an aggressive cancer. She died fourteen months later. "We don't know why God does these things and we do our best to reckon with them," he says.

When he and his wife started trying to have children again, they faced secondary infertility. "The whole notion that God may owe me something—it's a little simplistic. I don't know how God works, I don't know if he owes me." Intellectually he knows that, but emotionally he sometimes feels otherwise.

"I can still be angry and questioning and not understanding of the very same God I still ask for things and believe in," he says. "Faith helps, in a sense," he says. "I think He provides in ways I did not understand, with the people around us, the community around us, and in each other."

Three years of trying to get pregnant resulted in a miscarriage and an ectopic pregnancy. Two rounds of IVF were unsuccessful. And then they took a break. "We were stopping for a moment and playing it by ear," he says. "We couldn't keep doing that to ourselves."

That's when his wife got pregnant.

"To me the greatest testimony to God's presence in our lives isn't whether he sent us this or that miracle—it's how those who are committed to him conduct themselves, how supportive they can be," he says. "I don't see [our baby] as a miracle, but as a gift."

When Miracles Do Come True

Others do believe in miracles.

Miriam always wanted to be married with children. Still single at thirty-seven, she felt her Jewish faith was not helping her. "I was battling with God. I felt like, how did I end up in this situation in my life? If God wanted me to get married, then why am I not married?" She decided to freeze her eggs, but the night before the cycle, the clinic canceled the treatment because she wasn't responding well to the meds.

"I completely fell apart, it was horrible," she says. She reached out to her rabbi. "I was begging for validation not to do it again." But her rabbi advised her to try another round of egg freezing. "You're show-ing God how much you want this," the rabbi advised.

Miriam got married four years after that rabbi told her to freeze her eggs. She and her husband soon got pregnant, but miscarried. They tried IVF, with terrible results. They'd already started exploring using donor eggs when they thawed her frozen eggs. Only one out of the ten eggs she had frozen made it.

"Don't have a lot of hope," the doctor warned her when they trans-ferred the embryo.

Her healthy son, conceived using the egg the rabbi convinced her to freeze, was born when she was forty-four years old.

Chapter 17

Baby Envy: Living with the Green-Eyed Monster

During the time when I was grieving over my pregnancy loss or struggling with fertility issues, every joyful, expectant baby announcement felt like a tiny stab in the heart. It's not that I wasn't happy for these people, but I would think, *Why are these shiny, carefree, fertile women so easily able to do what I cannot?* And then I'd immediately feel guilt and shame for harboring that jealousy . . . I've always been one to keep my eyes on my own paper, but when it came to having a baby, that proved to be a challenge.

—actress Melissa Rauch

The phone call should've been a clue.

Who actually *called* anymore instead of texting? Especially for something as silly as asking me to get a pedicure. It's not like Helaine and I were particularly good friends—we had a good friend in common who'd moved away, so we were good enough friends to get a mani-pedi, but not to chat on the phone.

"Sorry, I can't go today," I told Helaine. Solomon and I were cleaning house—well, he'd cornered me into cleaning house. He was an anti-hoarder long before Marie Kondo, but instead of asking me what "sparked joy," he was pulling things out of the closet, asking, "Do you really need four pairs of sneakers?"

I stepped out of the messy room to hear Helaine saying she'd been wanting to talk to me. ". . . and I wanted to tell you that I'm pregnant. I know you're having some difficulty and I wanted to tell you in person I was pregnant but since you can't make the manicure . . ."

I stood in the hallway, tears streaming down my face, stifling sobs. Why was she telling me this? Why did she need me to know she was pregnant? And why the *F* was she going to tell me in person? Did she want us to sit there getting our *nails done,* where I wouldn't even be able to wipe my eyes, let alone my nose, which had also started running, adding to this symphony of misery?

Solomon came out into the hallway holding a pair of beat-up tennis shoes, but dropped them as soon as he saw my raccoon face, nodding mechanically into the phone. Helaine was saying something about doctors' visits and being nervous but I couldn't hear her. All I could hear was my doctor saying, *It looks like there's no heartbeat.* I gestured to him to help.

"Um, Amy—I need you here," he called as if he were in the other room. "Now!" *God bless his soul,* I thought.

"Helaine, I'm so sorry, gotta run, let's get that manicure soon!" I said in a cheery voice that any real friend would know indicated trouble. "And congrats, great news," I managed to squeak out before collapsing onto the messy bed, sobs coming in heaves.

Solomon rubbed my back. "I cannot believe she called me!" I said to him.

"That was . . . considerate?" he offered.

"Really? Why was it considerate? She just wanted to rub it in my face!" I said. "And I can't believe she's pregnant anyway. Isn't she, like, forty?" I sat up, finally mad enough to start folding all the clothes on the bed. I would give them away, every single one of them. I would give everything away, *everything*, if I could just have a baby.

"Just lucky, I guess," Solomon said tentatively. He knew if I was folding clothes, I was really pissed.

"Yeah, that baby will be lucky, with parents like *that*," I spat out. Helaine and her partner were both successful and gorgeous but always traveling for their high-powered jobs. I couldn't believe they got to be parents and we didn't.

"It's not like there are a limited number of babies in the world and they're taking one away from us," Solomon said. "Why can't you be happy for her?"

Happy for her?

Happy for *her*?

"Well, you're a better man than I," I said, throwing all my folded piles of clothes on the floor then storming out of our apartment.

As I walked, the bitter winter wind froze the tears on my face and I thought I would even give *him* up to have a baby.

Is Everyone but Me Pregnant?

I've always considered myself a generous person, wanting the best for everyone: *He got a movie deal? Great. She's marrying a billionaire? Fabulous.*

I wished that was how I felt about other pregnant women.

But it was not. I was not happy for them. I was so very, very sad for myself and my non-family, and therefore, I was sad about their pregnancies. To be honest, I was *mad* about their pregnancies. Their easy, no-charting, no-doctor, no shots, no-house-down-payment, "oops, we were barely trying" pregnancies.

When you're trying to conceive, when you're $30,000 in the hole with no end in sight, let me tell you: It's going to seem like every single person in the universe is with child but you. And everything will remind you of your situation:

- **Your friend, your sister, your sister's friend?** Check. They're all going to be having babies and they *are going to want you to be happy for them.* More on that in a hot minute. But let's take a moment to have some emotions.

  AAAAAAAAAAAAAAAAAAAAAAAAAA! When you're diagnosed with infertility, your world stops. Plans stop. Your once certain future stops. Your present has even stopped: Instead of girls' nights out and steamy sex with hubby, your calendar is filled with tests, appointments, and long phone calls with your insurance provider. So it would seem like the rest of the world should stop. Guess what? It doesn't. And that sucks. It's not like you want everyone else *not* to have a baby, but you fervently wish they would Just. Wait. Until. You. Do.

- **Celebrity magazine covers?** Check. Back when I was in my twenties, trying *not* to get pregnant, stars didn't flaunt their baby bumps and the tabloid covers weren't made on "Is Jennifer Aniston Pregnant?"(Nope!) These days, you can expect to read interviews with the Royal Gynecologist's nurse's sister, and female celebs Too Old for Any Romantic Lead who will be announcing their totally "genetic" pregnancy (yeah, right! I'm sure those are your fifty-two-year-old eggs).

- **Every movie or book?** Check. There was once a time that infertility was so taboo, it didn't even make a plot line in a Lifetime movie except as a ridiculous premise. You know infertility has come far when you come across a *male factor infertility* storyline . . . and it's accurate! This is fine when you're binge-watching by yourself at four A.M., but Not So Fine when you're sitting in your living room with your friends, trying to have a goddamned night off from your troubles, and then there's a *hilarious* scene of a desperate couple having loud sex, trying to get pregnant.

- **Social media?** Check. Remember when social media was new, and it seemed cool to add all those follows to Insta and FB? Ugh, now these virtual "friends" keep posting:
  -ultrasound pics!
  -pregnancy belly photo shoots!
  -newborn, I'm-not-wearing-makeup-but-I-really-am candids
  -and the extra worst: Mommy Complaining Memes ("an Instagram filter called 'before kids' that erases the dark circles under my eyes and makes it look like I've showered this week"). It's enough to finally make you go on that social media cleanse the whole world is bragging about.

- **The mail?** Check. If you thought the holidays were bad when you were single, with all the "What are you doing for New Year's/Valentine's" pressure, just wait till you're stuck in No Babyland. Now you're actually friends with people with kids, and you're going to be bombarded with sweet holiday cards featuring all of them dressed in matching holiday jammies.

Okay, I'm going to stop the list here because you get the point. Infertility and pregnancy are going to be everywhere now, and it will sucker punch you when you least expect it. The world hasn't stopped for us, and people are not going to stop being happy, getting pregnant, having babies, and celebrating *just because we aren't*. The question is: What to do about all of it?

It's Not Easy Being Me(an)

As women, we are trained to be good, to be positive, to be supportive. And we fear that the minute we aren't, we become certifiable. It all comes back to Solomon's question as I stormed out: "Why can't you be happy for her?"

The question should have been, why should I be?

When therapist Ellen S. Glazer hears clients suffering from infertility say, "I'm really happy for my friend that she's pregnant," she counters, "If I were you, I would not be happy for her pregnancy at all. I would wish it would go away."

Finally! Someone, somewhere, gets it! And she knows we're not wishing anything horrible like a miscarriage on anyone. Glazer simply empathizes with the desire to not have to deal with it. "I think it's a natural thing, it brings up a whole category of 'mean thoughts'" (she should copyright that!). "I think it just goes with the experience," she says. "Mean thoughts happen to nice people."

So before we decide on what you're going to do with all these mean thoughts, bad feelings, and kidnapping fantasies, the first thing you're going to have to do is honor them. Honor the green-eyed monster, allow it some space in your psyche—maybe even give it a Twitter account like these actual ones: @hilariouslyinfertile, @Womby McWombface, @unpregnantchicken, and @ballsdontwork. Engage in the "Who Deserves to Be Pregnant?" Olympics, make graffiti moustaches on those annoying holiday cards, and add a "Sorry, can't talk now! @ fertility clinic!" autoreply to your texts to that one annoying friend complaining of her pregnancy symptoms, so that maybe, just for once, she will get the hint.

Once you make room for those nonbeautiful thoughts, perhaps that monster will . . . well, it might not die until you have a baby, but maybe you can learn to live with it and tuck it away most of the time. And you can stop feeling so ashamed about it.

Show yourself some compassion: You feel bad. You're going through a hard time. You can't be there for everyone right now.

Think of it as one of the stages of grief—you're way past denial and stuck between anger and depression—but it's not your final destination.

Scientifically Speaking: *This* Is Trauma

Maybe some people think that infertility is not a big deal. After all, it's not *cancer* or another life-threatening disease. You're not dying. You still can do whatever you want—except, well, have children. Right?

WRONG.

"Recent studies have repeatedly associated posttraumatic symptoms with women's experience of pregnancy loss," one study begins.[1] Researchers examined the long-term psychological outcomes and reactions to pregnancy loss and infertility among almost three thousand women. Childless women with infertility report the "lowest life satisfaction and highest levels of depression despite a considerable period of time (seven years)." The study suggests that the "non-event" of involuntary childlessness is a big stressor.

Another study found that the distress of infertility "often reaches the severity found in sufferers from cancer or heart disease.[2] Another found that women with infertility felt as anxious or depressed as those diagnosed with cancer, hypertension, or recovering from a heart attack.[3]

Does this make you feel better? It should at least make you feel better about feeling bad. And let those naysayers know you're entitled to your pain.

When You Lose Friends Due to Infertility

The questions I hear the most often are of the "must I?" variety, as in, "Must I go to so-and-so's shower/bris/naming ceremony?" For example:

Q: Do I need to go to my friend's baby shower?

A: No.

Q: What if it's my best friend?

A: Still probably no, if you can get out of it. I'd like to say your best friend should understand, but she might not.

Plan B: Can you be out of town?

Plan C: Can you drop by?

Plan D: Can you take a Percocet left over from your last miscarriage and mix it with a bit of bubbly? (Sorry if you're cycling—see plan E).

Plan E: Can you lie with panache? Go for as short a time as possible, give your gift, be gracious and complimentary and hightail it out of there with a work/pet/house-flooding emergency.

Let me tell you, I went to almost everything and this is what it looked like:

SCENE: BABY SHOWER

CUT TO: CHILDLESS WOMAN WAILING IN THE BATH-ROOM STALL, SILENCING HERSELF WHEN ANYONE WALKS IN.

You get the picture: I went to quite a few baby namings, random holidays with pregnant women, and work parties where people announced their pregnancies. Attending them did not make me a better person.

If you think doing so will make you a better person, if you think you can handle it, if you think the relationship can't handle your absence, then go. But choose plan D or E.

Because you don't want to inadvertently fall on plan F: Go to the party against your better judgment because it's really important to your mom/husband/sister/frenemy, sit there like a zombie with a psychotic smile pasted on your face, and then *totally lose it,* brandishing the ketchup bottle like a weapon and splattering it all over the cute pink display.

No, you definitely don't want that to happen.

If You Can't Say, "I'm So Happy for You!" Say . . .

1. You must be so happy!
2. Well, isn't that nice!
3. That is such good news!
4. Wow! Just wow.
5. How do you feel?
6. Aren't you excited?
7. Amazing! When are you due?
8. Do you know what you're having?
9. Thank you for sharing.
10. Bless your heart.

How to Lose Friends and Alienate People

Everyone has their own shit to deal with. And it might not match up with your own.

"Why does anyone have children except for their own egos?" my once close friend Robin said after I told her about a failed cycle. I say "once close" because she'd been distancing herself for a while; I hadn't realized I shouldn't be complaining to my unmarried friend who was contemplating a child-free life. We drifted apart; she to her dreams of solo travel, me to my family. I hope we can become close again one day.

I know some people who are willing to burn everything down when they're trying to get pregnant. My friend Megan stopped talking to her family because they were so focused on her sister's pregnancy—and so pitying of her.

I get it. I really do. When my sister started telling me about her pregnancy symptoms, I oohed and ahhed like the best of them (plan E: lie with panache), and then I hopped on a plane to L.A., where all my friends had either already had their babies or were never going to.

I'm a terrible big sister, I should really be there for her, I admonished myself—and even got admonished by my own mother. But a person can only do what they can do. That's my life motto: Do what you can do when you can do it.

There've been times in my life that I've been an excellent older sister and performed superhuman acts for my siblings. But this was not going to be one of those times.

It's not that I wasn't happy for her. It's that I *did not have an ounce of happiness in me.*

My family wasn't sympathetic. One relative spent an hour on the phone telling me what she was getting my sister's upcoming kid *and* my brother's upcoming babe.

Do you really think I'm as strong as this? I thought as this relative blathered on. I should have stopped talking to all of them right then: my fertile siblings, my obsequious parents, and everyone else who was fluttering around the new babies like nothing else mattered.

Mean Thoughts (Where I Say Them So You Don't Have To)

1. Is their relationship really strong enough to handle a kid?
2. I guess if I married a guy for his money, I would be able to afford all those IVF cycles, too.
3. She really doesn't seem healthy enough to carry a pregnancy.
4. I bet he has like ten other children running around town.
5. I wouldn't want to have a mother with *those* genetics.
6. Well, she doesn't really seem like a career person anyway.
7. She's not kidding anyone if she thinks we think her pregnancy is genetic.
8. They better start a therapy fund for that kid.

I didn't, though. I held on by the skin of my teeth, nurturing my own pregnancy—which I announced well before the birth of my new nephew (February) and niece (April)—so by the time my own baby came along (July), these cousins could bond without any bad blood.

Infertility will put many of your relationships to the test. Some will survive, others won't.

How Can People Help You?

I'd like to believe my family was doing their best. I'd like to believe that all my family and friends felt bad for me and truly wanted to help me.

Now, maybe you don't want their pity, like Megan didn't want her family's. But what is it that you need?

Do you need space? Money? Do you need someone to complain to? Do you need sympathy? Do you need to not hear about every successful IVF story—or worse, miracle pregnancy—your mother has ever heard about? Do you need to be informed about pregnancies by email so you can have your own private reaction before the public one? Do you need to skip that quinceañera or toddler birthday party?

Tell them.

Also, know this: It can be hard for pregnant women to hear about your sadness. Physiologically speaking, happy hormones are coursing through their veins, making them want *everyone* to be happy.

Like Solomon, they also may not see their pregnancy as related to your lack of one. Or maybe they want you to be happy for them anyway. Or maybe you've been so good at putting on a brave face, *they don't know how down in the dumps you really are.*

Or maybe they do, but they can't handle it—and it may be time for a time-out.

Pop culture can often perpetuate the myth that female friendships are ride or die, through thick and thin, *Sex and the City, Girls,* etc. In reality, women's friendships are *rough,* especially during life changes, and extra-specially when one of us is pregnant and one of us is not but desperately wants to be.

Yet if someone else can make room for your infertility feelings, for your pain, for your fears for the future, then that's a relationship worth saving.

My oldest friend, Michelle—I still remember playing at her house when we were three—called me once to give me some news: "I just wanted to let you know that I'm pregnant," she began, knowing that our being the same age and this being her fifth was probably not the best news I could hear. "I don't expect you to be happy for me, I just wanted to let you know."

And that was the nicest thing anyone had ever said.

Dear Pregnant Girlfriend:

Thanks for sharing your pregnancy news! I know this is one of the happiest, most exciting times in your life—your first baby!—and I wish I could be there with you, exactly like we've been together through college (our awful frosh roomies!), junior year abroad (hola, Marco!), (naked) graduation, and our penny-scraping days living off ramen noodles in that crummy apartment. We even made it through being bridesmaids at each other's weddings!

You've been so wonderful through all my losses and disappointments, even letting me crash on your couch when I had that blowout with Solomon. He didn't get it, but you did.

And that's why I feel so, so terrible about how I reacted to your news. It took me by surprise.

In another universe, I would be jumping with joy, running out to buy gender-neutral booties, and registering for every damn item for your baby layette.

I value our friendship so much, so I'm just going to be honest: Right now, I can't seem to do that. I want it for you, but I want it for me, too, and your news just makes how far away I am from having a baby of my own hit home for me. I feel so, so ashamed of how I'm feeling—I wish I didn't feel this way, but there you have it.

I know I won't feel this way forever, and as soon as she's born (don't you think it will be a girl???), I promise to be the best auntie EVER! For now, I just need a bit of time and space, and to be there for non-pregnancy things.

Love you always,
Amy

Chapter 18

_____

I Will Survive: Perseverance and How to Keep On Keeping On

I was devastated when it didn't happen [again and again].
I had to remain hopeful and resilient and, "Okay, let's do
it again."

—Angela Bassett

Maybe I'm not meant to be a mother. Maybe I should just let this whole thing go. I'm sure there are plenty of people who are happy without children. I could be happy without children. Could I be happy without children? Could we be happy without children?

I was in a deep, dark winter. And I was only talking to people who could be with me in the messy muck. (Sorry, Mom, that's why I didn't return any of your calls that month.) One of those people was my dear friend Lisa, a businesswoman–turned–intuitive healer. She couldn't predict the future, but could sense what was going on in people's minds, hearts, and health. Although she did not predict my miscarriage, she'd been right about a lot in the past. And now she told me something that resonated.

"Do not give up on this. You are meant to be a mom. This is something that you *have* to be. You will not be complete without it," Lisa said. It was only by forging my own family that I would be able to move beyond my own difficult childhood, she forecast.

Was she right? Did I have to be a mother? Especially if it was going to be so hard?

Really, Really Want It

Some women are ambivalent about having children, saying, "If it happens, it happens." (I used to be one of those women!) But you can't be ambivalent when you do fertility treatment. If you're going to spend time and money and energy on treatment, you have to really want it.

Did I really want it that badly?

I thought about quitting. I thought about what life would be like without a baby. I thought I would have been okay—I *could* have been okay—if only I hadn't *gotten* pregnant. If only I hadn't seen the plethora of positive pregnancy tests, been to the OB and watched my baby floating around inside of me. At one point in my life I could have gone babyless, but not anymore.

Not with Solomon, anyway. I knew he was destined to be a dad. Like me, he was late to the game and hadn't known his whole life that he wanted to be a father, but by the time he'd gotten to me—his first marriage failed just as they started trying to conceive—he was ready. He'd already given up his itinerant musician life, and unlike me, he seemed certain about how to be a parent. (Little did I know then that he sounds certain about *everything*.)

I didn't think we would be fine, just us. We'd be a family, technically, but to me it didn't feel that way. I couldn't picture the script, the next scene, the dialogue, the plot points, the character arc. Just the denouement. The unraveling, the pretending we'd never tried to be together in the first place.

This is not to say that what came next was for him. It wasn't. It was for us. And for me. And for the me that was married to him.

When I was trying to learn to surf, I would always pull back the minute I saw the shadow of the wave hovering over my longboard. "You have to commit to the wave," one wise observer said.

And I kept that advice in mind as I continued after my failures: I was going to commit to this wave of being a mom. I'd do whatever it took to have a baby. But how?

Snappy Answers to Stupid Questions

WHEN THEY SAY	YOU SAY (OR THINK . . .)
1. Do you really think it's going to work?	1. Don't you think you should be more supportive?
2. I just think you should be more realistic.	2. I think you mean "pessimistic and hopeless."
3. Don't you think it's time you switched doctors/clinics/treatments?	3. Time I switched off my hearing aid? Yes!
4. I know someone who relaxed/adopted/traveled and got pregnant.	4. Why don't you hang out with her?
5. You can still be happy if you're not a mother.	5. I'll be happier when the only idiots I deal with are my children.
6. Don't you think you should quit?	6. Our relationship? YES!

Keep Calm and IVF

"Did you hear the story of the woman who just kept on trying and trying and finally got pregnant?" people would always ask me. Sounds like an urban myth—except that I heard this one with my own ears.

A top New York fertility clinic basically kicked "Beth" out after three rounds of IVF, telling her she was "past the age" where they thought they could help. She was forty-one.

She decided to try another clinic to do low-dose stimulation, which she thought would be better for her. Over the next three years, she did twenty retrievals.

Yes, you heard me, twenty. Twenty rounds of IVF in a period of three years—straight.

"I didn't want to take a break," she says. Some rounds she got only one or two eggs. "Making embryos for me was almost impossible," she says, explaining how she was going to bank them all to test them. Her clinic charged one bulk price for genetic testing the embryos, as opposed to some clinics, where they charge per embryo.

After all that, they had five embryos, two of which tested normal. They transferred one of them when she was forty-four, and at the age of forty-five, she gave birth to a healthy boy.

Beth is the ne plus ultra of fertility stories. An urban legend come true. (She offered to send me her receipts from the clinic as proof, but I have enough of my own paperwork, thank you.)

What I really wanted to know was, how did she persevere? How did she go on despite all that disappointment?

"There's nothing I ever wanted like I wanted this," the new mom says. Is she made of stronger stuff than the rest of us? No—she actually describes herself as a quitter in general. "I never really tried that hard at anything," she says. But this? This baby with her own genetics? "It became my life's work."

In fact, she quit her fifty-hour-a-week job in the restaurant business to pursue it. "It soon became clear that IVF was going to tamp down my work style, working late shifts at night." But then, after years of IVF, she realized she was miserable, with no life, so she started doing yoga and pottery.

So obsessive was she about her pottery (so much for her being a quitter) that they offered her a job of sorts, training kids for free studio space. "That became my sanity," she says. "IVF was a full-time job."

Now let it be said that not only could Beth *afford* to leave her job, but nineteen of those twenty rounds were covered by insurance!

Her patience wasn't endless. By that twentieth round—technically twenty-third, if you count her first clinic—she knew she had to test the embryos, like, *now*. "That was it. If we didn't have any embryos that were viable, I was quitting IVF," she says. "We were going to adopt."

"I was at my breaking point," she admits. "I was emotionally done. I could not bear any more."

Good thing she got pregnant when she did.

Nevertheless, She Persisted

Most women doing fertility treatment have to persevere, despite failure.

The big question is . . . how? How do you go on after trying for six months on your own, starting your IUIs all hopeful and excited, and proceeding to costly IVF, cycle after cycle?

Lainy thought IVF would guarantee her a baby when she started treatment at thirty-one. But four cycles and three years later . . . nada. During that time, she needed "persistence, and plenty of blood, sweat, and tears—literally and figuratively!"

Her friends and family would tell her, "You're so strong. I would've given up by now. How do you do it?"

She told them she wasn't ready to give up. "Something told me to keep going. Part of me was in denial: denial that it might actually *never* work. But something told me there would be a light at the end

Can Your Doctor Help You Persevere?

Many women describe their doctors as advocates.

That's what Erin Khar's doctor told her, after five miscarriages and two IVF cycles. The author of the addiction memoir *Strung Out: One Last Hit and Other Lies That Nearly Killed Me* already had a thirteen-year-old son, and desperately wanted another with her new husband. Despite a second-trimester loss (after going through labor!), Khar says what kept her going was "the carrot of moving forward with the next transfer or next round of IVF."

Her doctor told her, *We aren't going to give up. We're going to do whatever it takes.* "And I believed her: I believed we could do this together." Khar did Reiki, acupuncture, and meditation and learned how to sit in acceptance. "With all of that I had a new-found determination to move forward."

And it worked. She gave birth to another son.

Many doctors want to be supportive, whatever you decide.

"I give my patients hope to carry on by giving them encouragement, a friend to connect with on an emotional level and mental level," says Dr. Janelle Luk of Generation Next Fertility. "I really spend my time with them to understand how they feel, if they want to continue or not."

But she says she never pushes patients to keep going. The statistics may be against them, or their finances might be. "My job is to present them with enough information: The patient comes up with the answer and not me."

But the motivation, the drive to continue, the determination, she says, comes from within. "This is really all coming from the patient, from their passion and wisdom, from the voice in their heart that talks to them, that tells them to keep going."

of the tunnel and that someone would crack the code . . . and they did." Although many doctors had no answers or insight into her failures, "I simply refused to believe that I would not be able to create a baby and get pregnant." She says she kept pushing through. "Finding the strength and fight to carry on throughout this daunting process is incredibly challenging, but very possible," she says. Her fifth cycle at her fourth clinic was the magic number—she got pregnant.

No matter how much IVF a woman has done, she tends to gloss over the hard times, the sad times, the dark times. But it's important to note that they're part of the journey.

"Surprisingly, I never really got too dark, given all that was going on," says Lainy, surprising *me* since I had witnessed lots of her lows—when she was panicking, freaking out, depressed, despondent, unhopeful. Maybe it was the pregnancy hormones that made her forget.

When I was doing my time (yes! It's like prison!), I met a woman who gave me hope. Carla went through ten rounds of IVF over five years to have her son. Her IVF was also covered by insurance (that seems to be the recurring theme of persistence: the ability to pay for it . . .).

When I checked in with her now, she still remembers the hard times, even though her son is almost in middle school. "I look back at those five years, and they were so dark. I retreated from the Jewish community," she says. Seeing all the baby strollers on her Sabbath walks would make her cry. Synagogue was no better—not with the yentas nosily asking her, "So when are you going to start a family already?"

For her, the answer was to talk about it, to tell them it wasn't easy, to be very upfront with her struggles and to consider adoption. "The whole thing was so painful," Carla recalls.

She too describes her last round—lucky number ten—as the breaking point.

"Everyone's journey is so different, you hear of people who are devastated they have to do IVF at all, then they have success on their first try, and some people have to go through two, three, four—or more."

Her doctor is the one who gave her hope, switching protocols after each failure. By the last cycle, Carla told the doc: "This is the last time, I can't do anymore. Stim the shit out of me" (meaning give her as much medicine as possible). "I couldn't put myself through another disappointment or another cycle."

If she hadn't gotten pregnant on the tenth cycle, would she have continued to an eleventh one? "I don't know. That's when my insurance ran out," she says. But she also knows she might have stopped IVF and pursued adoption. "At the end of the day, I know there are many ways to have a baby—and it's just a matter of how you get through that challenge."

10 Ways to Build Resilience

(According to the American Psychological Association)

1. **Make connections.** Part of being resilient is having a strong support network within your family, friends, and community. "Accepting help and support from those who care about you and will listen to you strengthens resilience."

2. **Avoid seeing crises as insurmountable problems.** Stress is going to happen—but what's your response to it? "Try looking beyond the present to how future circumstances may be a little better." A little better is on the road to better.

3. **Accept that change is a part of living.** You can't always get what you want, the song goes. But can you get what you need? "Accepting circumstances that cannot be changed can help you focus on circumstances that you can alter."

4. **Move toward your goals.** What are realistic goals and small steps you can take? "Instead of focusing on tasks that seem unachievable, ask yourself, 'What's one thing I know I can ac-

complish today that helps me move in the direction I want to go?'"

5. **Take decisive actions.** Don't detach from problems, wishing them away. "Act on adverse situations as much as you can."

6. **Look for opportunities for self-discovery.** I don't believe infertility is a blessing, but you can learn something about yourself from it. "Many people who have experienced tragedies and hardship have reported better relationships, greater sense of strength even while feeling vulnerable, increased sense of self-worth, a more developed spirituality and heightened appreciation for life."

7. **Nurture a positive view of yourself.** You build resilience by gaining confidence in your problem-solving ability. "Trusting your instincts helps build resilience."

8. **Keep things in perspective.** "Even when facing very painful events, try to consider the stressful situation in a broader context and keep a long-term perspective."

9. **Maintain a hopeful outlook.** "Try visualizing what you want, rather than worrying about what you fear."

10. **Take care of yourself.** What do you need? "Taking care of yourself helps to keep your mind and body primed to deal with situations that require resilience."

The IVF Gamble

Those women who kept going to double digit cycles have resilience, I thought, wondering if I should have kept going, too.

"Resilience used to be thought of as traits of grit, determination and perseverance," says Linda Graham, MFT, a licensed marriage and family therapist, mindful self-compassion teacher, and author of *Resilience: Powerful Practices for Bouncing Back from Disappointment, Difficulty, and Even Disaster.*[1]

Perseverance is the "continued effort to do or achieve something despite difficulties, failure or opposition," according to the dictionary. "We persist because we believe that we'll meet our goal," Graham points out. And that is true of every woman I have spoken to, who has put her life, her body, her relationship, and sometimes her finances on the line in service of having a baby.

Not everyone is a hero, though.

"You can make the decision to do everything you can and you *still* might not get the result you want," Graham says. "Part of being resilient is being able to discern whether this is working or not working."

In fact, the American Psychological Association now defines resilience as "the process of adapting well in the face of adversity, trauma, tragedy, threats or significant sources of stress . . . It means 'bouncing back' from difficult experiences."

Resilience is not just about persistence, in other words. Because isn't the definition of insanity doing the same thing over and over and expecting different results?

Recognizing the difference between willfulness and willingness is also important during IVF, when considering whether to change protocols or clinics.

Take Tom: His daughter was born on their second round of IVF. So when it came time to try again, of course he and his wife went back to their doctor. And they kept going back, round after round, two, three, four, five times.

"I'm a firm believer in odds," says Tom, who works in finance and describes himself as a math guy. "Each flip of the coin doesn't affect the other coin flips." Because they were 1 for 2 on the first try, he figured 1 for 5 or 6 was a reasonable expectation.

"We always had one embryo to put in; it wasn't like zero/zero/zero." He says they were waiting for the "magic gumball." (I've heard many a reproductive endocrinologist describe our eggs/embryos as a gumball machine waiting for that one good one.) "You can't roll the dice twice and expect to win," he says. Their sixth try resulted in a pregnancy, so Tom was glad they stayed. But when that pregnancy miscarried, they finally decided to switch clinics, ignoring what Tom calls the "sunk costs," a finance term for irrecoverable costs that have already been incurred and therefore *should not be a factor in future decision-making.*

Sunk costs are what make many people continue down the wrong path. If you invest in a stock and it's losing money, you might decide to stick with it and hope it will turn around because you're already invested. Same with IVF—you might decide to stay with your doctor or clinic because you're already there, they know you, and you know them (and there is something to be said for that!).

Still, you have to periodically take stock, see what's working and what isn't, and do what will be most effective *in the future.*

How to Turn Worry into Hope

They say there are no atheists in foxholes, and infertility is certainly a foxhole. Even though I am no longer religious, I can tell you that when I was staring at a pregnancy test and waiting the excruciating two minutes for that second line to show up, I did send many a prayer out to . . . someone. Somewhere in the universe.

I don't believe there is one being out there overseeing my life and fertility (because if there were, S/He is doing a terrible job!). But there was something spiritual that did help me. I tried to turn my worries and fears into hopes, the way the hokey law of attraction might advise.

INSTEAD OF SAYING:	SAY THIS:
I'm so scared X ruined this cycle.	I hope this cycle works.
I can't look at another failed test.	I hope that I am pregnant.
I'm afraid I won't see a heartbeat.	I'm excited to hear a heartbeat.

As an investor, Tom wanted to make sure he had enough emotional and financial capacity to get to that future goal. "Gambling simulations clearly show that if you show up to the table without enough money, you're a lot more likely to lose," he says. "We wanted to make sure we had enough cash and enough emotional bandwidth for the next part," meaning finding a new doctor and switching clinics. The second clinic was the charm: They had their second child.

When is persistence just plain stupid?

"I see a lot of people who have really bad business ideas," Tom says. "It doesn't matter if they put in forty-hour workweeks or eighty-hour workweeks—if you're going down a bad path, it's not going to get better. At a certain point you need to start exploring new paths."

Obviously no one can make the decision to persist for you.

Take Beth: She'd quit her job and devoted herself to IVF and pottery. No doubt all her friends and family thought she was nuts.

Only you and your partner know what the right path is for you.

The Real Resilience—and How You Get It

I'd always thought of resilience as just plain grit, as soldiering on.

So where does a story like mine fit in? After four IUIs and eight rounds of IVF, producing no normal embryos, I decided to move to donor eggs.

Should I have continued? Did I fail because I did not continue with my own eggs and had a baby with a donor egg?

No, Graham says.

"Resilience is having some overarching self that says, 'The wise choice is this one. It's up to me to define what success is.' Part of being resilient is owning your own agency to decide what success is," Graham counsels me. "And your goal is having a child, deciding *that* option didn't work but *this* one did. That is being resilient and being successful in your choice of options."

As a therapist for the last twenty-five years, Graham says that building resilience is at the heart of her work with patients. "It's what we do all the time, helping clients cope with stresses and trauma and helping them find new skills and practices to cope better, more reflexively, adaptively, resiliently."

These days, I like to think of resilience not as blind persistence, but as a coping practice that anyone can learn. Because even after you have a baby, you will still have stressors to deal with. That's what neuroscience is beginning to show: We can create new neural pathways in our brain to cope with stress and trauma better. "We not only have the ability to be more resilient, we have the ability to strengthen our brain function," Graham says, calling it a "responsibility" to learn those skills so we can meet and deal with stress.

Here's the thing: We all have stress in life. And resilience is not measured by what happens to us (i.e., having to do twenty-three rounds of IVF like Beth), but by how we respond to it.

Graham says many people have a hard time dealing with the fact that bad things simply happen. "We can wind up thinking, 'This isn't supposed to be happening to me,'" she says.

Which is exactly how most of us feel when we get hit with an infertility diagnosis. Especially since it's often the first time (if we're lucky) that we're dealing with the medical system. (For many women, birth is the first time they're in the hospital.) But Graham, who is older, says she and many of her friends get health diagnoses all the time. "My friends don't say, 'Why me?' They're getting older. They say, 'Why *not* me? Let's get on and deal with it.'"

And that's what resilience is—getting on and dealing with it. The best way you know how.

Section IV

NEXT STEPS

Chapter 19

The Women in Waiting (Room)

Going into it, I thought I was going to get a little bit of negative pushback—kind of like, *Well, you already have a son, so be happy for what you have . . .* but I still wanted to tell the story because I had known of people who were going through secondary infertility but they didn't have a name to put on it. They were just having trouble having another child.

—*TODAY*'s Dylan Dreyer

Younger than me, older than me, prettier than me, richer than me.

It may be petty, but this was what was usually going through my mind when I was at one of my many fertility clinics. What else was I supposed to do during those endless waits?

Why is that woman here if she already has a baby? I'd think about the frantic female whose wild child was running circles around the waiting room, reminding the rest of us of our empty wombs.

God, that girl is so lucky, she can't be even thirty and she has so much time to figure out her fertility, I'd think about the fresh-faced millennial thumbing through her phone. Ditto the Prada-purse-carrying fancy ladies who would likely be able to afford as many treatments as their hearts (or uterus) desired—or so I imagined.

Really, you never know what someone else is going through. Those picture-perfect celebrity profiles and Instagram feeds are actually carefully crafted to showcase a happy family. Who knows what it took to *get* that happy family? A miscarriage or two? An IUI, multiple rounds of IVF, even a surrogate? Or, in the case of older celebrities, a donor egg or embryo?

Take me, for example: On the surface you'd see a woman who started later in life, but there are a million reasons why: I'd left a tight-knit religious community and was trying to find my own way . . . well, that's basically the main reason; yet pull on that one thread and you unravel a whole person.

When you're sitting in the waiting room, comparing yourself to others and fantasizing how their life—and fertility journey—is better than yours, you aren't seeing another person in all her complexity.

Here are their stories.

Young and Infertile

"You have time! You're so *young!*" friends, family, and medical professionals were always telling Zoe, who went off birth control shortly before her wedding at thirty-two so she and her husband, Adam, could get pregnant. She never did get her period, and after a few months, a gynecologist diagnosed her with hyperthyroidism, excitedly sending her straight to IVF. "You'll do really well there," the doc told her, like it was summer camp.

The fertility doctor even promised he'd have her pregnant by the holidays—a month later! But then Adam was diagnosed with male factor infertility, too. (See chapter 13.)

"It's so frustrating to be 'young': I'm just as desperate to get pregnant as anyone over thirty-five," Zoe says.

Anyway, her young age became "old news pretty quickly," she says. "My age didn't mean a thing in our case: We're young and *still* have severe, complicated fertility issues." Besides, if you're young at the fertility clinic, then the standard "it's your age" is not the cause. *Something is actually wrong.*

Zoe says having an "out of the box" case with no diagnosis was extremely frustrating: The fact that she has time means she could be doing it for another five years—not to mention spend an obscene amount of money. She felt like she did everything, from acupuncture to organic food to BPA-free beauty products, and still had no answers over many years. "I felt . . . hopeless. Alone. Doomed. As if someone is out to get me."

Some people started off fertility treatment "young," but then aged into the "old" category at thirty-five.

"I think at any age you try to have kids, you're surprised when it's not so easy," says Ben, who'd started trying when he and his wife were twenty-seven. They're now thirty-five.

"At almost every age, your friends are going to be having children." He told me how difficult it's been to watch people around them have kids—multiple times—over the years.

Older people in the waiting room have no idea what "young" people like he and his wife face. Actually, most doctors don't, either. Their first four clinics gave them the "unexplained infertility" spiel.

With time on their side, they had the liberty of switching clinics—but it didn't help. "Every doctor tells you they'll solve the problem," Ben says. Finally, at their fifth clinic, the doctor said he wasn't sure what the problem was, and that made Ben think, *This is the only person that listened to what we had done before and is not going to do it again.* Ben is now enrolled in a trial for a "three-parent IVF" outside the US.

When Ben sees older women in the waiting room, all he thinks is, "At least you don't have this condition inside you that's a ticking time bomb," he confessed. He says that people like me—older women— might have a host of reasons why we didn't start when we were younger —we're divorced, we're single, we're trying for a second kid; but it doesn't matter.

"It's almost all out of your control, and it sucks."

What's a Three-Parent Baby?

There's been a lot of talk in the news about the "three-parent baby," which is not exactly what it sounds like, plus, is only available for very, very few people.

"Techniques to create 'three-parent babies' seek to offer mothers a way to have a child without passing on metabolic diseases caused by faulty mitochondria, the structures that provide energy to cells. Researchers do this by exchanging the diseased mitochondria of a prospective mother with those of a healthy, unrelated donor: the 'third parent,'" a review in *Nature* explained.[1]

The way that Dr. John Zhang, founder of New Hope Fertility Center and progenitor of the technique explained it to me was that "it's like taking the egg yolk of one woman (the mother) and borrowing the shell of another (the donor.)"

Unlike using donor eggs, which is when the mother carries the DNA of another woman mixed with her partner's sperm, with this, the DNA is entirely from the mother—so not a three-parent at all, even though they're mixing two women's cells.

Dr. Zhang told *Nature* he'll test the technique for older women (forty-two to forty-seven years old) to see if mitochondria from younger donors would stimulate the older eggs' ability to be fertilized and develop normally.

A number of normal babies have been born using this technique but "we won't know the follow-up for many generations," Dr. Zhang said.

Secondary Infertility

Had I seen her in the waiting room, I probably would've hated Elissa Strauss: Not only is she younger, thinner, *and* prettier than me, but the CNN journalist sometimes took her toddler son with her when she went for fertility treatment (mostly on weekends).

Strauss had secondary infertility, a term that means a woman has had children (it doesn't matter if she's had one, two, or three or more, or if she previously did IVF to conceive) but is struggling to get pregnant again. (Primary infertility is when a woman is having trouble getting pregnant with her first child.)

With Strauss's first, she got pregnant naturally at thirty-two. After casually Trying for a few months, she decided to take a break and go on vacation. Lo and behold, she got pregnant with her son.

A couple of years later, she and her husband kind of, sort of started again. "I was super chill about it," she says. Even after four or five months, she wasn't "super worried" about it. But she was almost thirty-five, so her OB thought she should make an appointment at a fertility clinic. She could only get an appointment for six months (!) in the future, but assumed she'd be pregnant by the time she got there. But she wasn't. She had the appointment, and testing found . . . nothing. Two IUIs yielded nothing, so she started IVF at thirty-five.

IVF was really, really hard for her. At certain times during the process, "I was a mess. I was bawling, I was totally unhinged," she says. What was also hard was trying to navigate the process with a kid in tow.

"Practically, it's a nightmare," she says. "Figuring out the childcare, you have to get out of the house early, you and your husband work . . ."

For example, for one transfer on a Saturday morning at eight A.M., "They don't want children there because it's triggering, but you need your husband," so what was she to do? She understands why clinics don't want children in the waiting room. "It's coming from a really good place, but secondary infertility is really common," she says. "It's hard for a working person, period—never mind a working *parent*."

It can be hard on a marriage, too, she says, because while she was doing treatment, her husband had to pick up the slack with their kid. "I saw everyone else at the clinic with their husbands and I would feel resentful," she says. (I guess it goes both ways!) "I didn't blame him—you just get in the survival mode. There's only so much you can do."

Her husband—like many partners experiencing either primary *or* secondary infertility—didn't always get where she was coming from. "He was more like, 'Whatever happens, happens.' I was more like, '*I WANT ANOTHER KID.*'"

Did she ever have guilt about wanting another kid when she already had one?

"No guilt," she replies. "Just like you imagine yourself as a mom, I imagine myself as a mom of two kids." She is one of four and is "very tight" with her siblings, and "I really wanted my child to experience that," she says.

She knows that wanting a kid when you already have one is much easier than wanting a kid when you don't have one. She didn't experience the existential angst of, " 'I will never know what motherhood is like,' " she says. "I'd imagined a different *version* of motherhood, but I'm still a mother." During treatment, "it's better to go home to a child than go home to a quiet house," she muses.

Some moms who have dealt with infertility the first *and* second time around feel they're both hard in different ways.

"I think secondary infertility is just as hard—it's different, but it's also very painful," says Ayako, who was an only child herself and wanted her daughter to have a sibling.

The first time around, she wasn't surrounded by mothers or pregnant women. The second time, going through IVF, "I have a lot of mom friends and they're all having babies and I just look at them getting pregnant and think, 'Why not me?' "

Ironically, even though she's doing this for her daughter, she feels the mom guilt—that pervasive feeling that seems to seep into all aspects of motherhood, that whatever you're doing, you're not doing enough. "I don't spend enough time with my daughter because I'm doing treatment and recuperating," says Ayako.

Strauss, after one retrieval and two transfers (the first ending in unexplained early miscarriage), finally had her coveted second child. "There's no perfect version of family building," she says.

Causes of Secondary Infertility

Secondary infertility can be shocking, especially if you conceived easily the first time around.

Some studies show that if you had a C-section, it may make it harder to get pregnant the next time than women who delivered vaginally.[2] In one study, researchers found that C-section scarring can cause infertility due to "retention of bloody fluid in the uterine cavity and scarring."[3] They recommend "Endoscopic treatment, such as hysteroscopy or laparoscopy" to treat the scarring.

Other causes of secondary infertility might be due to lifestyle changes for both partners, such as smoking, drinking, hot-tubbing, or other environmental factors. Other risk factors include your weight, your medications, and the good old standby: your age.

Fertility Treatment for Cancer Patients

Melissa Thompson never *imagined* she'd have to go through fertility treatment, not after having her daughter with her partner when she was thirty-two.

But at six weeks postpartum, the public policymaker had breast-feeding problems. That's when she found out she had stage 3 breast cancer, specifically, pregnancy-associated breast cancer (PABC). She was told she would need chemo, which can compromise fertility, and if she wanted more children she should preserve her fertility now. "Chemotherapy and radiation therapy often result in reduced fertility," according to the ASRM ethics committee's opinion on oncofertility, which is fertility for cancer patients.[4] They recommend that oncologists discuss fertility preservation options before doing therapy. So does the American Society of Clinical Oncology, noting that healthcare providers should initiate the "discussion on the possibility of infertility" either with patients and or their parents even though patients may be focused on their cancer diagnosis.[5] The oncologist should discuss fertility preservation options, including freezing eggs, sperm, and embryos. Because fertility meds can have different effects on different cancers, it's essential for your oncology and fertility teams to work together.

Thompson didn't have the luxury, like other women, of deliberating over whether to freeze her eggs. "I started the next day," she says. "I had a newborn and cancer and I was asked to choose my future." She froze embryos with her partner's sperm. (Something she does not recommend, just in case you split up. Instead, she says, freeze just your eggs.)

As if life hadn't hit her with enough—a new baby, a faltering partnership, breast cancer, and chemotherapy—she got hit with a massive hospital bill. Her insurer had learned her "infertility" was linked to her cancer diagnosis, and so reversed its pre-authorization of the egg freezing.

Despite being a new mother, having a double mastectomy, and surviving brutal chemotherapy, Thompson didn't take her insurance bill sitting down. She was the driving force for Melissa's Law for Fertility Preservation, a Connecticut bill that requires insurance coverage for fertility treatment based on medical necessity, ensuring that people who have issues of medical necessity won't have to wait a year to qualify for fertility coverage. It was enacted in 2017, and other states are following suit.

Two years after chemotherapy, Melissa was the beneficiary of her *own* law, as she underwent another egg freezing procedure, due to a legal battle with her ex-boyfriend over their embryos (she wants them destroyed, he doesn't). "And it was covered by my bill," she proudly says. "This will give newly diagnosed cancer patients peace of mind."

Before her cancer treatment, she had twenty-two eggs retrieved; and after, at age thirty-five, six. "Post-chemo egg freezing *is* possible. I didn't know that," she says, noting that patients are often under the impression that chemotherapy is "sudden death" for fertility. "It's suboptimal but possible."

Going through breast cancer definitely helped Jennifer Lowright get through the vicissitudes of IVF. She'd been diagnosed with stage 2B breast cancer a mere six weeks after her wedding at thirty-four. Right after her double mastectomy and prior to chemo, she did a few egg retrievals, ultimately freezing nine embryos. But she didn't use them for a while, first doing fifteen months of chemo and then finishing the entire five-year regimen of Tamoxifen, an estrogen-blocking drug meant to prevent cancer recurrence. (Some people take it for three years, start their family, and then go back on for two years to finish the regimen.)

She was forty when she could start transferring.

Over the next three years, she had three failed transfers (including a chemical pregnancy) at two different clinics. "I had the same mentality I did with the cancer: what do I have to do next?" Just like with cancer, she says you have to have a "positive attitude" about IVF. "You can't go in thinking, 'This is not going to work,'" she says. Her fourth transfer, of their two last embryos, finally brought her a baby girl, right before she turned forty-four. "Nine years, nine embryos later, I had one baby. I am extremely blessed."

IVF for Genetic Reasons

Jean Hannah Edelstein wasn't actually infertile when she found out she'd need fertility treatment. At thirty-two, the writer and marketer learned she had Lynch syndrome, a rare hereditary genetic condition that has a high risk of colon cancer as well as other cancers. Finally, she understood her familial history—her father had died of lung cancer and his mom had died of colon cancer. She'd need to get a preventative hysterectomy at around forty. And her offspring would have a 50 percent chance of inheriting the disease.

"You can do IVF to avoid passing Lynch syndrome on to your kids," the doctor told her. She would have to do preimplanation genetic diagnosis (PGD) to test embryos for a specific disorder. (I'll discuss this more in chapter 20.)

"I wasn't thinking of having kids or IVF. I was thirty-two!" she says, noting her last relationship had ended at thirty. "I saw kids in my future—my mom had my sister when she was thirty-nine! And my mom was born to a mother who was thirty-nine."

Since she'd eventually have to do IVF anyway to obtain healthy embryos, it made sense to freeze her eggs as soon as possible.

Edelstein looked into freezing her eggs, but then met the man who would become her husband. "Are you with the man you want to have kids with?" her doctor asked her. She was, so they began the business of creating embryos for testing. "It felt unfair that we could get pregnant naturally and yet we had to do this convoluted thing," she says. During treatment, she'd be out in the world, for instance, at a yoga class, where a woman would say it took her a few months to get pregnant, and she thought, "I can't believe people have sex and have a baby—their journey is so different." On the other hand, she knows she's lucky. "On the flip side, I know people who struggle with IVF for years and never get pregnant." Also, she found a job that included IVF coverage (though the genetic testing was out of pocket).

After two rounds of IVF, they had seven embryos to test—and miraculously, none had the disease. "The genetic counselor was shocked," Edelstein says, noting she was glad she did it. What if I had a kid that had Lynch syndrome and he got sick?" she says. "I have the ability to prevent that."

Eradicate All Disease?

Elissa Strauss, who did IVF because of her secondary infertility, also screened her embryos for BRCA, a gene that when mutated, predisposes to breast cancer because her husband is a carrier of the gene. "I had so many embryos, it seemed like the minimum," she says, noting that she wanted to prevent having a girl who carried the gene.

The ASRM calls screening "to avoid the birth of offspring with a high risk of inherited cancer ethically acceptable."[6]

Some believe that genetic screening for disease is one of IVF's best applications.

"We are leaving the largest opportunity for IVF on the table, almost untouched," Dr. David Sable, a former fertility doctor and biotech investor, writes in Forbes.[7] "IVF's greatest potential contribution to medicine, its use for disease prevention using preimplantation genetic diagnosis, is a blip in the reproductive medicine marketplace," he says, noting that between four thousand and five thousand pregnancies in which the baby is at risk for having cystic fibrosis and more than seven thousand in which the baby is at risk of having sickle cell anemia are conceived in the US each year. "PGD could prevent all of these diseases—with an IVF procedure that is cheaper, safer and more effective than methods either in place or in development to treat them."

It's Not Easy Being Them

"If we all threw our problems in a pile and saw everyone else's," the saying goes, "we'd grab our own problems back."[8]

In the end, despite all my envy, it seems like the women in the waiting room had even bigger problems than I did. Because they were young, they actually had an issue: cancer, genetic disease carriers, unlimited time to spend all their money on something that might not work.

So next time you're in the waiting room coveting someone's youth/wealth/wardrobe, know that there is always more to the story than meets the eye.

What We're Thinking About
The Women in the Waiting Room

WHAT YOU'RE THINKING ABOUT HER	WHAT SHE'S THINKING
She's so young, she has no biological clock.	I can't miss any work at this early juncture in my career if I'm going to afford IVF.
She already has a kid—why is she even here? I'd be happy with *one* child.	I feel so guilty that I can't be with my son. And I feel so bad that he can't have a sibling.
Is she even twenty-five? She has all the time in the world to have a baby.	I can't believe I've just been diagnosed with cancer and have to start chemo next week.
Another mom, breastfeeding this time.	How do I prevent my next baby from having BRCA?
She has so much money, she can probably buy this clinic.	Well, at least I'm rich.

Chapter 20

The Whole IVF Toolbox: Trying Everything

Now there's so many different treatments and there's so many ways . . . I do think medicine has come so far but I think the emotional part is the same: It's just a struggle, it's so difficult, but talking about it, making women okay with it, embracing it, that's where we have come a long way."

—Molly Sims[1]

"I'll give you a million dollars if you can get me pregnant—and keep me pregnant."

I never said this to my doctor. First off, because I didn't have that kind of money (especially not after IVF) and also: I'm not sure it would be legal.

But go with me here for a minute: What if your doctor was really, really motivated to get you pregnant and help you carry to term? What if you were, for example, royalty or an A-list celebrity? What kind of tests would the doctors order, what kind of procedures would they perform, what kind of meds would they give if they were really under the gun? (That's another scenario: to threaten your doctor at gunpoint till they get you pregnant. Probably harder to carry out. Also, again: illegal.)

Doctors don't tell you that the first round of IVF is often a test round, or what they call diagnostic.

"It's fair to say we do learn a lot—you get to see the eggs and sperm in action for the first time," says Dr. Richard Scott, the founding partner of Reproductive Medicine Associates of New Jersey, noting that "it should not be a test round. There's no dress rehearsal."

What Can Go Wrong in a Cycle?

1. You can't start your cycle due to cysts, fibroids, or other uterine conditions.
2. Your cycle is canceled due to poor response. (But can you do a transfer anyway? And how much money do you save on canceling? Can you convert to IUI?)
3. They didn't retrieve any eggs ("empty follicles").
4. Your eggs failed to fertilize. (Did they do ICSI or emergency ICSI?)
5. Your transfer is canceled due to poor endometrial lining, or hyperstimulation of your ovaries. (Do they recommend another retrieval before transfer or frozen transfer next time? What can they do to improve your uterine lining?)
6. Your eggs fail to make it to day-3 or day-5 blastocyst.
7. The world is ending. (Can you do a transfer anyway?)

After a failed cycle, it's time to have your WTF Meeting.

Now is the time to sit down with your doctor for a follow-up to discuss what the hell happened and why the hell you're not pregnant.

(They usually schedule this meeting *after* your period so you don't go postal.) If you're simply freezing and banking embryos, you'll still want to know what could be better: more eggs, more embryos, better embryos, thicker lining, fewer side effects, different med protocol . . . something!

Now's the time to get practical, get aggressive, and change it up.

If the first cycle is indeed diagnostic, let's see what they've learned: For the next round, how do they adjust your meds, the timing of your trigger, and all the factors that go into a successful cycle? Because now is a "diagnostic" time for you, too: You'll learn how flexible your clinic is, or if they're a one-size-fits-all place. You'll begin to see if they're the right place for you in a way that you can't know when you're just starting out.

You're no longer a shiny penny, a newbie clueless about all things IVF, afraid of the shots, afraid to ask questions, afraid of your insurance bill. Now you're experienced.

So whether it's your second or seventh cycle, you want to do everything possible to ensure that your next cycle is a successful one.

You want them to use everything in their toolbox.

WTF Questions for the Doc

1. What went wrong?
2. What will you do differently?
3. Can we change my medicines? Trigger earlier?
4. Can you do an ERA (endometrial receptivity array)?
5. Do you have a special protocol for diminished ovarian reserve?
6. Can we do a fresh/day-3 transfer?
7. Do you test for endometriosis?
8. Will you do an immune panel to see if something's wrong with my body?
9. Will you transfer a mosaic embryo?

Mini IVF and DOR

I've never been a big medicine-taker, and I did not want to take a lot of drugs for IVF.

That's why I chose "mini IVF," which uses much lower doses of medicine "to provide a few quality eggs," says Dr. John Zhang, founder of New Hope Fertility Clinic in New York. (Other clinics call it "minimal" or "mild" stimulation.)

"With the development of modern lab technology, you really don't need many eggs to have a healthy baby—less medicine is much easier on the body," says Dr. Zhang, noting that 85 percent of eggs retrieved do not generate a live birth; plus, medicine makes people gain weight, "which women don't like." (He also offers needle-less IVF, prescribing only oral medication—like with IUI—and monitoring via saliva and urine instead of blood.)

But not everyone drinks the minimal stimulation Kool-Aid.

"Look at the outcome—for those under thirty, there was a thirty percent success rate compared to sixty percent success rate," says Dr. William B. Schoolcraft, from the Colorado Center for Reproductive Medicine. "Clearly less eggs is less eggs and less embryos and less chances."

In fact, in a study pioneered by Dr. Zhang and published in the *American Journal of Obstetrics and Gynecology,* out of more than five hundred couples with women under thirty-nine, half doing conventional IVF and half doing mini IVF, 49 percent had a baby using mini IVF and 63 percent of the couples using conventional IVF had babies.[2] With mini IVF, though, none of the women suffered from overstimulation of the ovaries (OHSS).

While minimal stimulation may be easier on a patient's body, Dr. Schoolcraft argues that putting a patient through many cycles—the time, the shots, the retrievals, the transfers—is harder on women than higher doses of medication for fewer cycles.

Many doctors, like Dr. Schoolcraft, *do* use minimal stimulation protocol on some women, like older women and/or women who don't respond well to a lot of drugs. "If you're a low responder, only getting two, three, four eggs on maximum with high-dose IVF, then a higher dose isn't going to help," he says. But he emphasizes that you are not getting *better* eggs with less medicine, dispelling the claim that medicine can ruin your egg quality. "It just doesn't seem to be true."

I started with mini IVF, then moved to conventional (and got the same results). Don't do that! I suggest starting with conventional high-dose IVF, and if that doesn't work, move to minimal stimulation.

You should consider mini IVF if:

- You're a poor responder to conventional IVF, or have a low AMH (which predicts that you may be a low responder to IVF).
- Your body can't tolerate a high dose of hormones.
- You're in danger of ovarian hyperstimulation.
- You want to spend less money (though it may come out the same if you need more cycles).
- You also might want to consider "natural IVF"—with no drugs to stimulate the ovaries.

Some docs believe that older women with diminished ovarian reserve need their own protocol.

"You have to treat older women differently because their whole physiology is different," says Dr. Norbert Gleicher, founder and medical director of the Center for Human Reproduction (CHR) in New York. "If you give them the same protocol and IVF treatment, you will not succeed."

Two months before a cycle, they pretreat older women with supplements to try to improve egg numbers and quality. They also retrieve eggs earlier in the cycle. "If we wait to retrieve eggs as long as we do with younger women, we'll get 'hard-boiled' eggs instead of soft-boiled; they'll fall apart at retrieval," says Dr. Gleicher.

Dr. Gleicher conducted a study, published in the *Journal of Endo-*

crinology, which showed that by triggering women when their lead follicle was 16 millimeters rather than 19 to 21 millimeters (i.e., a few days earlier in the cycle), older women had more and better embryos and clinical pregnancy rates.[3]

CHR recently announced some of the two oldest pregnancies conceived using the women's own eggs; both the women were almost forty-eight years old, and one of them went on to give birth to a healthy baby.[4]

"I'm old enough to remember when we didn't accept women above age thirty-eight because we couldn't get them pregnant," Dr. Gleicher says. "It took us over thirty years to get to forty-eight, and at some point we will hit the wall when it comes to age."

The Great Embryo-Testing Debate

Since your first cycle or two might be diagnostic, many start out doing retrievals, then transfers. If transfers fail or miscarry, then people might move on to genetically testing embryos.

Someone could write a whole book on whether you should genetically test your embryos, but that ain't gonna be me. I'm going to try to sum up the fierce debate dividing doctors across the globe. There are two camps:

- Yes, you *must* test embryos, so you can find the healthiest embryos and have a baby in less time and with less money, and avoid miscarriage (or get to failure faster).
- No, you'd be *crazy* to test embryos, because the testing isn't accurate, it doesn't favor women with poor ovarian reserve, and it results in discarding healthy embryos.

In order to understand the great embryo-testing debate, you have to understand that in the past, embryologists graded embryos by their morphology: their shape, structure, form, cell size—basically, their looks.[5] There was no way to definitively *know* which embryos were even chromosomally normal. That's why doctors used to transfer so many embryos (two to four) at a time, resulting in high-order multiples.

If only there were a way to know which embryos were healthy!

Enter genetic testing: Pre-implantation genetic testing for aneuploidy (PGT-A, sometimes just called PGT), originally used for screening embryos for specific diseases like Fragile X syndrome and cystic fibrosis, is also used to distinguish between chromosomally normal (euploid) and abnormal (aneuploid) embryos.

"There are other important benefits to PGT-A: Fewer clinical losses, less time to achieve an ongoing pregnancy, and reduced transfer order resulting in the near elimination of multiple gestation," Dr. Scott writes in "Fertile Battles," a hot-topic section of the journal *Fertility and Sterility*.[6] Basically, if you know which of your embryos are good, you can transfer the best ones first, and transfer fewer of them, too. Dr. Scott is a big proponent of elective single-embryo transfer (eSET), putting in only one tested embryo in order to reduce multiples. Also, he writes, testing is cost-effective in the long run because you aren't wasting time on transferring bad embryos, which might result in a miscarriage.

But, Dr. Scott says:

1. You need to have enough embryos (two or three) to do genetic testing. (You can test one, but it might not be cost-effective, since some clinics charge by batch rather than individual embryo testing.)

2. Since the pregnancy rate for even healthy tested blastocysts is 70 percent, you're going to need two or three healthy blastocysts to result in a child.

That means you're going to need *a lotta* eggs. Say you retrieve 9 eggs, and 6 of those fertilize; then only 4 of *those* make it to blastocyst stage, and in the end, only 2 are genetically normal.

This doesn't even take into account the discussion of "mosaics"— embryos that are in between, showing both healthy and unhealthy cell lines. "Mosaicism can also be identified as a result of technical limitations of the testing platform, in which an intermediate result is generated that resembles a mosaic profile," said the study "Mosaic Embryos Present a Challenging Clinical Opinion."[7] As testing technology has improved, the newer technologies "are capable of evaluating far more data points than has been previously possible," another study found.[8] Meaning, with a better microscope, you'll find more flaws.

"There's no such thing as normal and abnormal—an embryo is a spectrum of mosaicism," says NYU Langone Fertility Center's Dr. James Grifo, meaning *every* embryo contains a combination of normal and abnormal cells that can be found in embryo testing. Some doctors believe that's because the testing isn't accurate enough: Studies[9] show different labs report mosaicism in between 3 percent and 83 percent (!) of embryos tested, with an average of 15 percent.

"The test isn't perfect, but it's pretty darn accurate," Dr. Grifo says, noting that with newer technology like Next Generation Sequencing (NGS) the tests are getting more and more accurate.

He advises using PGT-A as a way to rate your embryos, then transferring the best, healthy ones first, and if there are mosaics, those in-between ones, transferring them after. "In our opinion, the detection of mosaicism is of great clinical value. It should be reported and used to help decide which embryo(s) should be prioritized for transfer. Mosaic embryos can be considered to represent a distinct category in terms of viability, lying in between euploid and fully abnormal embryos," Dr. Grifo and his colleagues concluded in a study of mosaicism.[10]

But opponents of genetic testing, who are dismayed at the high rate of those in-between mosaics and have seen healthy babies born from mosaics, do not even believe the "bad" embryos should be discarded. They believe, in fact, that the testing *itself* harms the embryos.

"We are totally opposed to it," Dr. Gleicher says. "We feel it harms thousands of infertile women if normal embryos are discarded." Scientifically, he writes in "Fertility Battles," testing "simply cannot work." Those bad embryos have been shown to self-correct in

THE WHOLE IVF TOOLBOX

mice and humans. "What, then, is the purpose of testing embryos on day 5, when aneuploidies [chromosomal abnormalities] disappear on days 6 and 7 further downstream?" he asks about abnormal embryos self-correcting.

Opponents believe that testing only helps those who have a lot of good embryos anyway (up to 25 percent more!), but hurts women with poor ovarian reserve, those who cannot produce blastocysts or get healthy ones.

So . . . should you test?

- If your embryos don't make it past day 3, if you can't make a lot of blastocysts, or if they result in abnormal after genetic testing, perhaps try a cycle or two without testing.
- If you keep getting chemical pregnancies, or if you keep miscarrying (and the miscarriage shows that the fetus was chromosomally abnormal, which we'll learn more about in chapter 21), you can bank embryos and test them. If you *are* testing, do it at a high-volume PGT clinic. Dr. Scott's clinic, Reproductive Medicine Associates of New Jersey, boasts a whopping 43 percent live birth rate in women over forty-two;[11] Dr. Schoolcraft's CCRM also boasts a 46.8 percent live birth rate in women over forty-two—presumably both with tested embryos.[12]

If you're considering testing, ask your clinic:

- Which PGT technology do you use?
- Do you disclose mosaics? (Some clinics just label embryos "abnormal.")
- Will you transfer mosaics? (In my opinion, if you only get mosaics, consider transferring them.)
- What kind of counseling do women need before a mosaic transfer?
- Will you transfer abnormal embryos?
- How many PGT-normal embryos do I need for a baby?

Maybe someday soon the technology will be flawless. For now, the American Society of Reproductive Medicine ethics committee concludes, "At present, there is insufficient evidence to recommend the routine use of blastocyst biopsy with aneuploidy testing in all infertile patients."

After I had a few miscarriages, I started testing my embryos. None were normal. So we did not transfer any. To this day, I wonder if any of those embryos could have resulted in healthy pregnancies.

Her Mosaic Baby

Jennifer Coughlin did three rounds of IVF with PGT after being diagnosed with diminished ovarian reserve at thirty-five. Her one normal embryo from the first round became her daughter. A few cycles produced some abnormal embryos and one mosaic.

"We thought there were two possible testing outcomes—normal or abnormal. Turns out, there is a third potential testing result. Mosaic means some of the cells tested had a chromosomal abnormality and some did not. In a world that we thought was black and white, we now had a gray area. And that gray area was very gray—in a quick Google search, we saw there was very little information about mosaic embryos available," she says. After consulting with some doctors, they decided to transfer the mosaic, even though they knew it could result in miscarriage or [birth] defect—or a healthy baby. They nicknamed their mosaic "Baby Mo."

Ten months later, their daughter was born healthy, and they named her Everly Maura, in homage to Baby Mo. "I can't help but wonder how many mosaic embryos have been destroyed because doctors won't transfer them, or because the patients do not understand the potential for a positive outcome."

Timing Is Everything

When genetically tested embryos don't result in pregnancy, or when perfectly good-looking blastocysts fail to implant, people want to know why.

The embryo isn't everything—even proponents of PGT will readily admit this. Timing might be the problem—specifically, "synchrony" between the embryo and the endometrium, the lining of the uterus to which an embryo attaches itself in the early days of a pregnancy. (Each month, your hormone levels rise in the weeks leading up to ovulation, causing the endometrium to thicken in preparation for a potential pregnancy; if conception doesn't occur, your hormones drop off and then your uterus sheds the endometrium—i.e., you get your period—after which the process starts again.)

Think about that timing: During a natural pregnancy, the egg gets fertilized and presumably moves into the uterus, where the endometrium is ready and waiting—the embryo is in the exact right place at the exact right time. But now . . . science.

Enter the endometrial receptivity analysis (ERA), which, according to one company that offers the testing, helps "avoid implantation failure by establishing the best day for embryo transfer." The company claims that three out of ten women have a "displaced window of implantation," meaning their endometrium is not at the right stage when the embryo attempts to implant (it's like moving into a house before the house is finished).

Here's the deal: In an ERA, you have to go through a "mock" cycle—a fake cycle during which you still take estrogen and progesterone, but instead of doing a retrieval and transfer, your endometrium gets biopsied on what would otherwise be your transfer day. The biopsy determines if your endometrium is at the right stage for implantation, or how "receptive" it is (hence the test name), and the results of the biopsy can help you and your doctor determine whether your transfer day needs to be adjusted for your next cycle.

The pros: If you only have a limited number of genetically tested embryos, this test will ensure you're doing everything you can.

The cons: ERA can be painful and expensive, and some clinics/states don't offer it. And you may find that you're already having your transfer on the correct day, meaning endometrium-embryo synchrony isn't the problem.

Are Two Retrievals Better Than One?

There are three phases to your menstrual cycle:[13] (No, they aren't Hungry, Bitchy, and Tired.)

- The **follicular phase** is the first phase, when your follicles are growing.
- The **ovulatory phase** is the LH surge (measured by those darn ovulation tests), which stimulates egg release (ovulation).
- The **luteal phase** occurs after you ovulate, preparing your uterus for pregnancy or menstruation.

Traditionally, fertility doctors use their magic to increase your egg count during the first (follicular) phase, inducing ovulation and retrieving your eggs.

But guess what? There are still follicles in the luteal phase. And some docs want to do two retrievals in the same cycle. "Recent evidence indicates that folliculogenesis occurs in a wave-like fashion, indicating that there are multiple follicular recruitment waves in the same menstrual cycle," Dr. Zhang writes in an overview of what is now called "DuoStim."[14] The second retrieval occurs two to seven days after your first retrieval *within the same menstrual cycle.*

Whether it produces better eggs and healthier embryos "remains to be determined," Dr. Zhang writes. But a 2018 review of 310 poor-prognosis patients in four fertility centers found that women doing two retrievals got one healthy (PGT tested) embryo 65.5 percent of the time, compared to 42.3 percent for the women who did just one retrieval.[15] Maybe two retrievals are better than one.

Your Own Blood

They say we are born with all the eggs we'll ever have—and it goes downhill from there.

Not so fast. Some researchers believe ovaries can either regenerate or have "sleeping" stem cells to create more eggs. "Recent studies suggest that the adult mammalian ovary is not endowed with a finite number of oocytes, but instead possesses stem cells that contribute to their renewal," noted an article in the journal *Fertility and Sterility*.[16] This would be the holy grail of fertility treatment: If we could regenerate eggs, well, we might not even *need* IVF for most diagnoses. Goodbye, DOR, POF, POI, and all those other annoying acronyms.

Experiments are underway to test the ability of the mitochondria,[17] stem cells,[18] and even a woman's own blood to either regenerate eggs—i.e., recruit senescent or resting eggs—or create new ones. I'm going to focus on platelet-rich plasma (PRP), since it's available at US clinics.

In PRP, the doctor draws your blood, concentrates the platelets three to five times as much as in normal blood plasma, then injects it back into your body. (PRP was created by hematologists in the 1970s for transfusion patients, and is sometimes used for dentistry, wound healing, inflammation control, sports injuries, and, most recently, skin rejuvenation.[19] Tennis star Rafael Nadal used it to heal his knee.[20])

"Even after a woman goes through menopause, she still has up to one hundred follicles within the ovary. The follicles slowly regress and disappear," says Dr. Konstantinos Pantos of Genesis Clinic in Greece—one of the first doctors studying PRP for ovarian use. "Many women who have infertility problems have problems with endometrial thickness, and we used [PRP] there and in the ovaries."

His clinic has performed PRP on some six hundred patients—half for fertility, half for health reasons (to postpone menopause). He theorizes that PRP works either by maturing the senescent eggs or *producing new follicles* from stem cells inside the ovary.

They use it on perimenopausal women, usually under fifty, and it may take a few months for results to show up. Benefits only last for four to five months, Dr. Pantos says. "It doesn't last forever."

Smaller studies[21] have shown that ovarian PRP has led to restored menstrual cycles (for those who had none),[22] better egg retrievals, improved hormone levels and blastocysts,[23] clinical pregnancy,[24] and birth level.[25]

"When you concentrate serum, PRP enhances the blood flow and may reduce inflammation, may add growth factors which may be responsible for increasing the blood flow and proper environment to help the remaining eggs," says Dr. Robert Kiltz of CNY Fertility Center, which also offers low-cost IVF. He thinks it most beneficial to thirty-seven- to forty-two-year-olds more than forty-three- to forty-five-year-olds, who might have more prolonged ovarian and cell damage. Dr. Pantos notes that if there's a genetic cause for early menopause—meaning it's not caused by aging—"you will not see results" from PRP.

Which Experimental Treatment Should I Use?

Trends in IVF change faster than fashion on the runway. One decade, everyone's promoting the endometrial scratch as a way to help with implantation and the next, a systemic review shows there's no benefit to it.[26] After spending weeks reading conflicting information on IVF treatments—no PGT, yes PGT, PRP is amazing, PRP is bogus—I feel like I've been bloodied in battle.

Why can't all IVF doctors just get along?

"That's the nature of medicine. In general, medicine takes any research and takes it apart," Dr. Kiltz says, rather candidly for a fertility doctor. "It's our nature to pick things apart rather than say that it's not easily defined—and when things aren't easily defined, we hold back until science has answered it clearly." He says he used to be one of those people, the "show me the prospective, randomized placebo, double-blind study" types, he says, referring to the types of scientific studies that can more conclusively prove cause and effect but are often difficult to produce in reproductive medicine. But then he began to be swayed by results in patients—results that didn't always have studies backing them up.

Patients with ticking clocks "don't have time until medicine answers clearly. You're desperate to try something," Dr. Kiltz says, "then amazingly it works." Think about it: All IVF was once experimental. Lesley Brown had blocked tubes, and after nine years of infertility, she allowed Dr. Patrick Steptoe to try IVF on her—and in 1978 the first "test-tube" baby was born.

I'm sure in the coming years there will be a dozen new therapies, procedures, and technologies on the horizon. But how can you discern between the experimental treatments and the quack science?

Do your research.

- **Is the doctor a pioneer in the field?**

  If you're going to use an experimental procedure, start with the doctor who pioneered the protocol or one who has a lot of expertise with it. You want someone who treats patients with your condition, not someone mimicking the doctor who does.

- **What are the risks?**

  With any surgery or medical procedure, there are possible risks—to you, to your embryos, to your future children. Embryo rejuvenation—which might use your own blood, mitochondria, or stem cells—is reputed to have fewer risks because it's "autologous," meaning it uses cells or tissue from your own body. Of course, if you're the first in the study, it's impossible to predict future risks.

- **Consider the evidence.**

  You're not a scientist—although at this point, you know a lot about reproductive medicine. What do the studies show? If there are few, know that you may be part of something experimental. Also, what does the anecdotal evidence show? Speak to other patients doing the treatment. They have no reason to lie. Many women on a PRP Facebook group have not seen improved results.

- **How much does it cost?**

  Of course, having a baby shouldn't be determined by cost. But by now you know: Show me the money! Ask your doc if there's another procedure or medicine that achieves similar results at a lower cost.

Confession: When it comes to experimental treatment, I'm pretty open. ("Gullible," some cynical husbands would say.) That's why, when I was thirty-nine years old—pre-Solomon—and I saw a friend ask on Facebook, "Who has really bad bags under their eyes and would like a free treatment to fix them?" I was the first to sign up. That Friday, I found myself in the swank Beverly Hills office of cosmetic surgeon Dr. Nathan Newman, having circles drawn around my floppy face like a clown. By Monday morning, I was undergoing a "stem-cell facelift," using stem cells extracted from my stomach and injected into my face (nineteen times!). It was only as I was recovering that it dawned on me, *What if something had gone wrong? Did I ruin my entire face?*

I did not. My face recovered beautifully, and when I moved back to New York City a few weeks later, it was as if the eight years I'd spent in Los Angeles had never happened. That's how young I looked: thirty-one.

One day, stem-cell therapy will become available for ovaries—and I'll be the first to offer my old ones up.

Chapter 21

Miscarriages: When a Pregnancy Ends

We've been trying to have a child for a couple of years and have had three miscarriages along the way. You feel so hopeful when you learn you're going to have a child. You start imagining who they'll become and dreaming of hopes for their future. You start making plans, and then they're gone. It's a lonely experience.

—Mark Zuckerberg

"You don't have to come with me to the doctor today," I told Solomon magnanimously. I could afford to be generous and let him go to work because I was pregnant—nine weeks! This was back before I started fertility treatment and was unaware of the long road ahead of me.

Everything was going swimmingly: After we'd returned from our honeymoon in Peru, I was pregnant again. *This* time I wasn't taking any chances, and we went to the OB right away.

She confirmed my pregnancy, and told me to come back to see the heartbeat: It was beautiful, a bright light blinking on the black-and-white ultrasound, the start of our little munchkin.

"Come back in a month," she said, cavalierly.

"A month?" I asked. That seemed like a long time. (Little did I know that most women don't even *go* to the OB till weeks 8 through 12.)

"Okay, two weeks," she relented. And that's why I was there, by myself, a few weeks after seeing the heartbeat. I wasn't one of those women who needed their husband to come to every single appointment. We had like, eight more months of this! Or so I thought.

I, too, was cavalier, scrolling through my phone as the OB gelled up my then flat belly. I was still 'gramming when she said in a deadpan voice, "There's no heartbeat."

Wait, what?

I put my phone down. "The fetus has stopped developing," she said, then told me to get dressed and meet her in her office.

It was awful. All of it. Every single moment.

I called Solomon, who came and met me, and we sat in the doctor's office while she wrote out a prescription for me to go get a D&C at an abortion clinic to scrape out my uterus. "It might be a party atmosphere in there," she actually said, "so just keep your head down."

Oh boy, was my head down. All I could think was, *What happened?*

Types of Early Pregnancy Loss

Miscarriage is "the spontaneous loss of a pregnancy before the fetus reaches viability," experts say, and early pregnancy termination is "any spontaneous abortion or miscarriage before 20 weeks of pregnancy." (In medical terminology, the word "abortion" is used apolitically: not the forced termination of a pregnancy but the spontaneous loss of one.)

There are a number of different types of pregnancy loss. Unfortunately, I've had many of them:

Chemical pregnancy: The first time I had a pregnancy end, I bled out into the toilet. Even though the OB had confirmed it ("Yup, you definitely *were* pregnant," she'd said cheerily, something that should have clued me in to what type of doc she'd be), I hadn't really considered myself pregnant. It was probably a chemical pregnancy, one that is only detected by rising hCG levels, within days after embryo implantation.

Clinical pregnancy: Technically, it could also have been a clinical pregnancy, which occurs several days or weeks after implantation "when ultrasound can detect a feto-placental unit," but I'll never know for sure since we never had an ultrasound.

Missed miscarriage: This second time, I hadn't seen a *spot* of blood. And I was certainly on the lookout for it, afraid to pull down my panties each time I went to pee, but nada. I should have been in the clear. Wrong. I'd had a missed miscarriage, where the fetus stops developing and the heart stops beating, but you don't see signs of it along the way.

Blighted ovum: Another type of loss. Also called an embryonic intrauterine gestation, it occurs when there's an empty sac (the embryo implanted but didn't develop).[1] The worst thing about a blighted ovum is that your hCG levels may rise normally, so you'll *feel* pregnant without actually really being pregnant with a viable embryo.

Ectopic or molar pregnancy. An ectopic is when the embryo implants in the wrong place and always ends in miscarriage. The placenta fails to form properly and instead forms a mass; molar pregnancy usually ends in miscarriage. Both can be extremely dangerous for the mother.

Doctors estimate that one in five pregnancies end in early pregnancy loss.[2] Somehow, that statistic never made me feel better.

After my miscarriage, I was talking to a friend experienced in IVF. "But it was healthy! I saw the heartbeat!" I was incredulous—outraged!—while she just nodded sympathetically and said, "It happens."

I couldn't believe she was so matter-of-fact. It reminded me of my early dating years, when I'd recounted the magical night I'd just had, how we'd stayed up all night talking and he made reference to a future—and then poof. I never heard from him again. (This was *way* before "ghosting" became a thing.) As I became more jaded, accustomed to the fact that good first dates were no guarantee of a future, I would nod sagely and sympathetically when a younger woman expressed shock when a date failed to live up to its promise.

My pregnancy had started off great, but it had ended. "It happens."

Miscarriage is common, even for women who get pregnant naturally. If you talk to almost any mother, you'll learn that she likely suffered a loss along the way—and still succeeded.

Women who are doing fertility treatment may be more aware of how many pregnancies they've lost than women who aren't in treatment. That's because when you're doing IUI or IVF, you know the minute you're pregnant, whereas women trying naturally may not be monitoring their status as closely.

"Between my two kids I had two chemicals," another one of my friends admitted. "But my OB just gave me progesterone." Indeed, early pregnancy bleeding can be treated with extra progesterone to save the pregnancy, one study found, noting that causes for early loss include "infection, hormonal imbalances, and uterine structural abnormalities," not to mention that sometimes it's just a bad egg, which is also known as aneuploidy. Chromosomal abnormalities cause a majority of early miscarriages, which increase with age.

Her Ectopic Pregnancy

"I knew something was wrong," author Judy Batalion wrote of her second pregnancy at thirty-six. As she chronicled in her memoir *White Walls: A Memoir of Motherhood and Daughterhood and the Mess In Between,* her hCG was low but doubling, but she felt tired and weak and fainted a few times, and "countless scans" didn't find anything. Finally, a gynecologist diagnosed her with an ectopic pregnancy.

In an ectopic pregnancy, the embryo implants outside the uterus—nearly always in a fallopian tube—putting the woman's health at risk. Ectopic pregnancies are rare in natural pregnancies (1 in 100) but can occur more frequently with IVF.[3]

You may be at risk for an ectopic pregnancy if you've had previous pelvic disease or scar tissue, used an IUD, or had an abortion. If you have pelvic pain and bleeding that lasts for a long time, and if doctors cannot find a pregnancy in utero despite rising hCG, you may have an ectopic pregnancy.

The earlier ectopic pregnancies are discovered and treated, the better[4]—if left to grow undetected, the embryo can burst the fallopian tube.

Batalion took methotrexate, a chemo drug, to get rid of her ectopic pregnancy, and didn't need to have surgery—"I was lucky," she says, because she'd likely have lost her fallopian tube.

After an ectopic pregnancy, there's a 30 to 40 percent chance of recurrence.[5] In her next pregnancy, Batalion was closely monitored until an "intrauterine pregnancy"—a normal pregnancy—was confirmed. She gave birth to her second daughter, and four years later, at forty-one years old, she had her third child, a son.

What to Do About Your Miscarriage

"My sorrow is so intense it often feels like it will flatten me," writes Ariel Levy in *The Rules Do Not Apply,*[6] her searing memoir about the loss of her pregnancy, husband, and home.

It doesn't matter how many people before you suffered a miscarriage and went on to have healthy babies: Loss is loss.

Still, before you can deal with the emotional aftermath of a miscarriage, you first need to know what you're going to do about it physically. First things first: Are you having a miscarriage? You have to be 100 percent sure that the fetus is not viable. Many women experience some bleeding during pregnancy—that doesn't mean it's over, or that nothing can be done.

A 2010 study in Ireland found that twenty-four miscarriages *had been misdiagnosed,* most of these between 2005 and 2010.[7] But after the country implemented new diagnostic criteria and better ultrasound equipment, there were no reported instances of misdiagnoses.

Put it this way: Even if a doctor says you have a blighted ovum, it is recommended you recheck it seven to ten days later to make sure. "The requirement to repeat scans will inevitably leave women in a state of uncertainty that may be distressing," an article[8] in the *BMJ,* Britain's premier medical journal, about redefining miscarriage criteria, understates. ("Distressing?" Can you imagine having to wait more than a week to see if you're miscarrying?) But they also say that doctors can tell you, based on measurements of the fetal sac and embryo, what the likely outcome will be.

If you are indeed suffering a miscarriage, there are a few options: Let it happen naturally (expectant care), take medicine to induce the miscarriage (medical management), or have it surgically removed (surgical).

During a miscarriage, some women just start bleeding on their own. The bleeding can last for days or weeks, depending on how early the pregnancy ends. With my first loss at five to six weeks, I bled and cramped like I was having a mild period. The doctor told me that if I saw a big clot, I could "collect the products of conception [POC]"—what they so lovingly call the fetal remains. But I could not and did not.

How to Collect Your Miscarriage[i]

If you've been told that you're going to miscarry or are already experiencing a miscarriage at home, there are things you can do to collect the products of conception for testing.

1. If you're less than eight weeks pregnant, everything will look like menstrual blood. If you're eight to ten weeks pregnant, there may be a discernable sac or more pink/gray material.
2. Find a sterile container: This can be a new Ziploc bag or Tupperware, or a specimen cup you may have from your clinic.
3. You can use a strainer in the toilet to separate the tissue (or take it out of the toilet).
4. Place the tissue in the sterile container. If you can't get it to the doctor's office immediately, store it in the refrigerator (not the freezer).[9]

i According to Natera, a genetic testing company.

Some doctors advise medicine to induce miscarriage, either misoprostol or a combination of misoprostol and mifepristone, which will likely induce heavy cramping and some bleeding.

Look, I am not a doctor, but this is the one time I give medical advice *from a patient's standpoint:* If you have the option to choose from expectant care, medical management, and surgical management, have the surgery. A D&C (dilation and curettage) is usually done in the first trimester and a D&E (dilation and evacuation) is done in the second trimester: both clean out the uterus.

One study of more than 1,500 women compared expectant care

("waiting for the miscarriage to finish on its own, and may involve bed rest, examination by ultrasound, and antibiotics") to surgical treatment (which "might cause problems such as trauma, heavy bleeding, or infection").[10] It found that almost a third of those who let nature run its course *needed surgery anyway*—and often also required blood transfusions.

Another study comparing all three methods found gynecological infection rates after each were the same, and if you took the pill or waited for the miscarriage to occur on its own, you were more likely to end up in the hospital for surgery anyway. Also, the pills are messy.[11]

"I feel like they're just a lie," says Latoya, a radio producer who took misoprostol/mifepristone pills to expel her twelve-week miscarriage. She wished the doctor had told her, "Look, there will be Jell-O-type clumps coming out of your body." It didn't work, anyway—she had to go in for not one but two D&Cs to clean out what is termed "an incomplete miscarriage."

Not everyone agrees with surgery as a first line of treatment.

Patients should talk to their doctors and see what works for them, says Dr. Zev Williams, chief of the Division of Reproductive Endocrinology & Infertility at the Columbia University Fertility Center, NewYork-Presbyterian Hospital. "Each approach has distinct risks and benefits." He says one disadvantage of a D&C is that the entire uterine cavity is scraped, which can leave scarring, or tissue from the pregnancy behind. Dr. Williams and his team pioneered a less invasive treatment for D&Cs. Ask your doctor if this treatment is available.

Among patients choosing between first trimester miscarriage management options, a 2019 study found that women made their decisions based on the anticipated level of pain, the amount of time it would take to get back to regular activities, the chance of complications, and the expected amount of bleeding.[12]

The first time, I was afraid to have a D&C because I was wary of going under anesthesia. So I opted for a D&E, during which you remain awake. Big. Mistake. I saw things I could not unsee.

After that, I always did a D&C.

After the Surgery

There's another very important reason to have surgery versus waiting to miscarry naturally or inducing miscarriage: so you can test the fetus. While a high percentage (60 percent) of early miscarriages are due to aneuploidy—chromosomally abnormal embryos—you'll want to know for sure.

Testing is not always informative. After one miscarriage, my test was inconclusive. Apparently, the mother's tissue can contaminate the results when the baby is a girl,[13] which I guess it was. I was hoping for a chromosomal abnormality.

At age thirty-nine, my younger sister had two miscarriages a few months apart. Thankfully, her doctor had the foresight to tell her to get the D&C. (Many doctors don't.) I told her to test the products. Both miscarriages came back chromosomally abnormal.

"That's great!" I wanted to tell her. Not the miscarriages themselves, but discovering that they were caused by chromosomal abnormalities meant she'd gotten pregnant with bad embryos—ones that would not have become healthy babies.

"If the miscarriage is chromosomally abnormal and the parents are tested and found to have no abnormalities, the chances that a miscarriage will happen again are almost the same as someone who did not have a miscarriage," Dr. Williams says.

"When I spoke to you, I felt better," my sister now tells me. She didn't really feel *better* better, but she felt better about it.

Can't Stop the Feeling

"I was obviously very upset and down," my sister says about her first miscarriage, which occurred at about seven weeks. In retrospect, it was nothing compared to her second miscarriage, which happened at about nine or ten weeks, after they'd heard a heartbeat. "My body just couldn't handle the second one," she said, adding that she felt flu-like symptoms. "I was much weaker and it was much harder to get over."

Research shows pregnancy loss *may* cause psychological damage. And why *shouldn't* you be depressed?

"The future I thought I was meticulously crafting for years has disappeared," Levy so poignantly writes in her memoir, "and with it have gone my ideas about the kind of life I'd imagined I was due."

One minute, you're planning your cutesy baby announcement (sign on dog: "Mom and Dad are getting me a human!"), and the next you're wondering how to tell people you're only chubby because you *were* pregnant.

By the way, after a miscarriage, you might gain weight. Think about it: Your body was basically *filled* with natural hCG—a hormone that some people actually inject to lose weight, counter to the FDA warnings[14]—and then the hCG starts plummeting. I think I gained five pounds each time I miscarried. Maybe it was the emotional aftermath (or the chocolate?), but I think it was my body: It had been through quite a roller-coaster ride.

I also got whiplash from the step-ball-change dance move: first experiencing a secret joy and terror, knowing Solomon and I would be parents, then discovering—*WOMP WOMP*—we weren't going to be parents after all.

I made Solomon swear not to tell anyone, especially not his family, who were celebrating a special occasion that weekend. Also, I didn't want to be one of those women who kept having miscarriages. I just wanted to be like my friend with the two kids who could mention it in passing, after the fact. *Oh yah, I once had a miscarriage, it was so long ago, I don't even remember it.*

And also, perhaps, I was a little bit ashamed. *Was it the day-old Chinese food I ate from our fridge?* I thought it might have caused listeriosis, a food-borne infection caused by bacteria that grows in raw cheeses, sushi, and . . . leftovers.[15] *Or was it because I kept up my running, like that dumb doctor said I could?*

Even though I wanted to be over it right away and move on, I couldn't help but blame myself. And I'm not the only one: "Miscarriage remains shrouded in shame and silence, even amongst friends and family, and its emotional impact has not been sufficiently investigated," begins the National Survey on Public Perceptions of Miscarriage, co-authored by Dr. Williams.[16] For the survey, more than one thousand men and women completed a questionnaire on misconceptions surrounding miscarriage. The authors of the survey found the following:

- More than half thought miscarriage was an uncommon event, occurring in less than 5 percent of pregnancies (it's 15 to 20 percent of clinically recognized pregnancies, the study says)
- 76 percent of the people who had a miscarriage thought it was caused by a stressful event
- 64 percent thought it was caused by lifting a heavy object
- 28 percent thought it was due to the use of an IUD
- 22 percent thought it was due to oral contraceptives

I've learned that people think differently about their losses. Some women call them "angel babies" and give them twee winged emojis in their "infertility signature." Some plan mourning ceremonies for them. Some view losses simply as pregnancies that were not meant to be.

I viewed each miscarriage differently: one as a very late period, another just a failed IVF cycle that didn't really get started. On the one where I had heard a heartbeat, I was devastated.

All feelings about it are okay.

In the survey on miscarriage perception, 37 percent of the people who had miscarried felt they had lost a child, 47 percent felt guilty, 28 percent felt ashamed, and 41 percent felt that they had done something wrong. But get this: When the cause for the miscarriage was found, only 19 percent felt they'd done something wrong.

I can tell you this now: You've done nothing wrong.

There's a saying: "Pain is inevitable, suffering is optional." With miscarriage, pain is inevitable—but you don't have to add suffering, judgment, blame, and regret to the experience.

In fact, that might be the only way to move forward.

Late-Term Loss

Technically, "miscarriage" is any loss before twenty weeks, according to the CDC.[17] After twenty weeks, a loss before or during birth is called a stillbirth, a term applied to 24,000 babies or 1 percent of all births each year in the US (the same number that perish in the first year of life).

"Losing a baby at forty weeks was the worst day of my life," says actress Jaime Ray Newman (of Marvel's *The Punisher; Midnight, Texas;* and *Bates Motel,* among others). Newman had a totally normal pregnancy with her husband, Israeli filmmaker Guy Nattiv, but when she went into labor at forty weeks, the umbilical cord was wrapped around their daughter's neck. After, Jaime was "in a fog" for a long time, but a TV show filming in Chicago (ABC's *Mind Games*) distracted and saved her.

At their next pregnancy, everything seemed normal—all the early maternal blood tests were good, etc. But at her four-month ultrasound, the OB gave their baby a 5 percent chance of being born healthy. *WTF, how is that possible?!* she thought. They had to terminate. With all that, how did Jaime go on?

"After that I had to keep my head down," she says. She started IVF, suffered another miscarriage, and then gave up on carrying a pregnancy herself. "I figured, we're taking me out of the equation," she says. "The benefit of being married to an Israeli who was in the military is that he's like a commander in a war," she says of her husband, noting that his attitude was, "We're driving the tank, the goal is to win the war, but there will be losses."

Her surrogate gave birth to their daughter.

"It's been the craziest year of our lives," Newman says. Not only because of her miracle baby, but because *Skin,* a short film that she and her husband produced (and which he co-wrote and directed) and filmed in New York while her surrogate was pregnant in California, won the 2018 Academy Award for Best Live Action Short.

How to Help Someone After Miscarriage

1. **Express sorrow for their loss.**
If you're not sure how they feel about it, if it was an early or late loss, the best place to start is with sympathy. "I'm sorry for your loss."

2. **Listen for cues.**
Some people want to talk more about it, giving you details of how far along they were or what they did for their loss, and others just want to pass on the information and then move on without an inquisition. Follow their lead.

3. **Save your optimism.**
You might be tempted to express optimistic sentiments, like "better off next time," or "I'm sure you'll have a baby soon," but moving on to the next step feels like a betrayal of their current loss. (Ask any grieving pet owner who's told to buy another dog.)

4. **Make it about them.**
This is not the time to share stories of others' failures or successes, nor is it the time to express disbelief about their journey ("I didn't even know you were trying"). This loss is about them. See if you can attend to their emotional and physical well-being.

5. **Ask what you can do to help.**
Offer to send over dinner, take them out for a drink or spa date, or watch their other kids.

Trying After Loss

Many women want to know when they can start trying again after a loss.

It really depends on a number of things:

- How far along did you miscarry?
- What was your post-miscarriage treatment?
- What is the state of your health now?
- What is your emotional state?

Obviously, you should ask your doctor. Recommendations are all over the place, with the World Health Organization advising waiting as long as six months before starting again. But a study of more than one thousand women, published in the journal *Obstetrics & Gynecology*, found that "there is no physiological evidence for delaying pregnancy attempt after an early loss."[18]

Most doctors, especially fertility clinics, will want you to get your period first. That shows that your body has returned to baseline. Yeah—it's annoying, waiting, again. First you pray for no blood, then you pray for blood. (Make up your damn mind, infertility!) Just as you once monitored your rising hCG, now you are watching for it to decrease. If your hCG doesn't decrease (to less than 5) or you do not get your period within a few months, you might need a D&C. And after surgery, your doctor must give their clearance before you have sex and/or try again (I mean with a petri dish).

After my first miscarriage, I waited a month. We got pregnant the very next month.

Which brings up the question, does fertility *increase* after a miscarriage?

Evidence is mixed. The study in *Obstetrics & Gynecology* showed that women who started trying within zero to three months after miscarriage were *more likely to achieve live birth* than those who waited three months (53.2 percent versus 36.1 percent), with a shorter time to getting pregnant!

The thing is, before you get your period, you will ovulate, so you *can* get pregnant before you get your period again. (That is, *if* you can get pregnant naturally.) My nonscientific theory is that the people who have sex for just, well, sex purposes, aren't aware that they're ovulating, so, *whoops, it's an accident!* Also, if you have a successful surgery (if you can think of a D&C removing your baby as "successful"), it may clear out the system.

The bottom line is, is your body ready?

Fertility clinics will make sure your hormones, uterus, and reproductive system are ready. If you're getting alternative treatment, your practitioners will also be able to help.

My sister—who was so weak after her second miscarriage—went to acupuncture. She got pregnant with my nephew a few months later. "I was nervous the entire time," she says, "but that's my personality."

Getting pregnant after a miscarriage is nerve-wracking. Many people just wait to exhale after they pass the point at which they miscarried last time. The good news is that the risk of miscarriage after a first aneuploidy (when the cause is a bad embryo) is about 15 to 20 percent—the same as it was with the first pregnancy. "The vast majority of women who have one loss will go onto have a normal baby," Dr. Williams says.

Now, hear me loud and clear: If you have a second miscarriage, especially if it's a chromosomally normal one (with tested embryos or results from a post-miscarriage test), please read the next chapter about repeat pregnancy loss.

Chapter 22

Repeat Pregnancy Loss: Do You Have Immunological Issues?

After marrying Alex I had only one thing on my mind—having another baby. I'd love to have another four, in fact. But by April 2010, after we had been trying for eight months, I became so worried we made an appointment with a fertility doctor.

—British media personality Katie Price[1]

"Keep trying," the doctor said to me after he performed a D&C to get rid of my fourth miscarriage.

KEEP TRYING?! WTF?!

It's a good thing we weren't in the operating room anymore because if I had had a sharp utensil, I might have stabbed him in the uterus . . . oh wait, he DIDN'T HAVE A UTERUS. He had *no idea* what it was like to have your insides scraped clean, your body ravaged, and any last bit of hope you had pulverized to nothing.

He also had no idea what it was like to lose a pregnancy with a donor egg—the "sure thing" doctors had advised me to move on to, assuring me that using a twenty-five-year-old's oocyte would solve all my miscarriage problems. Since day 1 (or the day I was forty-one and had a second miscarriage), they'd been telling me that it was my eggs, my eggs, my eggs, my age, my age, my age that was causing all the trouble.

And they were wrong. Man, were they wrong. Tens of thousands of dollars and three years of my life wrong. I'd started this at forty-one and was now nearing forty-four, the natural end of my fertility. I probably couldn't use my eggs anymore because I'd listened to them. All of them.

To say I was mad was an understatement. After my second and third miscarriages, I'd been sad and disappointed. When my own eggs had tested abnormal at forty-three, I was *devastated*. But to discover now, after I'd moved on to accept that I'd need to use a younger woman's eggs to have a baby, that the doctors had been wrong all along?

I was livid.

What Is Repeat Miscarriage?

There are few things worse than a wanted pregnancy ending.

Except when it happens again.

And again.

And again.

It's enough to send anyone into a deep depression (as researchers found in a study with the self-explanatory title "Depression and Emotional Stress Is Highly Prevalent Among Women with Recurrent Pregnancy Loss").[2]

"I distinctly remember early in my fertility practice calling one of my patients with a positive pregnancy test and hearing a deep sigh followed by heavy silence," Dr. Lora Shahine writes in her book *Not Broken: An Approachable Guide to Miscarriage and Recurrent Pregnancy Loss*,[3] adding that she was surprised by the patient's atypical reaction, especially when the woman then said, "Here we go again." After Shahine hung up, though, "It hit me like a ton of bricks—this test was the patient's fifth positive pregnancy test and for her, this was just the beginning of the limbo, waiting, and anxiety until she knew whether this would be a successful pregnancy or not."

Repeat pregnancy loss (RPL), sometimes called recurrent loss, is a phenomenon little understood by fertility doctors, obstetricians, and gynecologists. If that sounds like I'm quoting a highly academic study, I'm not. I have a terrific sample of one to prove my point. (Don't fret; I've talked to plenty of professionals, too.)

RPL applies to anyone who has suffered two clinical miscarriages, the ASRM has finally acknowledged. (It used to be three, but the guideline changed sometime between my third and fourth miscarriages.) The European Society of Human Reproduction and Embryology defines it as any three losses—including chemical pregnancies (unlike clinical ones, no ultrasound has found a sac).[4] RPL affects 2 to 4 percent of reproductive-age couples.[5]

Lucky me!

When I'm feeling less than generous, I say that doctors don't care about repeat miscarriage. Or repeat failure of any sort. If they did, why would they tell women to "keep trying"? (Other phrases you might hear: "It's just bad luck," "It's nature's way," or "You only need one.")

If you get Solomon in on it, his Israeli cynicism would say it's a money-making business. In fact, that's what one young doctor at the ASRM fertility doctors' conference told me when I asked him, "Why don't fertility doctors just send miscarriage patients out to specialists?!"

"Moola," he said, rubbing his fingers together in the universal sign for cold, hard cash. (Some doctors actually get bonuses based on the number of IVF cycles they bring in.) "Also, it's such a small percentage of the fertility population," he said.

But is it really?

How many women miscarry without knowing it *before* they get to fertility treatment? How many suffer chemical pregnancies in treatment? What about my transfer whose beta hCG came back at 8? I was desperately hoping it would be one of those miracle beta stories, but my clinic wasn't too upbeat. And they were right! The next test fell to 5. But now I wonder: What *was* that? An implantation that could have been helped along . . . with . . . *something?*

And what about patients who experience repeat implantation failure (RIF)—when you undergo IVF transfers with no resulting pregnancy—which the fertility community is only just beginning to recognize as three failed IVF attempts with "good quality embryos."[6] (Although they will no doubt quibble over the exact definition—"Are the embryos genetically tested?" "How old are the women?" etc., etc., etc.)

I spoke to a woman who, after having five transfers of genetically tested, chromosomally normal, *near perfect* embryos fail to implant, saw her general practitioner who diagnosed her with lupus, an autoimmune disease (more on that later). After starting treatment for lupus, she got pregnant at a different clinic during her next cycle. I mean, how can you miss that?

The incidence of patients who suffer from repeat pregnancy loss or repeat implantation failure is no doubt higher than mainstream fertility doctors recognize. Especially since many RPL patients *aren't even in treatment,* just losing natural pregnancies on their own.

As I tried to explain to my "keep trying" doctor that this pregnancy loss with a donor egg was not supposed to happen and I was at the end of my rope with trying, he said snidely, "Are you going to try *'reproductive immunology'*?" (He actually put air quotes around the phrase.)

Despite his sarcasm, by then I knew what reproductive immunology was, and I was ready to give it a try.

When Your Body Rejects the Embryo

Reproductive immunology is a subspecialty of fertility medicine usually practiced by regular fertility doctors who also study immunology, the science of the immune system and immune responses.

In layman's terms, reproductive immunologists treat immunological causes of pregnancy loss (those not due to chromosomal abnormalities or cervical/uterine problems). Often, a woman's body cannot tolerate a pregnancy, treating it as a foreign body and rejecting it. This is much like how the body of someone who's received an organ donation cannot tolerate the foreign liver, heart, or lung, and reproductive immunologists try some of the same treatments used in transplant immunology. An RI will often modulate a woman's immune system so her body will "accept" the "foreign" embryo.

The field was founded by Dr. Alan E. Beer, an OB/GYN with a fellowship in immunology and genetics, who started publishing on immunology as early as the 1960s.[7] (He established the Alan E. Beer Medical Center for Reproductive Immunology in Los Gatos, California, in 2003.) Reproductive immunology is one of the *most* controversial topics in fertility—which is saying *a lot,* since it's a pretty contentious field already (which you'll discover when your doctor speaks ill of other clinics, labs, and even other fertility doctors).

"Many studies have suggested that women with pathological pregnancies such as recurrent miscarriages have signs of generally exaggerated inflammatory immune responses both before and during pregnancy," a review of reproductive immunology explained.[8]

I wish I could describe reproductive immunology to you completely objectively: lay out the options, the pros and the cons and the in-betweens, and allow you to decide for yourself. I will do that, but with one caveat: I was treated by one of the top reproductive immunologists in the field, Dr. Jeffrey Braverman of Braverman Reproductive Immunology (BRI), and after I had four miscarriages, I went to him and he got me to *stay* pregnant with my daughter. So I might be a wee bit biased.

According to Dr. Braverman and his partner Dr. Andrea Vidali, you might consider consulting an RI if:[9]

1. If you have two or more early miscarriages before a heartbeat was detected (for example, a chemical pregnancy or a blighted ovum).

2. ANY pregnancy loss after the fetal heartbeat was detected—unless testing of the pregnancy after a D&C showed a genetic abnormality.

3. Any stillbirth (a pregnancy loss after twenty weeks). Although many patients are told there is no explanation for their stillbirth, the majority of these "unexplained" stillbirths are most likely due to undiagnosed immune issues. It is *rarely* caused by a cord around the neck.

4. Any failure of a donor egg or donor embryo cycle.

5. Any patient with an autoimmune disease who has experienced an early pregnancy loss or late pregnancy complication (such as preeclampsia).

6. If you have failed IVF cycles despite the transfer of good quality/genetically tested embryos.

7. If you're under the age of forty and were told you may need donor eggs or have unexplained poor egg or embryo quality.

8. If you have endometriosis with recurrent pregnancy loss and/or IVF failures.

9. If you have a low AMH or elevated FSH that cannot be explained by your age.

10. If you have a diagnosis of PCOS and have experienced multiple miscarriages or late pregnancy complications. PCOS has a strong negative effect on the immune regula-

tion of pregnancy. This includes patients with a diagnosis of PCOS who have:

   a. Greater than twenty eggs retrieved in an IVF cycle

   b. A history of gestational diabetes during pregnancy

   c. A strong family history of diabetes

11. Anyone who has had preeclampsia, placental abruption, or preterm labor (which are strong signs of an autoimmune issue) in a prior pregnancy followed by ANY miscarriage or other reproductive failure.

12. Birth of a son followed by multiple pregnancy losses. (Having a boy can cause secondary recurrent miscarriage.)

Causes of RPL and Treatment

When we were looking for repeat loss specialists (I hadn't known it was even a thing until after my fourth miscarriage when I had the idea to Google the phrase), I came up with a few in New York, and we met with two. "I want to go to the most scientific one," Solomon said. I deferred to him, since I hadn't done such a stellar job in choosing docs before this—and besides, Dr. Braverman had spoken to me on the phone for longer than his ten-minute free consult . . . stretching it to an hour . . . while I was in Israel!

You know you've been in the Trying Game too long when you hope the doctor will come up with a diagnosis. Any diagnosis. *Anything.* And so it was a relief, a month after meeting with Dr. Braverman and telling him our story and giving him what felt like all of my blood (it was only twenty-seven vials), when he had plenty to say about my miscarriages. He handed us a six-page, single-spaced consult report, replete with graphs and even red color-coding for the worrisome part. The problem was, I didn't understand it.

In his report, some of the red lines stated that I was "in the highest risk category" and my "immune system could be contributing to failure to initiate or maintain pregnancy," and I might have "an inability to appropriately establish maternal immune tolerance to an embryo or fetus." "You had a little bit of everything," says Dr. Vidali.

In other words, I was screwed.

Dr. Vidali told me that without treatment, I'd have only a 20 percent chance of carrying a pregnancy to term. And that's *after* the struggle of getting pregnant itself, which I already had a low chance of doing (depending on the age of the eggs I would use). But also, it didn't matter if I used my own eggs or a donor's—because of my immunological issues, adding a third party wouldn't change much, since I'd still be carrying the baby. As Dr. Vidali says, "Donor eggs are not a treatment for RPL."

The causes of RPL, per Dr. Vidali, include:

- The presence of autoimmune disease, such as lupus, rheumatoid arthritis, or antiphospholipid antibodies (antibodies to the fatty molecules on the surface of a cell), which can cause clotting.[10]

- The woman's immune system reacting against the sperm, the embryo or fetus, or even the pregnancy tissue around it. She may have antipaternal antibodies (known as HLA) or natural killer (NK) cells, a type of immune cell that provides a rapid response to infection.[11] Dr. Vidali points out that there is a distinction between regular NK cells and uterine NK cells: "Testing NK cells in the peripheral blood has no bearing on what's going on with the uterine NK cells," he says.

- Thrombophilia and other clotting disorders, which are "not exactly immune issues," Dr. Vidali says, but have to be ruled out.

- Systemic inflammatory conditions, including endometriosis and PCOS.

Is Endometriosis Ruining Your Fertility and Pregnancy?

Endometriosis affects some 7 million American women. The average time to diagnosis is 6 to 10 years.[12]

Usually detected by laparoscopy, there is a new test, ReceptivaDx,[13] which detects inflammation associated with endometriosis.

Endometriosis is more frequently diagnosed in patients with infertility than in a normal population, according to the study "Endometriosis, Recurrent Miscarriage and Implantation Failure: Is There an Immunological Link?"[14]

The study found evidence linking endometriosis to recurrent implantation failure. The condition could create "autoimmune" antibodies. "Infertility in endometriosis patients may be related to alterations within the follicle or oocyte, resulting in embryos with decreased ability to implant."

A 2017 study titled "Endometriosis Doubles Odds for Miscarriage in Patients Undergoing IVF or ICSI" basically found exactly what the title says.[15] A 2018 study published in the journal *Human Reproduction* found that endometriosis was associated with adverse pregnancy and birth outcomes including placenta previa, C-section, preterm birth, and low birth weight among women doing IVF (and for women who conceived naturally just placenta previa and preterm birth).[16] Recurrent pregnancy loss may also be caused by endometriosis.[17]

Many women do not know they have the condition.

April Christina got her period when she was nine—but thought nothing of it because her cousins (from her dad's twin) also got it young. She also didn't know the heavy bleeding and cramps were abnormal. At fifteen, a pediatric gynecologist put her on birth control, and she spent her teens and twenties switching oral contraceptives . . . and suffering. "It was extremely hard to function." Finally, at twenty-eight, she got diagnosed with endometriosis. The health and wellness blogger, who also writes about endometriosis, was angry because it took so long to be diagnosed. "I had a season of depression because I felt isolated and during that time there wasn't a vast community of people where I could emotionally express my feelings." But she was also "relieved," because she always knew something was wrong. "I was glad that I didn't stop listening to my body to find the accurate answers—no matter how long it took."

"The majority of [my] patients have not a single painful symptom of endometriosis. In fact, one of the first symptoms that we see is infertility and recurrent pregnancy loss and pregnancy complications," Dr. Braverman said in "Outsmarting Endo—Diagnosing Silent Endometriosis," a speech he delivered to the Endometriosis Foundation of America in 2014.[18] He said he came up with the term "silent endometriosis" after seeing all his patients with complications (he was first an OB, delivering some five thousand babies). "The funny thing is, it is silent to most people but to me it just screams."

Clues that a woman might have endometriosis despite not having painful symptoms of it include a family history of the disorder, poor egg quality in younger women, unexplained outcomes with IVF, unexplained low AMH, unexplained high FSH, brown discoloration of the eggs, and adenomyosis (when the inner lining of the uterus breaks through the muscle wall of the uterus).

A laparoscopy is the most common procedure to diagnose and remove endometriosis.[19] Done under general anesthesia, the procedure usually takes under an hour.

After a few miscarriages, Ana Sofia did two years of treatment with Dr. Joanne Kwak-Kim and no results. She had a laparoscopy, where they removed stage 3 silent endometriosis that had damaged one of her tubes and was covering her ovaries. She conceived naturally a few months later.

These are some of the treatments offered by various reproductive immunologists for different diagnoses:

- **IVIG**—"Intravenous immunoglobulin (IVIG) is a preparation made of purified plasma of thousands of healthy donors," a 2005 study explained.[20] It shields the embryo from the mother's immune system, according to Dr. Braverman. IVIG can be expensive. (At CNY,[21] a low-cost center, they price it at $1,500 per treatment, not including nursing costs of $500—and most patients require many infusions.)

- **Intralipid infusion** is an emulsion of fatty acids composed of egg yolk, soybean oil, glycerin, and water (one of my skeptical doctors called it "mayonnaise") given intravenously at home or in a doctor's office, before and after transfer and during pregnancy. (I had it at eleven and fifteen weeks, sitting at the doctor for two hours each infusion.) According to Dr. Braverman, Intralipids have a suppressive action on certain components of the mother's immune system, essentially safeguarding the embryo from the immune reactions that might otherwise result in a miscarriage. Intralipid infusions are much cheaper than IVIG, but work for different diagnoses.

- **G-CSF (granulocyte colony-stimulating factor) medicines** like Neupogen (filgrastim) cause the body to generate neutrophils, a type of white blood cell that plays an important role in the immune system, according to Dr. Braverman. G-CSFs may work when IVIG has failed. They can also improve egg quality or the uterine lining, he said.

- **Anticoagulants** like heparin or Lovenox can be injected during the first trimester or throughout pregnancy. "The goal of anticoagulation during pregnancy is to safely balance the maternal risk of thromboembolism and hemorrhage," one study found.[22]

- **Metformin**, a common medication for type 2 diabetes, "appears to improve reproductive function in some women with polycystic ovary syndrome (PCOS)."[23]

The Case Against Reproductive Immunology

"The concept of 'Reproductive Immunity' and its role in the field of IVF is one of the hotly debated and controversial elements of screening and therapy for IVF treatment," reads the introduction to a survey by Dr. Joanne Kwak-Kim, the director of Reproductive Medicine and Immunology for Rosalind Franklin University, and Professor Simon Fishel, managing director of CARE Fertility in the UK.[24] The survey found that while 93 percent of fertility doctors said they thought understanding reproductive immunology is important, 66 percent thought it was not easy to find information on it in the infertility network, 15 percent don't check for *any* immunological or blood clotting problems, and almost *a third* don't know which of their RPL patients have abnormal immunological tests.[25] Most interestingly (infuriatingly?), when an IVF miscarriage is chromosomally normal, 39 percent of doctors surveyed *repeat the same protocol*.

In other words, "keep trying."

Aside from the fertility doctors ignorant about immunological treatment, there are a vast number of doctors who are opposed to it. Most doctors against RPL treatment believe the testing doesn't work and some of the treatment can be harmful for patients, especially since there is not enough research into reproductive immunology.

"The testing available to prove a dysfunctional immune system has little value," Dr. Shahine writes in *Not Broken*. She doesn't offer any of the immune treatments such as IVIG, Intralipid, and steroids. "I am very humble. I believe women's bodies are working and they're not broken," she writes. "Patients with RPL are desperate for answers and it's comforting to find an 'answer' and address an 'issue' when testing and treating immune dysfunction. . . . Focusing on the immune system attacking the embryo and causing RPL plays well into women's inherent ability to feel guilty and blame themselves for miscarriages." Her center, like some others devoted to repeat loss,[26] offer "expectant management," looking at structural, hormonal, and genetic causes of miscarriage, and prescribing meds like aspirin and blood thinners, as well as telling patients to genetically test embryos, but do not offer real immunological treatment.

Dr. Vidali says that when perfect embryos don't result in pregnancy, some doctors feel powerless, knowing *something* needs to be done. "That something, unfortunately, has been giving a nod to immunology by doing very superficial and often inaccurate testing," he says. They then give some sort of treatment to patients "in inadequate dosage or low dosage," which really is just to "appease" the patient demanding the immunological therapy. "In reality, more often than not, it's nothing more than window dressing."

This happened to me: One of my skeptical early doctors threw some immunological treatment at me—in the form of 5 mg of steroids (nothing compared to the 30 to 40 mg I was on during my successful pregnancy). I miscarried anyway.

"Probably a chromosomal abnormality due to age," that doc guessed. But it was not. His half-hearted treatments, borrowed from immunological experts, didn't fix my issue.

On the subject of reproductive immunology, it's hard to find an objective doctor who isn't totally for or against immunological treatment. "I believe that this debate is actually a philosophical one rather than a scientific one," writes Australian IVF doctor Gavin Sacks in "Enough! Stop the Arguments and Get on with the Science of Natural Killer Cell Testing."[27]

Dr. Sacks discusses the charge against immunological treatment, with some doctors opining that it has a "lack of scientific rationale,"[28] that treatment is given to patients based on a uterine NK cell "myth," and called for "stricter regulation" of immunotherapy because "it is clear that the potential risks and costs of these therapies outweigh any benefits."

But . . . but . . . where does that leave patients like me?

"Patients have real problems that need pragmatic solutions rather than theories," Dr. Sacks concludes, noting that more education is needed, as well as more research and a more open and two-way relationship between doctors and researchers. Dr. Sacks looked at my immunological report, and said, that with more than 350 data points, it was too individualized to extrapolate a general treatment for others. (*Isn't that a good thing?* I wondered. *Don't we want individualized medicine?*) Still, I understood what he was saying: More clinical studies needed to be done before immunology would be accepted by most fertility doctors.

"If, for whatever reason, women with high NK cell levels benefit from immune therapy, we need to understand why," he writes. As to the call to ban or restrict immune therapy, he says, "How can that approach possibly be of benefit to anyone, including their own research? In the words of Abraham Lincoln, 'He has the right to criticise, who has the heart to help.' "

It's Not the End

I'll tell you who had the heart to help me: Dr. Braverman. I saw him every week of pregnancy until my second trimester; throughout, he kept doing blood tests and adjusted my medication accordingly. During one appointment, he had to excuse himself, because he was crying about another patient he'd just seen. "She failed again," he told me later, apologizing for his absence.

Tragically, about a month before I finished this book, Dr. Braverman passed away from cancer at fifty-nine. The news gutted me. This was not just some doctor who died. It wasn't even enough to say "my baby's doctor died." It was as if my baby's father—one of them, anyway—had passed away. Think about it: I'd been through so, so many doctors, from that mean OB who wanted to send me to an abortion clinic to the Israeli one who told me he treated infertility as a battle: "This is a war. We have to send in all our ammunition." (And

Do You Have an Autoimmune Condition?

Nearly 30 million women are dealing with an autoimmune condition like rheumatoid arthritis, Hashimoto's thyroiditis, inflammatory bowel disease, celiac disease, endometriosis, or type 1 diabetes, writes Aimee Raupp, MS, LAc, in *Body Belief: How to Heal Autoimmune Diseases, Radically Shift Your Health, and Learn to Love Your Body More*[29]—and that doesn't include all those with an undiagnosed autoimmune condition. "It is estimated that one in nine women between the ages of 20 and 45 will be diagnosed with an autoimmune disease," she writes, noting that autoimmune diseases occur when "the body begins attacking healthy tissue because it begins to see it as unhealthy tissue, and this reaction creates inflammation and illness in the body."

The incidence of autoimmune diseases have tripled over the last forty years, according to the American Autoimmune Related Diseases Association (AARDA), affecting women—specifically women of reproductive age—75 percent more often than men.

She provides a list in her book of about one hundred symptoms of immune disease. Some of these are common to many conditions, but if you check three or more symptoms, you may have an autoimmune condition.

"Seventy percent of your immune system is in the tissues surrounding your gastrointestinal (GI) tract," she writes, and for some people, certain foods can trigger an immune response. She recommends following her "Body Belief" plan, an eight-week elimination diet. The aim of the Body Belief plan is to rid the body of chronic inflammation, "which is at the root of [all] autoimmune diseases," says Raupp.

these are the doctors I *went* with—forget the ones I interviewed and decided not to see!) Finally, we got to one who told us we weren't crazy, it was never my age but my body, and he really, really believed he would be able to help me.

I didn't believe it, but he did. At every moment—before my beta, before the heartbeat appointment, before my sixteen-week nuchal appointment—I was sure I would lose the baby. With a rigorous regimen—including such a high dose of steroids that I felt like I wanted to kill my husband once a day ("Only once a day?" Dr. Braverman joked)—I made it through the first trimester, past when I'd lost all the other babies; I made it through the second one, too, still under Dr. B's care, concurrently with my OB.

I even spoke to him when I was forty weeks pregnant. I was on the subway platform, on my way to my OB, who was constantly monitoring me for high blood pressure. Dr. B wanted me to be induced already, but I felt like my baby girl was going to come out at any moment. "We've worked too hard for this, for too long, to risk anything," he told me.

Dr. B couldn't make our daughter's baby party, but he got to meet her and hold her at the annual ASRM fertility conference four months later. She was probably just another bald, big-eared infant to him, one of thousands he had helped bring into the world. But she was our future: he gave us our family.

He gave many other women their families, too—including Zoe, who was one of those women in the waiting room, "young and infertile" when she started at thirty-two. Even though her first doctor diagnosed her with hyperthyroidism, she didn't get any special IVF treatment. There she underwent four IVF cycles, retrieving sixty eggs (!!), but only a few fertilized, and her one transfer there resulted in nada. She was ready to move on to donor eggs when someone put her in touch with me, and I made her go to Dr. Braverman. "What do you have to lose?" I said. He diagnosed her with endometriosis, PCOS, insulin resistance, and a mild clotting disorder.

"I felt a smidge of hope when Dr. Braverman diagnosed me so easily, telling me he sees this all the time," Zoe says, noting that while she felt "relieved," she also felt "incredibly cheated" at the same time. "I had already been through nearly three years of failed treatments with ZERO answers and had just been told to look into adoption."

She had a laparoscopy, went dairy- and gluten-free, and took immune-suppressing drugs, and her first retrieval yielded fifteen eggs, then four day-5 embryos (that's four more than she'd ever gotten). Her first transfer didn't work, but her second did.

When she was seven months pregnant, she said, "Of course I'm happy to be experiencing this chapter of life, but my husband and I still hold SO much resentment toward the doctors who never thought to dig a bit further or help us really find some answers and diagnoses." Her son was born in October 2019, and is one of the last Braverman babies.

Dr. Braverman's work lives on. His partner, Dr. Vidali, carries on the work, with a full research team of reproductive endocrinologists who consult with fertility doctors around the world, unafraid to admit what they don't know or don't specialize in.

He's not the only one. There are a handful of reproductive immunologists around the country, and your own fertility doctor might even work with one.

I am mostly agnostic about all things fertility: I don't care if you do acupuncture or positive thinking or a gluten-and-dairy-free diet, if you freeze your embryos or genetically test them. But I'm not objective about this: If you've had chromosomally normal losses, long-term losses, or implantation failure with perfectly good embryos, and if you have any immunological disorders or suspect endometriosis, you need to see a reproductive immunologist.

You can thank me later. I owe it all to Dr. Braverman.

Chapter 23

Donor, Where Art Thou? Donor Eggs, Sperm, Embryos, and Surrogacy

I'm a single mother who had a baby through a gestational carrier, and I know that people had opinions about how it was done. . . . And I think it's really important that people also embrace that it's not about those details, it's about how you carry on from the point of having your child and loving your family.

—Lucy Liu[1]

"Do you want to be pregnant right now?" the Israeli doctor asked me. I was interviewing doctors abroad to see if they thought that after three miscarriages and four rounds of IVF, I should give up on using my own eggs.

We'd always had what Solomon called our "escalation plan"—a road map for our fertility journey: how many cycles we would try, how much money we would spend, etc. Somewhere before "bank-ruptcy" and "I'm going to kill myself if I have to do any more hormone injections" were donor eggs. Between you, me, and the random strangers reading my *New York Times* column, I never thought it would come to that. I was sure I'd be the one to defy the odds. We were in Israel because IVF was free for citizens forty-five and under.

The doctor told me the success rate for donor eggs was over 50 percent—as opposed to the single digits I was facing at age forty-three. Solomon was ready to sign on the dotted line then and there. (*Easy for you to say,* I hissed, *it's still your genetics.*)

"The good thing about donor eggs is they're not going anywhere," the doctor said. "You have time." Like most new doctors, she believed

Snappy Answers to Stupid Questions: Donor Baby Edition

STUPID QUESTION	SNAPPY ANSWER
1. "But who is the mother?"	1. "Um, me! You mean who is the donor?"
2. "I'd love to go out with your sperm donor!"	2. "It's a sperm-donating site, not a brothel."
3. "Oh, you're so lucky you don't have to be pregnant and get sick."	3. "Oh, you're so lucky I don't punch you in the face."
4. "Aren't you taking advantage of some poor woman?"	4. "No, I paid her handsomely, not that it's your business."
5. "We shouldn't mess with God's plan."	5. "So I guess your heart operation was a mistake?"
6. "Maybe you're just too old to have kids."	6. "Maybe you're just too insensitive, but that hasn't stopped you!"

her protocol could have a shot. I did, too. I wasn't ready to give up on my own genetics and move on to donor eggs.

What *Is* a "Donor," Anyway?

I once assumed "third-party reproduction" meant baby-making was between me, my partner, and the embryologist growing our future baby in the lab. The "third party" is actually someone else's eggs, sperm, embryos, or uterus.

And that word "donor"? A euphemism. Sperm, eggs, and wombs are usually paid for—unless a family or friend is generous enough to actually step in and help for free.

Your situation will determine whether you need:

- **Donor Sperm**
  Men with low sperm count or no sperm left, as discussed in chapter 13, may need to use donor sperm. Single moms and lesbians often use sperm donors, too. Donors are usually under forty. Men give sperm (the old-fashioned way) to sperm banks around the country—with clinics often advertising near colleges with cheeky slogans like "Get Paid for What You're Already Doing!"[2] Sperm is frozen for at least six months and then delivered for an IUI or IVF cycle.

- **Donor Eggs**
  Women who are older, or younger women with diminished ovarian reserve, repeat miscarriage (like me), or "unexplained infertility" may use donor eggs. Gay men also use them to create embryos. Donors are usually under thirty. If you do need donor eggs, the process is like splitting up a regular IVF cycle, with the donor doing the first, more complicated part—everything leading up to retrieval, such as monitoring and drugs—and you doing the second

half, easier part: the transfer. After the donor eggs are extracted, the viable ones are fertilized with sperm, and some of the resulting embryos are transferred to your uterus. Donor eggs have higher success rates because it's the age of the eggs (i.e., the age of the woman providing the eggs), not the age of the uterus (the woman carrying the baby), that predicts fertility.

- **Donor Embryos**

  Couples who need both sperm *and* egg donation may choose donor embryos. Some people create their own embryos using both donor eggs and donor sperm, resulting in a genetically unique embryo. Others may choose embryos that have already been created; these are actually donated by a couple doing IVF who (for any of a variety of reasons) will not use them. In the US alone, there is a surplus of some 1 million embryos. Only 6 percent of couples donate embryos—most are reluctant to, because the resulting child would be fully genetically related to them and their children (unlike embryos created from separate-donor sperm and eggs). Embryo donation can be cheaper than buying donor eggs, although there are still associated IVF costs. (Although the term "embryo adoption," is often used interchangeably with "embryo donation," embryo adoption programs have some of the same legal protections as regular adoption: "home studies, legal contracts, post-adoption support and education—are applied to the embryo recipient/adopter," according to the Embryo Adoption Awareness Center.[3]

- **Gestational Carrier (Surrogate)**

  In addition to gay men, women with health problems or uterine issues or who experience repeat miscarriage and/ or stillbirth may need to use a gestational carrier, also called a gestational surrogate, someone who carries a baby but did not provide the eggs. An embryo is created and transferred into the gestational surrogate. Surrogate laws vary by state, so make sure you choose a surrogate in a state friendly to the genetic/intended parents.

Tips: What to Ask Donor Egg Programs

1. How long will the process take from start to finish?
2. What kind of screening do you do for your donors?
3. What kind of screening do you do for the intended parents?
4. What is the matching process like?
5. What guarantees do I get (how many eggs, embryos, sperm, cycles), and what happens when a cycle fails?
6. Is this process anonymous or open?
7. What are the legal processes and contracts necessary?
8. What are the total costs (medical and nonmedical), such as legal fees?

Deciding It's Time to Use a Donor

In Israel, we did four rounds of extremely high-stimulation IVF—I'm talking dizzy days of so much medication I could barely see straight—and none of my embryos tested normal. "I'm not saying you have a *zero* percent chance of having a baby with your own eggs," that once optimistic doctor said, defeated, "but I will say you have a less than one percent chance."

It wasn't the number that convinced me to move on. I just knew I was Done, with a capital D: I could not go through any more days being loopy from hormones, moody from treatment. I remembered her question from a year earlier: "Do you want to be pregnant now?" I was almost forty-four, and the answer was yes.

Some people don't have a choice in the matter. "They ruptured my last remaining ovary during the retrieval," Daisy told me, when I'd asked her how she decided. "So donor eggs were a no-brainer for me."

Carolina, a single woman who went through fourteen rounds of IVF (she had really good insurance), was offered a donor embryo. "It didn't pay for me to move on to costly donor eggs since I was already using donor sperm—I decided to try using a donor embryo," Carolina told me when she was fifteen weeks pregnant.

Although donor sperm are cheaper than donor eggs—a few hundred dollars as opposed to tens of thousands—the decision to use either is not an easy one.

After Mary's husband, Chris, went through an operation to extract sperm and those sperm did not fertilize her young eggs, he finally agreed to a sperm donor. But he was not pleased about it. Unlike us mothers, who get to carry the embryo from its very first days as tiny cells and nurture it before it comes into the world even if we've used donor eggs or a donor embryo, Chris felt that his sperm were the only thing he had to give to their child. Of course, once their twins were born, he realized he had lots to give: diapers, bottles—and tons of love.

Some people know themselves and what they can handle. "I can't go through nine months of pregnancy again to suffer through that," Heidi confessed after a full-term stillbirth. She and her husband are searching for a surrogate.

Sometimes it takes awhile to decide. "I really hoped IVF would work," said a former colleague, who got married at forty-three. In her voice, I could hear all the pain of the discarded needles and disappointing phone calls, the eggs that failed to fertilize and menstrual periods that meant no child was on its way. She took some time off after her IVF. "It took me a year or more to decide to do it," she said. "I started to realize that it was either donor eggs or no children. Kids or no kids. So I chose kids."

For a while, the choice for me was between my own eggs and donor eggs. But later on, it was really just, *Kids or no kids?*

The Grief of Letting Go

Infertility is an exercise in letting go of your expectations: that you'll get pregnant quickly, easily, and cheaply. Having to use a third party for help is yet another wrench in the plan, forcing you to let go once again—this time, giving up your or your partner's genetic role in creating your child.

"It's a grieving process—with the keyword being 'process,'" says mom-via-donor-egg Marna Gatlin, who heads Parents Via Egg Donation (PVED), an online community of thousands, and is the co-author (with Carole Lieber Wilkins) of *Let's Talk About Egg Donation: Real Stories from Real People*.[4] "Everyone is different, and they're going to grieve and process in their own way—there are no real rules in regard to grieving—and grief, as you know, has its own timetable." For her it came after her ninth miscarriage, when her doctor told her that her best chance to carry was through a donor egg. "Honestly, it was a hard pill to swallow."

The grief may even flare up for the partner who gets to use his/her own genetic material.

"I married Margie and I wanted a baby with Margie's eyes, her hair, her personality," Charles told me when the couple was considering donor eggs—ironically, it was Margie pushing for it and him resisting. "This was not what I signed up for," he confessed.

Using a donor "can feel like a death and is equated to the death of the fantasy child, the image of your future child and how he/she would fit into the image of yourself and your partner," Phyllis Martin, a licensed professional counselor in Fairfax, Virginia, and host of the *Fertility Forum* radio show, advises on RESOLVE's website.[5] Using a donor can mean giving up the genetic traits that would make your child resemble you—height, nose, athletic ability, musical talent—and that might make the choice difficult.

I never really thought of it that way—of letting go of my own (lack of) height or schnoz. Maybe that's because I didn't feel I inherited much from my own parents—not my mom's beautiful painting talent, nor my dad's height. And yet the more we learn about genetics, and specifically epigenetics—where the environment shapes gene expression, turning on and off certain traits—we see how much pregnancy can influence lifelong temperament and health, says psychiatrist Thomas R. Verny, author of *The Secret Life of the Unborn Child*, who is widely credited with launching the field of pre- and perinatal psychology. A fetus bathed in the roiling hormones of maternal stress will have different gene expression—a different brain—from a child gestated in calm. "The personality might be very much influenced by the first nine months," he says, noting that some studies have even found the genetic mother's stem cells in her donor-egg baby.

Couples who are able to create an embryo using their own genetic material but who must use a gestational carrier for the pregnancy have some mourning to do, too. The mom must give up on the idea of carrying a baby, bonding with it while it's in utero, giving birth, and, often, nursing.

"I think if, in year one, I learned I couldn't carry, it would've been much different than learning it in year seven of trying to have a baby," says Pregnantish founder Andrea Syrtash. "By then, I had experienced surgery, pregnancy loss, failed treatments . . . I was so depleted and had a feeling I had to pursue a new option." She says it was a "relief" to have genetically healthy embryos and the doctor telling her, "You have a strong chance of meeting your baby if you don't use your body." After two gestational carriers fell through, Andrea's first cousin volunteered to carry their baby. When Andrea's daughter was born, "I had the first skin-to-skin contact with her," she says. "I never felt less connected to her because I didn't carry or deliver her."

"You're making the best-worst choice," says Gatlin. "Everything is going to be a compromise. But you have to choose something in order to move forward."

Moving forward. That's the name of the game—getting out of the Infertility Club and moving into the New-Parent Club.

Choosing a Donor

Making the decision to use a donor is just the beginning of yet another process: the who, what, when, and where of third-party reproduction.

When choosing a sperm donor, "I looked for someone tall, thin, and well-educated," says Emily, the single mom we met in chapter 4. She confessed that looking through the men's profiles at sperm banks was *not* dissimilar from online dating. "I picked a man who looked like he would be a good date—and a good father."

Information on egg and sperm donors varies from clinic to clinic: Some show you a baby picture, others a current photo. Some give you a voice recording, others give you current video interviews! Some hand you a thirty-page booklet of information, others just sit you down for a verbal discussion. One friend told me she saw no picture of the donor, but the clinic told her "what celebrity the donor resembled." Most require extensive psychological screening for the donor and often the recipient, too.

"You have to jump through so many hoops to get donor eggs," Blaine told me while nursing her newborn donor-egg baby and caring for her (own-egg) toddler. "You can be a complete psycho to be a mom [naturally], but you have to go through so much counseling to become a donor mom," she says, noting that her sessions included coming up with a game plan on what she and her husband planned to tell their baby about its conception.

What do clinics look for in an egg donor? The website of Reproductive Partners in Beverly Hills states, "We usually recommend obtaining eggs from an anonymous donor who is selected because of physical characteristics similar to the intended parent, her young age and her excellent ovarian reserve. The characteristics used to match a donor to a recipient are usually primarily ethnicity, hair and eye color, and, in some cases, education. The recipient couple can ask for any set of criteria, but the stricter their criteria, the less chance that they will find a suitable donor."

Just like in dating, where searching for the "perfect" partner can be fruitless, you should be wary of searching for the "perfect" donor. "I've got clients who will only consider donors with extremely high academic test scores. Sure, I *can* find a donor with an ACT of thirty-one or higher, but that doesn't mean she will be the right donor for them," says Michelle Laurie at Donor Concierge, a matching agency. "Agency databases do not have a revolving door of extremely attractive, incredibly fertile donors with SAT scores off the charts, studying for master's degrees at Ivy League universities. Of course these young women exist, but they may not be choosing to donate their eggs. Limiting your criteria so strictly will only rule out donors who could be 'the one.'"

There are other considerations when choosing a donor: Do you want a "proven" donor—one whose sperm, eggs, or uterus have successfully produced a baby? Do you want to buy a "shared" egg cycle—in which the eggs from a donor's retrieval are split between you and others—or an exclusive one, where you get all the woman's eggs from that particular cycle? (Donors are usually limited to a total of three or four cycles—so if you buy an exclusive it's only for one cycle.) Do you want to use fresh or frozen eggs?

I have friends who have spent so long poring over donor profiles, they could be grandparents by now. Because we did donor eggs abroad, we did not get to choose our donor—we just requested some basic choices (hair color, height, education level) and the clinic selected a donor. We are all so focused on hair color, eye color, skin color, and height—but what I always tell everyone to look for is facial structure. Solomon has a long face (why the long face?!). I have a heart-shaped one. And our daughter? Round as the sparkling sun she is. (Some new companies, like Fenomatch, provide facial recognition software to clinics to find donors.)

"It's like an organ donation—you should only care if the donor is healthy," my nurse said. "Emotionally, psychologically, and physically."

Once I finally moved on to the idea of using an egg donor, I was in a hurry to be pregnant. So, her words were comforting to me.

Should You Travel Abroad?

The main reason people go abroad for third-party reproduction, especially for donor eggs and embryos (and sometimes surrogates), is cost.

For example, donor egg cycles at a clinic in the Czech Republic start at around 4,500 euro ($5,000), and donor embryos cost 1,400 euro ($1,600) and up. Here in the US, donor eggs and embryos can start at $10,000, and eggs can cost up to $30,000.

"There's a big surge in people traveling for embryo donation," says Sue Taylor, the founder of IVF Traveler, a California concierge service that helps arrange IVF abroad. The most popular countries for fertility tourism are Spain, Greece, and the Czech Republic, she says.

You also have to take into account ancillary costs, such as travel, lodging, time off from work, and the hassle of arranging it all. As if IVF isn't disruptive enough, there's tons you need to arrange abroad, from your cycle monitoring and medications to traveling with said meds. "For some people, the complexity of going abroad isn't worth it," Taylor says.

Also, she notes, "If you want to be in control, then going abroad for donors may not be for you." Due to the strict donor-anonymity laws in many countries, you get much, much less information on the donor. You may also get fewer eggs than in the US, since some countries limit the amount of stimulation donors (and IVF patients) can receive.

Of course, there are good things about traveling abroad: Some people looking for donors of specific ethnicities might find a different selection abroad. Also, clinics catering to IVF patients from abroad can actually be quite organized, with English-language websites, comprehensive price lists (more often than here!), and even door-to-door transportation and accommodation. Plus, you *do* get to travel. Take a nice trip to Prague, Madrid, or Athens, drop off your sperm, have an embryo transfer, and return home, possibly pregnant.

Relationship to the Donor

God, there are so many considerations when doing third-party reproduction. Will your surrogate be healthy while she's pregnant? (Do NOT watch the Tina Fey–Amy Poehler movie *Baby Mama* on that subject.) Was your sperm donor truthful on his self-submitted questionnaire? What about the embryo's grandparents—do you think they were drinkers? You can stay up all night driving yourself crazy with all these questions. Or you can move forward and decide what kind of relationship you'll want with the donor. Sperm donation is usually anonymous. If you're using a gestational carrier, can you be around for the surrogate's pregnancy so you can try to bond with the baby in utero? A New York woman recently told me her surrogate was in Idaho, since California and New Jersey were in such high demand.

Will you have an open donation, where you and the donor stay in touch? Or one where the relationship opens up after the child is eighteen? (England outlawed anonymous egg and sperm donation, and ruled that donor-conceived children have the right to find their genetic parent at age eighteen—resulting in a precipitous drop in all donations and fertility treatment.)

Know this: There's no such thing anymore as true "anonymous" donation. With the proliferation of genetic mapping and websites like 23andMe and Ancestry.com, donor-conceived children are finding their genetic donor parents and genetic half siblings ("diblings") conceived using the same donor.

Which brings many to the question: Should you use a family member or friend as a donor, referred to as a "known donor"? A known donor has many benefits: You may share genetics, it can be easier to find one, and it can be less expensive (although it's still costly when you're using a known egg donor, because clinics charge you as they would for a regular IVF cycle—for screening her, monitoring her, and retrieving her eggs). But it can also create fraught family dynamics. "My hubby and I are looking forward to having our second child and this time we will need to use a sperm donor," Vasyatka wrote on Babycenter, an online fertility board. "My mother-in-law asked us if we'd considered talking to my brother-in-law (my hubby's brother). And both my husband's and my reply was *NO*."[6]

Some people don't consider using family—or any open donor relationship. "We wanted it to be as anonymous as possible," Blaine says, discussing why she chose her clinic, which matched her with a donor. "But that doesn't mean it's a secret." Blaine has already mentioned the egg donor to her older daughter (who was conceived using Blaine's own eggs), telling her, "We wanted a baby so badly, Mommy had to borrow an egg."

Her daughter said, "Oh, okay," and ran off to play.

These days, most people believe it's important to be upfront about a child's genetics. It's essential to tell your children about their conception story, Gatlin says. "Tell your children early and often," she says. "It's something they should always know about themselves. Every day I get phone calls and emails from panic-stricken parents who say, 'OK, my kid is now a teenager and I know I need to tell them, but I have no idea what I should say—I put this off for so long,' or 'My child learned by accident that they were conceived via egg donation and she's very angry with me, what should I do?' "

I was pretty open about using donor eggs—telling everyone around me when my first try failed. (Even though we think of egg donation as a sure thing, it's only 50 percent successful—which, unfortunately means, 50 percent failure.)

But after I was heavily pregnant, the reality hit me: There's a baby inside of me. And she's going to grow up to be her own person, with her own thoughts and feelings and need for privacy. I can't go around telling everyone the story of her conception! That's her business.

Most celebs and other high-profile people do not disclose whether they used donors. "While I'm incredibly open about sharing almost anything in my life, our decision whether or not to use donor eggs was ultimately ours to make and keep," Christene Barberich, co-founder of Refinery29, wrote on the website.[7] "If we did choose to use donor eggs, I would have to think about the privacy of the child whose life the egg and donor made possible. And if I didn't use donor eggs, I wouldn't want women my age feeling ashamed or angry that I somehow struck some elusive lottery that they didn't. It is the one

Fresh vs. Frozen Eggs

FRESH EGGS	FROZEN EGGS
1. You must coordinate your cycle to the donor's, which can be stressful and take a long time to find a match.	1. You can do it at any point in time, when it's convenient for you. It's much easier to find a match.
2. You don't know what you're getting—you may be primed for the cycle but no good eggs are produced by the donor.	2. You know exactly how many eggs you're getting at the start (but you don't know how many will fertilize).
3. You can buy an exclusive cycle—meaning as many eggs as the donor produces in one particular cycle. (But she may have donated before.) Or you can share the eggs from one cycle with another recipient.	3. You are probably sharing the cohort of eggs.
4. Success rates for fresh eggs are higher, at 53.5 percent.	4. Success rates for frozen eggs are lower, at 38.5 percent (although this varies by clinic).
5. It's more expensive—$37,550 at the World Egg Bank.	5. It's much cheaper—$22,500 at the World Egg Bank.

piece of our process I feel private about—it's our business. And, well, now it's our baby," she wrote of her daughter.

"There's a difference between secrecy and privacy," Blaine explained to me, admitting that she felt the same way as soon as her daughter was born. "I think secrets are detrimental to a family, but certain things can remain private."

Had I known how many people would be commenting on my daughter's looks, I might have taken more care in choosing a donor who looked like me. But then I'd have Blaine's problem: "Everyone says the baby looks exactly like me, and she does! But I had to stop blurting out it was a donor egg, because it's not every stranger's business," she says. "I had to learn to smile and say thank you."

Keeping Up with the Kardashians

Women are always judged for their choices. If you have kids too young, you're selfish for not considering how you'll support them; if you focus on your career or finding the right partner, you're selfish for waiting too long.

"As a mother via egg donation and surrogacy, I stay away from regular infertility spaces because I know I'll be shat on, however subtly, for not having a baby in the way other infertile women all seem to want to," says Alexandra Kimball, author of *The Seed: Infertility Is a Feminist Issue*.[8] "In fact, I'm not even sure if I can say that I ultimately 'succeeded' infertility-wise because I know most other women would rather kill themselves than have a kid the way I did."

There will always be people who have things to say about our reproductive choices. But remember, IVF babies were once called "test tube" babies, celebs like Jimmy Fallon weren't talking about their surrogates on late-night TV, and no one had two daddies. So who knows what the future will bring?

While I don't think there are many good things about IVF, it does actually force us to reevaluate what it means to be a parent. If you don't get pregnant naturally, contribute your own genes, carry a baby in your body—does it mean you're not a parent?

"The baby you have is the baby you are meant to have," says Gatlin. And as scholar Joseph Campbell wrote, "We must let go of the life we have planned so as to have the one that is waiting for us."

Chapter 24

The End of the Road: Life After No Baby

I wanted that stomach. I wanted to know what nine months of complete togetherness could feel like. I was meant for the job, but I didn't pass the interview. And that's OK. It really is. I might not believe it now, but I will soon enough. And all that will be left is my story and my scars, which are already faded enough that they're hard to find.

—Lena Dunham[1]

I normally love my birthdays: throwing giant parties, getting lots of presents, reading every anodyne "happy b-day, Amy!" message on social media.

But at forty-four, I turned off my Facebook wall, went out of town, and left my phone at home. Although the previous three babyless years in treatment were no picnic, forty-four marked the end of my natural fertility.

It's when all the statistics suddenly stopped. BAM! Like Wile E. Coyote dropping off a cliff. "Assisted reproductive technology has a reasonable chance for success (>5%) up until the end of the forty-third year," is the generally accepted view.[2] Even my paltry insurance ended at forty-four, and I was beginning to feel like so had I.

I was at the end of my rope.

I'd just had my fourth miscarriage, while my lovely younger sister was pregnant with her first and my brother's wife with their fifth.

I. Could. Not. Deal. Not with my birthday, not with anything. I had run out of time. I had run out of hope. I felt isolated, embittered, unraveled, a stranger to myself.

The me who began this undertaking was not the me I was now.

I never, ever thought I would come to the end of the road. Not after my first miscarriage, not after my third. When I started fertility treatment, I hadn't considered how it would change me. And how circumstances would change. I did not know that there would come a time I would feel different about having a baby: I still wanted one, but not at any cost.

I was tired of Trying. I wanted to have a morning where my moods weren't tied to a future treatment, a week where I wasn't waiting for anything. I wanted to be a person again who thought about something other than fertility. I *felt* like I was done.

I wasn't, though.

Dr. Braverman got me pregnant. But had that transfer failed, had that pregnancy ended like the previous ones, I might have called it quits.

Is This the End?

Some people stop treatment because they just don't have it in them emotionally. Others stop because they've run out of time. And many people simply run out of funds.

No one can tell you when to stop treatment—or indeed if, when you take a break, you are actually stopping.

A week before Pamela Mahoney Tsigdinos turned forty, her clinic informed her that she'd be considered "high risk" and would have to change protocols for her third IVF round. "It was the final straw for me," says Tsigdinos, who had been trying to conceive for some ten years. "We were emotionally spent and out $60,000."

But she actually was *not* done then. Her husband was—actually, he'd have been happy stopping a few years earlier. "I think for men it's easier because biology is not in their face every twenty-eight days," she says, referring to her menstrual cycle. "For women it's really hard to walk away. You wake up in a panic, thinking, 'Maybe I didn't give it my best college try,'" she recalls.

So when she was forty-one, she went back to the clinic for two more IUIs—a "compromise" over more invasive IVF. But this time she had a different perspective. "My expectation wasn't high—and I also knew this was truly the last run."

And it was. At forty-two, she went back on the pill ("I needed to assure myself I was *done* done"), stopped looking at fertility treatment protocols, and unsubscribed from medical newsletters on the topic.

Yet saying you're done and *being* done are two completely different things, as she chronicles in her book, *Silent Sorority: A (Barren) Woman Gets Busy, Angry, Lost and Found.*[3] She'd been trying since she was twenty-nine years old. "I felt like my thirties were put on hold, and the rest of my life went by while I was trapped in this loop," she says. Not that she blames herself, all these years later. "Part of the challenge is that the IVF industry does a good job of controlling the narrative, with the message, 'If you stick with it long enough, you're going to succeed.' And that's not necessarily true for everyone." Tsigdinos founded a website, ReproTechTruths.org, as a forum for women with unsuccessful treatment and a platform to bring accountability to the industry.

Infertility is a long, hard road, but so is deciding to end treatment.

How Do You Know It's Time to Stop Treatment?

"How much more are you willing to endure?" says New York psycho-therapist Dr. Marni Rosner, who specializes in infertility and grief counseling. Rosner felt ambivalent about being a mother until, newly married at thirty-eight, an endocrinologist told her she had a "one in a million" chance of getting pregnant. "I couldn't believe how devastated I felt," she says. "From the minute you're born you're supposed to be a mother," she says society tells us, and most women internalize it on a "cellular and unconscious" level. "For me to be told I couldn't have a baby wiped out an entire paradigm I didn't even know I was carrying." She went through her own grieving process and wants to help others.

She says when deciding if you're going to stop treatment, you should evaluate your relationships: Do you feel isolated, unhappy, disengaged from your usual activities? Is the process "sapping you of your happiness and enjoyment for life?" Also, you need to evaluate if you and your partner are still on the same page, or if you have a lot of conflict around trying.

Basically, she wants you to remember life before infertility: You *could* get back to that place, she says, "but it may require getting off the treatment roller coaster."

How do you know if you should go on or stop? Dr. Rosner says that each treatment cycle failure can be experienced as a trauma "and numerous failed cycles (or miscarriages) can have a significant cumulative impact."

After my fourth miscarriage, I had to know I was doing something different—not just "eating pineapple core" or "going on bed rest" different, but something *radical*—for me to even muster the energy for another cycle. If you're going into another cycle thinking it will produce the same results, then it could be time to stop.

Looking back, Tsigdinos says, she would have established some kind of time frame, decided, "These are the gates I'm willing to go through." When a new cycle has a "fairly big ask" such as interviewing a new clinic or adding an extra procedure, that's a good time to check in and ask:

- Have things changed?
- Are we getting in over our heads financially?
- Is our relationship in a good place?
- How much more can I take?
- What's my prognosis?

Then you can decide if it's a go or a no go.

Moira and her husband knew when they were done with treatment. After three IUIs, they agreed they'd do three rounds of IVFs—which was what insurance covered. "When we got to the final round, I thought *this* would be the one." But a few weeks later, she got the call that it hadn't worked. "You're not really a candidate for another round of IVF," the doctor told her.

They stopped treatment but are still casually trying (yeah, like, sex). "If a miracle happens, we'd be thrilled," she says, now forty-six, two years after stopping.

It's not an easy decision, ending treatment. "Letting go of the hope for a biological child and the experience of pregnancy is life-altering," Dr. Rosner says. "But remaining trapped in what can feel like a state of endless failure can take all the joy from life. Sometimes deciding to stop can restore it."

For her, it was the right decision. "At this point, I'm actually happy I don't have kids: My brother has young girls and I have unfettered access to them. I just adore them, and I love saying goodbye. We have a really nice life, and it's worked out for the best."

Stopping treatment can sound appealing—no more doctor's appointments, sex only for pleasure, travel with no obligations—but then you also have to let go of being pregnant and having no baby *forever*. That's its own process.

Quiz: Are You Done with Trying?

1. When your clinic calls to make an appointment do you:
   a. ignore the call.
   b. answer, but put them on hold for twenty minutes as an act of revenge.
   c. engage the receptionist in an hour-long conversation about what you've missed.

2. When someone asks if you'd like some pineapple do you:
   a. say, "No thanks, I'm not ovulating till next week so I don't need help."
   b. throw it at the host and walk out of the house.
   c. run to the kitchen to squirrel away the core in your purse.

3. If your partner asks to clean out the medicine cabinet do you:
   a. let him put it all in a box in the closet.
   b. allow him to only if you can use all the syringes on him.
   c. tape up a spreadsheet for every vitamin, pill, and crème you must take.

4. When you're invited to a baby shower do you:
   a. bury the invite at the bottom of your to-do pile.
   b. burn the invite.
   c. start knitting a tiny hat for the upcoming tyke.

If you answered mostly A:

You seem ambivalent about treatment. Maybe you're on break, maybe you're done—only time will tell. And your checkbook.

If you answered mostly B:

Oh, girlfriend, stick a fork in it, 'cuz you are Done. Or you have a lot of unexpressed rage you should work through before you return.

If you answered mostly C:

Clear your calendar, cancel all plans. You'll be cycling again in no time.

How to Get Over—or Beyond—Fertility

For people who've been mired in fertility treatment for years, it's not so easy to let go.

"I was in the midst of zombie grief," Tsigdinos said.

So are most people going through infertility—yet they'd put it on hold, round after round, year after year, until they finally have a baby.

But what happens if you don't have that baby? What do you do with all that suffering?

"If you put it off or put it away it is going to find a way out—in unhealthy ways," she says. "As painful as it is to face grief and anger, if you don't address it, you do yourself harm." She advises people to let the emotions surface, talk it through. "Own your story." Only then can you move forward.

Lisa Manterfield wishes she could write down "ten easy steps" to making peace with being childless (not by choice), "but the answer isn't that simple," says the author of *Life Without Baby: Surviving and Thriving When Motherhood Doesn't Happen*[4] and the eponymous website. What helped her make peace? Writing down her journey, venting about injustices on her blog, drawing a line in the sand and saying, *This is where that chapter of my life ends and this is where I start healing*.

"Frankly, telling myself a big fat lie that I was better off not being a mother actually helped me to realize that in many ways I was," she explains. It helped her set new goals, to appreciate the benefits of not having kids, and allowed herself to feel "bitter and badly treated" when she needed to.

Make a place for yourself where you can feel safe, she says. And be flexible! "There's no prescribed timeline for getting over it and no linear path to follow. It's definitely a journey of making forward progress and dealing with inevitable setbacks.

Tips: Heal from the Heartbreak of Childlessness

Here's how Jody Day, founder of Gateway Women, the global friendship and support network for childless women, and author of *Living the Life Unexpected: 12 Weeks to Your Plan B for a Meaningful and Fulfilling Future Without Children*,[5] says to heal:

1. **Understand that you're not crazy, you're grieving.**
Day didn't understand that when she'd "been in hell for two years"—that that was grief. She was relieved to realize it, that it was a "process" that she'd come out of and that she wasn't "going mad."

2. **Your grief needs company.**
She says that you can't grieve alone. "It wasn't until I had others to talk to about it (who didn't shut me down with miracle baby stories) that things started to shift for me."

3. **Give up trying to explain yourself.**
She says childless women are often "misunderstood, disrespected or shamed by others," including family and friends. Don't try to explain yourself to these people.

4. **You're allowed to say NO.**
Day gives permission to decline invitations to baby showers, children's birthday parties, and work social events that suddenly turn into family picnics, and to not be "delighted" about others' pregnancies. "And if anyone tells you you're being selfish, agree with them. You are allowed to be selfish! You are grieving a momentous, lifelong loss."

5. **Face aging without children.**
There's a lot you can do about preparing for the future. Get to know some older childless women, she says. "You'll find that they're a lot more interesting, intriguing and powerful than you may have realized."

6. **Recovering from childlessness changes everything.**
She says that this "identity transformation" will change everything. "Once we've been through the fire and floods of grief,
we're not the same person as we were before. We have to have a
lot of faith that at some point, things will make more sense."

But she is at peace. She's closed the door on having children, "and
most days I'm good with it." Some days are better and some days
there are reminders of what she lost and that flicker of *what if.* "The
truth is, in many ways, I expect this healing to go on forever. The
experience of infertility has changed me. It is one of the most significant and life-changing events of my life, and I don't think the reper-
cussions of that will ever stop reverberating. It doesn't mean I won't
find harmony and even happiness in this new life—I already have—
but I don't expect this journey of coming-to-terms to ever fully end."

One of the most difficult challenges? Assimilating back into society again. After Tsigdinos mourned—"patched herself up"—she had
to find herself again. They were not going to have children, and for a
time, she sought out people who also did not have children. She told
her friends with kids, "I'll see you without your children." She didn't
want to sit around talking about breastfeeding or potty training (who
does?!!), feeling like she was going to have a panic attack. "You stair-
step your way back," she says about inching her way forward, slowly
allowing children back into her life. "You bring people back in when
you have the emotional capacity to be there for other people."

Tsigdinos says there are triggers that pop up, like going into a
business meeting and seeing three pregnant women there. Another
challenge was how much to share with other people. One time she
was at a party and a mother told her she was "sooo lucky" she didn't
have kids. Tsigdinos could picture other times in her life when this
comment would have sent her off the rails, but instead she gently
said, "I'm just going to tell you right now that that's not an appropri-

ate thing to say to someone who has lived my experience. We tried very hard to have children and never made it through pregnancy."

Some people take the question more humorously. Moira, who had a less traumatic time stopping treatment, says her husband tells people, "Maybe we'll adopt when we're fifty." When people ask if she has kids, she sometimes jokes, "No, but I'm an awesome godparent!"

Scientifically Speaking: Finding Meaning After IVF

The Chinese have a saying: "Behind every gain is a loss; behind every loss is a gain." A recent small study of men and women who did IVF—where nearly 65 percent remained childless, some 21 percent adopted and 14 percent conceived naturally—found that people who see their negative experiences of IVF in a constructive light can more easily move on with their lives.[6] Even though everyone saw infertility as a loss, they also gained a lot, too.

1. **Everyone experienced personal growth:** Parents and non-parents alike learned about a character trait in themselves by experiencing infertility, including inner strength, a sense of humility, and being a survivor instead of a victim.

2. **Most improved their relationships:** Even if infertility was hard and sad, this medical experience made most people feel closer to their spouses. Meanwhile, those who already had a kid learned not to take their children for granted. Seventy-five percent of the women got crucial support from friends.

3. **Infertility changed everyone:**[7] Everyone had a changed outlook on life, from learning how to not sweat the small stuff to how to grow from adversity and even how to accept childlessness. Two-thirds experienced a change in identity from being a service recipient to a helper.

Other times she may volunteer, "We tried IVF, but who knows, maybe we'll get lucky!"

Still, Moira hates the pitying look from others after they ask if she has kids. "I think it's obnoxious. It's a cultural thing—we haven't evolved to understand how personal a question it is."

For Tsigdinos, now that time has gone by—it's been almost fifteen years since she closed the door on that chapter of her life—she has a better understanding of the social component. People are not giving the kids question deep thought, it's more like, "how's the weather?" If someone really wants to know why she doesn't have kids, she might say, "It didn't work out for us."

Circumstantial Infertility

Life doesn't always work out for people in the way they expected it to. Some people don't have children because they never found a partner to have children with.

"Finding love and being a mom was everything I expected for myself," says Melanie Notkin, the author of *Otherhood: Modern Women Finding a New Kind of Happiness*.[8] "I always expected to have children—there was never a doubt in my mind. When I was ten I imagined I would have twins. When I was twelve, I bought a baby name book."

She terms being childless not by choice "circumstantial infertility"—the pain and the grief of not being able to have children because you don't have the finances, or perhaps because you met a partner too late in life, or never met one at all. Although women like her haven't done fertility treatment, they still experience "disenfranchised grief," a grief unrecognized by society.

The grief over not having children can last for a decade, Notkin says, noting that it's only gotten worse as science has extended how long a woman is able to have a child. "It used to be that as a woman got into her forties, she'd grieve and move on," she notes. But now with celebrities on the cover of magazines having children into their fifties (probably with donor eggs), it can serve as a reminder to people of what they don't have. She says some people find it difficult to grieve and move on because "there's always a chance."

For Tsigdinos, it got easier after menopause. "Knowing that the uterus and ovaries are shut down can trigger a lot of emotional identity issues for women going from fertile to barren—but I'd done all the emotional gymnastics at forty-two. By the time I hit menopause, I was like, 'Yes! I'm done!' "

Adoption After Infertility

Not everyone is *done,* done with the idea of children, even after they end treatment.

Maggie thought she was taking a break from IVF in order to save up more money for treatment. The forty-three-year-old branding consultant looked into adoption, but got overwhelmed by all the different options—international versus domestic, private versus foster-to-adopt.

"It seemed like *so* much physical and emotional work—it seemed insurmountable to me," says Maggie. Then she met an adoption consultant who walked her through the process. "I hadn't come to terms that I wasn't going to have a baby physically," Maggie says. "It was a big change—I felt sad I couldn't be pregnant."

On her forty-ninth birthday, she decided to work with the consultant and it all went pretty quickly after that. Not smoothly, though. The birth mother was addicted to opioids, skipped some doctor's appointments, agreed to rehab, and then fell off the wagon. "That's when I had a moment wondering if I would stay with them or move forward," Maggie recalls. But the bio mom gave birth a month early, the baby was drug free, and Maggie flew to Louisiana to meet her daughter. "I didn't feel good about the decision until she got here, when I felt that connection and love."

"Once I got to the other side of it, I never looked back. I never felt sad anymore that I didn't have a bio child. Part of that is moving forward day to day—you're trying to take care of a human—you don't have time to wallow in your own stuff."

Maggie is amazed now that it was such a hard decision to make. But it was not an easy process, especially going from fertility to adoption. "Going through fertility treatments made me feel like at least I tried, even though I knew going in it was a slim chance—at least I had made the effort." Now, comparing the two processes she says the risks, cost, and time commitment are similar. "It's a very similar emotional roller coaster."

In the end, she says, as a single mom with a lack of familial support, adopting was a better solution for her. Not to mention that "the child I adopted is the perfect fit for me."

More than half the women diagnosed as infertile consider adoption, and women who have used fertility services are ten times more likely to adopt than people who have not, according to the CDC.[9] Which would explain why a large number of adoptive parents had fertility issues.

Before moving on to adoption, it's important to grieve the loss of being pregnant and having a biological child. "Couples must reach the acceptance stage before pursuing adoption," advises American Adoptions, a domestic adoption agency. "Consult a local infertility or grief and loss specialist to help you move on from infertility and get excited about growing your family through adoption."

Yet some women pursue adoption even after having their own bio child. Three months after Sasha gave birth to her (naturally conceived) son, she had to have a non-cancerous tumor removed from her brain. Even though doctors told her it was safe to get pregnant again, she and her husband decided against it, worried for her health. They also decided against using a gestational surrogate to carry their genetic baby.

"I don't feel passionately about having a biological child—the genetic thing doesn't resonate with me, pregnancy doesn't resonate with me." Besides, she says, "I always wanted to adopt, ever since I was thirteen years old."

Not that her adoption path has been easy (it rarely is). After supporting a matched birth mother throughout the pregnancy, meeting her, playing with her other children, shortly after the mom gave birth, she disappeared—she didn't answer her phone while the couple was in state. Her only text to them was, "You can have the baby, but it's already in state care." Sasha is now pursuing another adoption.

"Adoption needs to resonate with you: You need to feel like you can love a baby that's not genetically yours, that needs to speak to you. I one hundred percent know I will love someone as much as I love my son (who doesn't look anything like me). There's so many ways to have a baby," she says.

Getting to Happiness—Either Way

Adoption is not an easy process. Journalist Farai Chideya endured three failed adoptions in her quest to be a mother. "This idea that people say, 'I will just adopt,' is a complete myth. I think adoption is beautiful. I think the industry has a very ugly side, though," she told NPR.[10]

Adoption is not for everyone. Third-party reproduction is not for everyone.

When the doctor told Moira and her husband to stop treatment and to consider moving on to donor eggs, she balked: "I had a visceral reaction to that. It wasn't the experience I was looking for," she says. She discussed it with her husband and they both decided they didn't connect to the idea of donor eggs or adoption.

"I had made a commitment to trying, and I would have loved to experience that—but it won't define my life," she says, noting that her happy marriage is what is most important.

For others, happiness is harder to come by.

"The most important lesson that I took away from all of this is not to be trapped in someone else's definition of normal," Tsigdinos says. "We live in a society that has lots of messages about what a happy life is, so the more I spent time—and some of it was introspective—understanding what brought me happiness, and how I could leave a substantial legacy of my own without children, I started opening up."

All of us—with or without children—have regrets: about not marrying sooner, Trying sooner, seeing a specialist sooner, maybe even quitting sooner.

But Melanie Notkin doesn't believe in looking back. "I don't see a reason to live in the past. I don't know that I did anything wrong, and if I'm living in the past, I won't be present to meet *him*," she says, referring to her future mate.

She says that people can't imagine what their life will be without children, but "our imagination is simply a repository of stories we tell ourselves." She says to tell yourself a great story. "I love my life and I'm living in the moment. I have come out the other side and am doing great. I'm a happy woman."

EPILOGUE
Pregnancy and Motherhood After Infertility

Congratulations! You're pregnant! Really, really pregnant, this time. You've passed those damn doubling betas, you've heard the baby's heartbeat (or *heartbeats*), and you might just be sailing out of your nauseating first trimester, seeing emails about the fruit or vegetable shape your baby resembles. (Pregnancy newsletters are weird.)

Whether you've been through one cycle or ten, three pregnancies or one, you deserve not only a baby but free diapers for a year. You won't get the diapers but you will get a *lot* of extra space in the medicine cabinet and closet after you get rid of all your meds, supplements, and supplies. You'll also get a whole lot more time in your schedule and brain—all of which will be taken up by your pregnancy.

It's unbelievable to finally be there after all this time.

"We had a deep appreciation for being pregnant," says Naomi Less, a singer/songwriter, ritual leader at Lab/Shul, and infertility advocate, who was trying for seven years, with two lost pregnancies, five IUIs, and eight rounds of IVF and two donor egg cycles. When she was pregnant, she and her husband would think, "I can't believe we're here. Did we really go through what we went through? Did this really happen?" She felt "astonishment and disbelief," but also immense gratitude. "I did not feel guilty for being pregnant," Naomi says. "I felt emboldened to advocate more now; I have privilege, I have to continue to not get sucked up in '*woo hoo! I'm pregnant!*' to continue to hold space for people who are not."

If you're one of those people who feel absolute gratitude about being pregnant, and you want to jump into planning your baby registry and decorating the nursery, more power to you. Join an expectant mothers group and never look back! You deserve to be happy.

Are You Happy Yet?

But if you're like me and so many other women whose road to motherhood was as bumpy as a bouncy castle, you might not exactly have the pretty pregnancy you always dreamed of. You may no longer have the desire to post a cutesy "bun in the oven" GIF on social media, have a gender reveal party with a pink or blue cake, or endlessly debate baby names.

First of all, you might not want to do all that out of sensitivity to all your friends who are still at it. Second, you might be too nervous.

I myself had been pregnant so many times that at first I couldn't believe *this* fifth pregnancy was the one that was going to stick. When Dr. Braverman first told me my beta was 55, my initial excitement was quickly tempered by the niggling thought, *Well, we've been down this road before.* Even after my betas doubled appropriately, I wasn't as happy as I once thought I would be. Shouldn't I be beaming 24/7?

With the heartbeat came relief—but only momentarily. A few days later I was back to worrying again. After all, I'd heard a heartbeat once before and that pregnancy ended—maybe because *I hadn't been paying enough attention.* Now I was paying attention, to every swallow, twinge, flutter. Always nervous when I wasn't feeling anything in particular. Pregnancy was so, so tense.

Even when I passed the in utero blood tests for major diseases and moved into my second trimester, I still couldn't relax. I couldn't be happy, not for longer than two minutes.

What was wrong with me?

Can't You Just Enjoy This Pregnancy?

I was having what I later realized was Infertility PTSD.

Post-traumatic stress disorder (noun): a condition of persistent mental and emotional stress occurring as a result of injury or severe psychological shock, typically involving disturbance of sleep and consisting of vivid recall of the experience *with dulled response to others and to the outside world* [emphasis mine].

- "Sleep disturbances?" Check. I woke up countless times in the middle of the night sure my pregnancy was over. I woke Solomon, crying. He bought me a home heartbeat monitor but only if I promised I would use it just *once a day.* And I lived for that moment in the evening, where he'd lube up my belly (oh so sexy) and play doctor and we could finally hear her, even though I hadn't felt a thing all day. For just that one moment in time, I could actually feel pregnant.
- "Vivid recall of the experience?" Check. Every time I went to do an ultrasound, I had a flashback to the previous times I had heard nothing.
- "Dulled experience to the outside world?" Check. During pregnancy, I was like two different people. I was a regular pregnant lady going to my appointments at a high-risk OB/GYN, but also a secret worried infertility warrior (worrier?), always keeping myself slightly at a distance from my pregnancy till the very end.
- "Persistent mental and emotional stress?" Check. I called Dr. Braverman numerous times so sure it was the end be-

cause I couldn't feel anything inside. "You'll only be happy when you are holding your baby in your arms," he said. He understood.

Other people, you will not be surprised to learn, do not.

"Just enjoy this!!" they counsel you, among a thousand other "helpful" tips they give to pregnant women. Non-IVF moms may lay off the pregnancy advice, but they still don't understand your caution: They're frustrated that you can't "just be happy, finally." (The *just* always kills me.)

That's another thing that infertility and repeat pregnancy loss robbed me of: the ability to enjoy a carefree pregnancy. Blaine's husband told her, "You have to be happy now! You have to accept something good is happening." But she couldn't. "I was just waiting for something to happen throughout my pregnancy. Because I had always left the doctor with some bad news," she says. "You're waiting to be happy because you just don't know when that's going to be."

For her, happiness only came after having the baby.

For some IVF mamas who never lost a pregnancy, the early weeks are fraught, but it becomes easier. "I feel like the whole thing comes in waves: I had moments of doubt and fear that if I did something, the pregnancy would go away," says Clarissa, who leapfrogged over using her own eggs and got pregnant with donor eggs. She took it "day by day, ultrasound by ultrasound." It wasn't until her second trimester that she began to feel like a "normal" pregnant woman. ("Whatever normal is—I don't think anybody goes through their pregnancy not worrying about a thing," Clarissa said.)

Knowing that she worked hard for it and that she was in the right place in her life made her feel so much better. "I'd been pregnant before and chose to terminate. And I'm in the right place now: I have a partner, we're married, we have a home, and we're starting a family. This is a place I want to be for a long time."

When I learn someone is pregnant after infertility, I temper my congratulations. "How are you feeling?" I say, trying to follow their cues. If they're in the elated camp, I'm elated with them. If they're cautious, changing the subject to frivolous non-pregnancy-related topics, I'm happy to do that, too, and to reassure them.

Hopefully you are a better pregnant woman than I, Charlie Brown. Maybe it's because you were never pregnant before, or maybe you are so hopped up on those happy hormones that it's obliterated all memories of Trying.

Some other not-quite-joyous feelings, left over from infertility, may emerge after the babe is born.

New Baby After Infertility

"I just thought I would be in love and elated all the time, but that's not how it was," Naomi Less says, a few months after her daughter was born. "I suffered from severe postpartum anxiety, would chastise myself because I wasn't over the moon with being a mom and still having to give myself [blood thinner] shots even after the baby was born."

IVF does not increase risk of postpartum depression, studies show.[1] But many women may suffer from infertility PTSD.

We IVF mamas were so intent on persevering—on seeing the most follicles, retrieving the most eggs, growing the best-grade embryos—then waiting, waiting, waiting, for a period, a retrieval, a transfer, a pregnancy test, a beta double, a heartbeat, that we didn't take time to process. To breathe, to feel.

"I went from intensive, fragile pregnancy to full-blown motherhood responsibilities with a massive drop off of hormones: I'm frankly surprised I survived," Naomi says, noting that almost two years later, "it still seeps out."

Solomon always used to tell me, "Keep your eye on the ball." I kept my eyes on the ball so much, I ignored the game. I didn't let myself take the time to wallow in my grief, my confusion, my anger, my frustration. I was onto the next treatment. It was only *after* I was in the safe zone (that's a sports metaphor, right?) that all those emotions started coming through. Which is what happens to many people in traumatic situations: They only feel everything when it's over.

That's another thing people don't talk about. Although more and more people discuss infertility and IVF these days, we're all so #grateful for everything we fought for, we do not discuss our mixed feelings.

I'm not talking about the feeling of being scared shitless, the excitement and terror that comes with knowing you're about to be first-time parents. I'm talking about the leftover infertility feelings from the past, mixed in with the awesome anticipation and enjoyment of your child.

When I used to train for marathons, I piled on the miles, curtailed drinking, and set my sights on the big day. When I was done? I *relaxed*. Yet when this marathon of Trying was over, what awaited me? A new baby. Which is everything I always dreamed of, but as relaxing as the construction outside my apartment.

I wasn't as overjoyed at I thought I would be.

"I loved her from the moment I laid eyes on her," is what I told everyone who asked.

But I was nervous and scared and afraid to be in love. I think it took me a few weeks to feel that unfettered joy about my baby. Sure, I was recovering from major surgery, trying to exclusively breastfeed (The Second-Hardest Thing in the World, after infertility), to subsist on negative sleep, to entertain Every Foreign Family Member Flying in, but I think I was holding myself at a bit of a remove. I couldn't relax. I couldn't understand she was here to stay. That she was *mine*.

"Mama?" the doctor's receptionist would say a few times before I understood she was talking to me. *I am the mama.*

Yes, I ran in to check on the baby every 5.4 seconds in the middle of the night. I watched her on the video monitor even when I was outside for a twenty-minute break. Maybe all new moms do this. But I was also still running from my feelings, like I had during infertility. I was still unable to relax into motherhood.

Now whenever I look back on early motherhood and even pregnancy, I know I wear rose-colored glasses. My eyes mist up when I see the first baby album or even find a stray newborn sock or hat. In reality, though, it was hard. It was harder than "new mother" hard, too, because I had expected it to be like the end of a marathon: only celebratory. Emotionally, it seemed like the first time I could finally stop pretending everything was okay. I hadn't had any time to process those feelings.

The remove did dissolve, though. My fear of the baby not waking up one morning was overwhelmed by an eagerness to see her, to see what another day with her would bring. That early dread was crowded out by love.

How Infertility Changed Me

Sometimes I wonder, *What if I'd gotten pregnant, stayed pregnant, gone to one doctor and poof, had a baby some nine months later, just like in the movies? What if I'd never lost those babies, never had to go to multiple doctors, clinics, countries, and been made entirely and completely a lunatic from all the desperate wanting, hoping, and failing?* I'd surely be richer, younger, and a little less insane. But what kind of mother would I have been?

You see, infertility changed me. I used to be a happy-go-lucky optimist, certain that things would always work out. Book a trip at the last minute? Definitely. Lost my luggage? No worries, we'll just figure it out—*and* get a whole new wardrobe. Give up my life in L.A. in order to meet a guy in New York? Sure! I was game for anything and everything.

And yet, losing pregnancy after pregnancy, going through unsuccessful IVF cycles made me pessimistic. The medical journey—charting ovulation, planning sex, revolving my entire being around IVF, made me less carefree. Not only did fertility treatment turn me into an anxious worrier, it also made me into a planner, a think-ahead type-A personality instead of a "let's wait and see" type B.

"Is there more pressure to do everything right because you spent so much time and energy on this?" a "regular" mother asked me. God, there is so much pressure to do motherhood right (I could say "parenthood," but that's a blatant lie—Solomon thinks he's a great dad when he gets her outfit on right-side up) that it's hard to imagine something creating even more pressure. "I Did IVF and All I Got Was This Lousy Kid," the souvenir T-shirts should say. Except she's not lousy, she's wonderful. "You the best mama," she says to me.

So maybe infertility wasn't *all* bad for motherhood. By now you must know that I'm not one of those people who searches for silver linings in everything, so there's no way I'm going to be grateful for my struggles to have a baby. But I will say that it made some of early motherhood less daunting. "Oh my God, I lost my life, I have no self!" some new mamas complain. Ha! I long ago lost myself in Hormone City, and spent years at a full-time job called "Waiting in Line at the IVF Clinic."

"I can't believe I have to take all this stuff for the baby just to go on a trip to the grocery store," others complain. For years my head had been so filled with medicine schedules and prognosticating for every possible outcome that packing for an eight-pound baby's outing to Midtown was nothing.

And yes, while I did engage in The Great Stroller Debate of 2016, the stakes were so much lower than IVF that it felt like I was doing it just to belong to the Regular Moms Club.

Once, at my friend Emily's baby shower (she was the single mom doing IVF we met in chapter 4) as everyone went around in a circle to give her a toast or advice, I said, "After years of IVF, nothing will be as hard." Although the moms of teenagers rolled their eyes, no doubt thinking, *You ain't seen nothing yet,* the point I was trying to convey is that infertility is difficult because you don't know if you'll ever succeed. Parenting is challenging, but you have the reward of a kid. And what a reward that is.

No Complaining, IVF Mama!

I will never, ever complain about parenting, I promised myself during those long years of Trying. "Oh, you don't know what tired is until you have kids," an exhausted mom would say, rolling her eyes. "Your body will never be the same," another said, pinching her pouch. "Can't wait to go back to work. These vacation days are killing me," another posted on Facebook.

Of course I never responded to those parents—those ungrateful, insensitive, unappreciative people who didn't know how lucky they were to have kids to complain about. I would have given up all my vacation days just to spend it with my kid.

Or so I told myself.

And then I had a baby. So what if my breasts weren't producing enough milk and my C-section scar wasn't healing and my mother-in-law didn't want me to let the baby cry it out and I would never ever sleep again? I was *NOT* going to complain.

HA!

I mean, seriously. How long can a vow like *that* last? I'll tell you: six months. At half a year I was losing my mind from a baby who wouldn't take a bottle (yup, that meant I couldn't go anywhere for more than three hours) and the sheer exhaustion of it all.

I was ecstatic to have a daughter and be off the IVF train, but I needed to vent, to let off steam, to rant and rave at Solomon or whoever else might have been in a hundred-mile vicinity. Also, isn't that a part of motherhood? Infertility shouldn't steal another rite of passage: complaining. In the age of social media, it seems like an essential part of motherhood.

When I was interminably single, I promised I'd never complain about my spouse, either. But then I got one. *Hello!* I'm human.

I do complain at times about marriage, motherhood, life itself, but I try to do it only to the right people. Just like I don't bitch to my single girlfriends about my husband, I try not to complain to the childless, either.

Going through infertility has made me more sensitive to others because I remember what it was like. I don't remember every hCG beta, every embryo count, every medical protocol. But I do remember the pain, the frustration, the desolation of not having a child.

Having a child—this child, this wonderful, beautiful, adorable person ("I'm not cute, I'm smart!" I've trained her to tell strangers)—is beyond amazing.

"She's incredible," Solomon constantly tells me. Doesn't every parent feel that way? Or just those of us who went through hell and back to get here?

The other day, we took our daughter to the pool and saw her swim, without floaties, for the first time—and she's not even four! A giant balloon of tears welled up in me: I don't care if she becomes a ballerina, goes to Harvard, or cures cancer. That she had so much of me and my love of water in her, that she had achieved so much in such a short time, made me so proud, so incredulous that I get to shepherd her into the world.

There were so many dark days and long nights when I never thought I would get here. I didn't know whether I would recover from a pregnancy loss. I didn't know that I could start fertility treatment, take so many drugs, uproot my life and move across the world, witness the world getting pregnant and moving on without me—me, who was denied the one thing I wanted. I did not know what would become of me, of Solomon, of us together.

Yet here we are, with our curly girl in a mermaid bathing suit flopping around like a fish. Most days the gratitude is too gargantuan to acknowledge, and I have to just pretend to be a regular mom in a regular family. I guess we are a regular family. Regular parents. Regular (extraordinary) kid.

I hope you are all lucky enough to be a parent. You deserve it.

ACKNOWLEDGMENTS

They say that writing a book is like having a baby, but due to my difficult infertility journey and my wonderful writing support network, thankfully birthing this book was a *wee* bit easier.

I can't imagine what it is like to know your every word and fight may be chronicled in a book or in *The New York Times,* so Eyal (*Al P. Solomon*) my love, my shark, thank you for giving me such great material—editorial *and* genetic. (Now let's see if Lily becomes a writer or a musician . . .)

As a journalist, I've always said I need to really look up to *and* like my team in order to produce good work: Allison Hunter, your sharp business sense and self-assured presence has kept this excitable writer in check from signing through auction. (Now if only I could get invited to Seder!) Sara Weiss, I always picture your red pen "marks" dotted with your gorgeous smile: your questions (and Elana Seplow-Jolley's) made this book so much better. Emily Isayeff and Kathleen Quinlan, you've rocked this book to the TOP!

My writing community supported me almost as much as my doctors, so I'll start with the incredible and prolific Sue Shapiro, writing godmother to all (and her invaluable Thursday night gang, Lisa Lewis, Alice Feiring, Rich Prior, Kate Walters, Brenda Copeland, et al.). Dear Abby Sher and Judy Batalion, sorry that you had to watch me cry through every miscarriage.

To My LMWG: Naomi Rand, I could literally not have done this without you, a veritable stranger handing me that list of agents, and telling me *every* step of the way to "just keep writing!" I love how *you* keep writing and can't wait to read it all. Erin Khar, who, by the time this comes out will probably be too famous to read this, but your upbeatness and willingness to hear my downbeats have been invaluable.

To my work wife, Melanie Notkin, I will never talk quietly but I thank you for listening. And to my gay husband, Jeff Leavell—are we there yet??!

Infertility sucks but the support from other people who went through it slays me, as in how much you give back, Jennifer "Jay" Palumbo, Andrea Syrtash, Jake Anderson and Deborah Anderson Bialis, Naomi Less, Angela Le, and the doctors who took my last-minute queries even while doing the more important IVF work: Dr. Aimee Eyvazzadeh, Dr. Janelle Luk, and Dr. Eric Forman.

Dr. Braverman and Lisa O'Brien, I hope you're reading this from Heaven.

"Can I stop talking about infertility now?" is probably what all my friends (fertile, infertile, or never even started Trying) have been thinking forever: Jessica Morgan Richter, Susan Josephs, Yariv Hofstein, Dana Trobe, Keren Goldman, Lisa Barr, Jessica Steinberg, Adeena Sussman, Devorah Blachor, and Danielle Berrin—the answer is NO. But thanks for reading all my drafts of *everything*. Charlotte Crawford (and baby Charlotte) thanks for the great shoot.

And to my dear family, Grammy, and especially Penny Klein Levy, I couldn't ask for a better sister—and without you guys babysitting, these pages would be stained with Bamba and tears.

If you have contributed your story to this book, as a patient, therapist, doctor—your generosity will surely help so many others.

And if you're still Trying? My fingers and toes are crossed for you, wishing "magic baby dust" to all.

NOTES

Prologue

1. Amy Klein, "A Fertility Diary's Happy Ending: Was It All Worth It?," *New York Times,* August 25, 2015, https://parenting.blogs.nytimes .com/author/amy-klein/?_r=0.

1. Oh Shoot, Am I Infertile?

1. U.S. Department of Health and Human Services, Office on Women's Health, "Infertility," WomensHealth.gov, https://www.womenshealth .gov/a-z-topics/infertility.

2. Diana Mansour et al., "Fertility After Discontinuation of Contraception: A Comprehensive Review of the Literature," *Contraception* 84, no. 5 (November 2011).

3. Kurt T. Barnhart et al., "Return to Fertility Following Discontinuation of Oral Contraceptives," *Fertility and Sterility* 91, no. 3: 659–63.

4. American Pregnancy Association, "Pregnancy Symptoms: Early Signs of Pregnancy," AmericanPregnancy.org, http://americanpregnancy .org/getting-pregnant-ebook/p7M7O0q1c71703C/gettingpregnant .pdf.

5. Samantha Pfeifer et al., "Optimizing Natural Fertility: A Committee Opinion," *Fertility and Sterility* 107, no. 1: 52–58.

6. Ibid.

7. Eliahu Levitas et al., "Relationship Between the Duration of Sexual Abstinence and Semen Quality: Analysis of 9,489 Semen Samples," *Fertility and Sterility* 83, no. 6: 1680–86.

8. Rachel Gurevich, "Detecting Ovulation with a Basal Body Temperature Chart," VeryWellFamily.com, November 30, 2016 (updated October 30, 2019), https://www.verywellfamily.com/ovulation-on-body -basal-temperature-chart-1960284.

9. David Dunson et al., "Increased Infertility with Age in Men and Women," *Obstetrics & Gynecology* 103, no. 1 (January 2004).

10. Korula George and Mohan Kamath, "Fertility and Age," *Journal of Human Reproductive Sciences* 3, no. 3 (2010).

11. Jerome Check et al., "Improvement of Cervical Factor with Guaifenesin," *Fertility and Sterility* 37, no. 5 (May 1982).

12. Ibid.

2. Woman, Know Thyself: What You Can Do Before Starting Treatment

1. Elisabeth Rohm and Eve Adamson, *Baby Steps: Having the Child I Always Expected (Just Not as I Expected)* (Boston: Da Capo, 2013).

2. Bat-Sheva Maslow et al., "Lifestyle Factors Do Not Meaningfully Impact Age-Based AMH Levels in Non-Infertile Women," *Obstetrics & Gynecology* 133 (May 2019).

3. S. Deb et al., "Quantifying Effect of Combined Oral Contraceptive Pill on Functional Ovarian Reserve as Measured by Serum Anti-Müllerian Hormone and Small Antral Follicle Count Using Three-Dimensional Ultrasound," *Ultrasound in Obstetrics and Gynecology* 39, no. 5 (May 2012).

4. Anne Z. Steiner et al., "Association Between Biomarkers of Ovarian Reserve and Infertility Among Older Women of Reproductive Age," *JAMA* 318, no. 14 (2017).

5. Judy Rollins, "The Power of Family History," *Pediatric Nursing* 39, no. 3 (August 2013).

6. Centers for Disease Control, "STDs & Infertility," CDC.gov, https://www.cdc.gov/std/infertility/default.htm.

7. PCOS Awareness Association, "Can I Still Get Pregnant with PCOS?,"
    PCOSAA.org, http://www.pcosaa.org/gettingpregnant.

8. Sebastiano Campo et al., "Adenomyosis and Infertility," *Reproductive
    BioMedicine Online* 24, no. 1 (January 2012).

9. Stephan Krotz et al., "Prevalence of Premature Urinary Luteinizing
    Hormone Surges in Women with Regular Menstrual Cycles and Its Ef-
    fect on Implantation of Frozen-Thawed Embryos," *Fertility and Steril-
    ity* 83, no. 6 (June 2005).

10. L. A. Wise et al., "A Prospective Cohort Study of Physical Activity and
    Time to Pregnancy," *Fertility and Sterility* 97, no. 5 (May 2012).

11. Ibid.

3. Mind/Body/Soul/Baby: Is the Alternative Route for Me?

1. Caralynn Lippo, "A Definitive Timeline of Kim Kardashian's Preg-
    nancy Journey, In Her Own Words," *Redbook,* April 14, 2017.

2. "Hard to Swallow," *Nature* 448, no. 106 (July 2007), https://doi.org
    /10.1038/448106a.

3. Daoshing Ni and Dana Herko, *The Tao of Fertility: A Healing Chinese
    Medicine Program to Prepare Body, Mind, and Spirit for New Life* (New
    York: HarperCollins, 2009).

4. "Herbology—Herbalism," Crystalinks.com, http://www.crystalinks
    .com/herbology.html.

5. Zack Andrade, "Nutraceuticals vs. Supplements and 'Functional
    Foods'—What's the Difference Anyways?," SpinacaFarms.com, https://
    spinacafarms.com/nutraceuticals-vs-supplements-functional-foods
    -a-subtle-difference/.

6. Rebecca Fett, *It Starts with the Egg: How the Science of Egg Quality Can
    Help You Get Pregnant Naturally, Prevent Miscarriage, and Improve
    Your Odds in IVF* (New York: Franklin Fox Publishing, 2019).

7. Sedigheh Ahmadi et al., "Antioxidant Supplements and Semen Param-
    eters: An Evidence-Based Review," *International Journal of Reproduc-
    tive Biomedicine* 14, no. 12 (December 2016).

8. Ibid.

9. Ibid.

10. Ibid.

11. Ibid.

12. D. E. Morbeck, "Air Quality in the Assisted Reproduction Laboratory: A Mini-Review," *Journal of Assisted Reproduction and Genetics* 32, no. 7 (August 2015).

13. Mu Yuan et al., "Environmentally Relevant Levels of Bisphenol A Affect Uterine Decidualization and Embryo Implantation Through the Estrogen Receptor/Serum and Glucocorticoid-Regulated Kinase 1/Epithelial Sodium Ion Channel α-Subunit Pathway in a Mouse Model," *Fertility and Sterility* 109, no. 4 (April 2018).

14. Jorge Chavarro et al., "A Prospective Study of Dietary Carbohydrate Quantity and Quality in Relation to Risk of Ovulatory Infertility," *European Journal of Clinical Nutrition* 63, no. 1 (October 2007).

15. Jill Mahrlig Petigara and Lynn Jensen, *Yoga and Fertility: A Journey to Health and Healing* (New York: Demos Health, 2013).

16. Amanda Rice et al., "Ten-Year Retrospective Study on the Efficacy of a Manual Physical Therapy to Treat Female Infertility," *Alternative Therapies in Health and Medicine* 21, no. 3 (February 2015).

17. Eliahu Levitas et al., "Impact of Hypnosis During Embryo Transfer on the Outcome of in Vitro Fertilization–Embryo Transfer: a Case-Control Study," *Fertility and Sterility* 85, no. 5 (May 2006).

18. James Schwartz, *The Mind–Body Fertility Connection: The True Pathway to Conception* (Woodbury, MN: Llewellyn Publications, 2008).

4. I Did It My Way: Single Mothers, LGBTQ Paths to Parenthood, and Freezing Future Fertility

1. Perez Hilton, "My Family. My Words," Huffington Post, October 21, 2017, https://www.huffpost.com/entry/my-family-my-words-perez -hilton_b_59ea9ffae4b02c6e3c609b08.

2. "How to Inseminate," Sperm Bank of California, https://www.the spermbankofca.org/how-to-inseminate.

3. Nicole Vermeer, "Coming to Terms with the Limits of Lesbian Conception," Offbeat Home and Life, January 17, 2011, https://offbeathome .com/lesbian-conception/#comment-1827367.

4. Arielle Yeshua et al., "Female Couples Undergoing IVF with Partner Eggs (Co-IVF): Pathways to Parenthood," *LGBT Health* 2, no. 2 (June 2015).

5. "Same-Sex Couples and Assisted Reproductive Technology," Carlton Fields, November 8, 2013, https://www.carltonfields.com/insights /publications/2013/same-sex-couples-and-assisted-reproductive -technol.

6. Angela Leung et al., "ART Outcomes in Female to Male Transgender Patients: a New Frontier in Reproductive Medicine," *Fertility and Sterility* 109, no. 3 (March 2018).

7. World Professional Association for Transgender Health, *Standards of Care for the Health of Transsexual, Transgender, and Gender Nonconforming People,* version 7 (2012), https://www.wpath.org/publications /soc.

8. Ethics Committee of the American Society for Reproductive Medicine, "Access to Fertility Services by Transgender Persons: An Ethics Committee Opinion," *Fertility and Sterility* 104, no. 5 (November 2015).

9. Tolga B. Mesen et al., "Optimal Timing for Elective Egg Freezing," *Fertility and Sterility* 103, no. 6 (June 2016): 1551–56.e4.

10. Kylie Baldwin et al., "Reproductive Technology and the Life Course: Current Debates and Research in Social Egg Freezing," *Human Fertility* 17, no. 3 (August 2014).

11. Ruthie Ackerman, "Don't Put All Your (Frozen) Eggs in One Basket," *New York Times,* June 19, 2009.

12. Natalie Lampert, "A Modern Woman's Burden," *New Republic,* March 19, 2015.

13. Suzanne Moore, "It's Not a Perk when Big Employers Offer Egg-freezing—It's a Bogus Bribe," *Guardian,* April 26, 2017.

5. Regrets and All the Feels: Getting Your Emotional House in Order

1. Ellen Sarashon Glazer, *The Long-Awaited Stork: A Guide to Parenting After Infertility* (New York: Lexington Books, 1990).

2. Kristin Rooney, "The Relationship Between Stress and Infertility," *Dialogues in Clinical Neuroscience* 20, no. 1 (March 2018).

3. Luba Sominsky et al., "Linking Stress and Infertility: A Novel Role for Ghrelin," *Endocrine Reviews* 38, no. 5 (October 2017).

4. A. J. Massey et al., "Relationship Between Hair and Salivary Cortisol and Pregnancy in Women Undergoing IVF," *Psychoneuroendocrinology* 74 (December 2016).

5. T. L. Ben-Shaanan et al., "Modulation of Anti-Tumor Immunity by the Brain's Reward System," *Nature Communication* 9, no. 2723 (2018), https://doi.org/10.1038/s41467-018-05283-5.

6. J. Boivin et al., "Emotional Distress in Infertile Women and Failure of Assisted Reproductive Technologies: Meta-Analysis of Prospective Psychosocial Studies," *BMJ* 342, no. 7797 (February 2011).

7. Catharina Olivius et al., "Why Do Couples Discontinue In Vitro Fertilization Treatment? A Cohort Study," *Fertility and Sterility* 81, no. 2 (February 2004).

8. J. Jones, "Who Adopts? Characteristics of Women and Men Who Have Adopted Children," *NCHS Data Brief,* February 2009.

9. Katy Lindemann, "Infertility and the Tyranny of Positivity," Medium, September 8, 2018, https://medium.com/@katylindemann/infertility-and-the-tyranny-of-positivity-79b7a96597cb.

6. So Many Doctors, So Little Time: How to Find the Right Clinic

1. Allison P. Davis, "Gabrielle Union Can't Believe She Just Said That," *The Cut* (2017), https://www.thecut.com/2017/10/profile-gabrielle-union-on-her-new-book.html.

2. "Why I Left My Fertility Clinic," Pregnantish survey, https://www.surveymonkey.com/r/pregnantish-patient-experience.

3. Andrew D. A. C. Smith et al., "Live-Birth Rate Associated with Repeat In Vitro Fertilization Treatment Cycles," *JAMA* 314, no. 24 (2015).

4. "Find a Clinic," Society for Assisted Reproductive Technology, https://www.sart.org/clinic-pages/find-a-clinic/.

7. Money, Money, Money

1. *O, The Oprah Magazine,* "*Real Housewives*' Kenya Moore: 'Fibroids Scarred My Uterus—but I Still Got Pregnant at 47,'" October 29, 2018.

2. "Components of IUI Cycle Cost," FertilityIQ, https://www.fertilityiq .com/iui-or-artificial-insemination/the-cost-of-iui#components-of -iui-cycle-cost.

3. Jeanne Sager, "Money over Medicine: 86% of Couples Say No to Fertility Treatment," CoFertility, October 2, 2019, https://cofertility.com /fertility-survey-costs/.

4. "Talk to HR," Progyny, https://progyny.com/talktohr/.

5. "State Laws Related to Insurance Coverage for Infertility Treatment," National Conference of State Legislatures, June 12, 2019, http://www .ncsl.org/research/health/insurance-coverage-for-infertility-laws.aspx.

6. Sager, "Money over Medicine."

7. CCRM Colorado, "Colorado Insurance Program," CCRM Fertility, https://www.ccrmivf.com/colorado/insurance-participation/.

8. Tarun Jain MD, "Socioeconomic and Racial Disparities Among Infertility Patients Seeking Care," *Fertility and Sterility* 85, no. 4 (April 2006), https://www.sciencedirect.com/science/article/pii/S0015028205043256.

9. https://www.sart.org/news-and-publications/news-and-research /press-releases-and-bulletins/ivf-treatments-not-as-successful-in -african-american-women/.

10. Ibid.

11. Ethics Committee of the American Society for Reproductive Medicine, "Disparities in Access to Effective Treatment for Infertility in the United States: An Ethics Committee Opinion," *Fertility and Sterility* 104, vol. 5 (November 2015).

12. L. A. Bishop et al., "African American Patients Experience Reduced Pregnancy, Higher Pregnancy Loss, and Lower Live Birth from IVF Embryo Transfers Despite Producing More Oocytes and More Transfer Quality Embryos Than Caucasian Patients," *Fertility and Sterility* 110, no. 4 (September 2018).

13. William L. Schpero et al., "For Selected Services, Blacks and Hispanics More Likely to Receive Low-Value Care Than Whites," *Health Affairs* 36, no. 6 (2017): 1065–69, https://doi.org/10.1377/hlthaff.2016.1416.

14. Karen Purcell et al., "Asian Ethnicity Is Associated with Reduced Pregnancy Outcomes After Assisted Reproductive Technology," *Fertility and Sterility* 87, no. 2 (February 2007).

8. Are You There, Doc? It's Me, Your Patient: What to Expect on Your First Visit

1. Faith Brar, "Anna Victoria Gets Emotional About Her Struggle with Infertility," *Shape,* https://www.shape.com/lifestyle/mind-and-body/anna-victoria-struggle-infertility-video.

2. Practice Committee of the American Society for Reproductive Medicine, "Effectiveness and Treatment for Unexplained Infertility," *Fertility and Sterility* 86, suppl. 4 (November 2006), https://www.asrm.org/globalassets/asrm/asrm-content/news-and-publications/practice-guidelines/for-non-members/effectiveness_and_treatment_for_unexplained_infertility-pdfnoprint.pdf.

3. "The Fertility Solution," Dr. Attila Toth, MacLeod Laboratory, http://www.fertilitysolution.com.

4. Practice Committee of the American Society for Reproductive Medicine, "Obesity and Reproduction: a Committee Opinion," *Fertility and Sterility* 104, no. 5 (November 2015): 1116–26.

5. Susan Sam, "Obesity and Polycystic Ovary Syndrome," *Obesity Management* 3, no. 2 (April 2007).

6. Samuel J. Chantilis, "Tipping the Scales for Reproduction: a Weighty Problem," *Fertility and Sterility* 111, no. 2 (February 2019): 254–55.

7. Phillip A. Romanski et al., "Effect of Class III and Class IV Obesity on Oocyte Retrieval Complications and Outcomes," *Fertility and Sterility* 111, no. 2 (February 2019): 294–301.e1.

8. Mohammad Reza Sadeghi, "Unexplained infertility, the controversial matter in management of infertile couples," *Journal of Reproduction & Infertility* 16, no. 1 (2015): 1–2.

9. Nora Pashayan et al., "Cost-Effectiveness of Primary Offer of IVF vs. Primary Offer of IUI Followed by IVF (for IUI Failures) in Couples with Unexplained or Mild Male Factor Subfertility," *BMC Health Services Research* 6 (June 2006).

10. Georgina Chambers, "Women Now Have Clearer Statistics on Whether

IVF Is Likely to Work," Conversation, July 23, 2017, https://the conversation.com/women-now-have-clearer-statistics-on-whether -ivf-is-likely-to-work-81256.

11. Reed Tucker, "Sorry, Ladies, There Really Is a Man Shortage," *New York Post,* August 25, 2015, https://nypost.com/2015/08/25/hey-ladies-here -are-8-reasons-youre-single/.

9. The Turkey Baster: The IUI First Try

1. Jon Gosselin, Kate Gosselin, and Beth Carson, *Multiple Bles8ings: Surviving to Thriving with Twins and Sextuplets* (Grand Rapids, MI: Zondervan, 2008).

2. "ASRM 2015: Sperm Count and IUI Pregnancy Rates," Shady Grove Fertility, October 20, 2015, https://www.shadygrovefertility.com/blog /why-shady-grove-fertility/sperm-count-iui-pregnancy-rates/.

3. Laka Dinelli, MD, et al., "Prognosis Factors of Pregnancy After Intrauterine Insemination with the Husband's Sperm: Conclusions of an Analysis of 2,019 Cycles," *Fertility and Sterility* 101, no. 4 (April 2014), https://www.sciencedirect.com/science/article/pii/S00150282140 00399#!.

4. Ibid.

5. Richard H. Reindollar et al., "A Randomized Clinical Trial to Evaluate Optimal Treatment for Unexplained Infertility: The Fast Track and Standard Treatment (FASTT) Trial," *Fertility and Sterility* 94, no. 3 (August 2010): 888–99.

6. Marlene Goldman et al., "A Randomized Clinical Trial to Determine Optimal Infertility Treatment in Older Couples: The Forty and Over Treatment Trial (FORT-T)," *Fertility and Sterility* 101, no. 6 (June 2014).

7. Patsama Vichinsartvichai et al., "The Influence of Women's Age and Successfulness of Intrauterine Insemination (IUI) Cycles," *Journal of the Medical Association of Thailand* 98, no. 9 (September 2015).

8. S. Babbar et al., "A Comparison of Intrauterine Insemination (IUI) Versus In Vitro Fertilization (IVF) in the Era of Pre-Implantation Genetic Testing for Aneuploidy (PGT-A): An Analysis of Efficacy and Cost," *Fertility and Sterility* 110, no. 4 (September 2018), supplement, e203–e204.

10. The Two-Week Wait

1. Shevach Friedler, MD, et al., "The Effect of Medical Clowning on Pregnancy Rates After In Vitro Fertilization and Embryo Transfer," *Fertility and Sterility* 95, no. 6 (May 2011).

2. "Progesterone," WebMD, https://www.webmd.com/vitamins/ai/ingredientmono-760/progesterone.

3. Jen Jones Donatelli, "Weathering the Two-Week Wait After IUI or IVF," *Redbook*, April 30, 2015.

4. "hCG (Human Chorionic Gonadotropin): The Pregnancy Hormone," American Pregnancy Association, http://americanpregnancy.org/while-pregnant/hcg-levels/.

5. "How Early Can You Take a Pregnancy Test?," Early-Pregnancy-Tests, https://www.early-pregnancy-tests.com/early-pregnancy-test.

11. Next Up, IVF: What to Expect During Your First Cycle

1. "Why Tamron Hall Is Being So Open About Her Experiences with IVF," *Allure*, September 17, 2019.

2. Norwegian Institute for Water Research, "Infertile Snails Have Recovered Along the Norwegian Coast," Phys.org, November 29, 2018, https://phys.org/news/2018-11-infertile-snails-recovered-norwegian-coast.html.

3. Anatte E. Karmon and Danielle Y. Sullivan, "Good Outcomes in Small Babies, and the Elephant in the Room," *Fertility and Sterility* 111, no. 5 (May 2019), 887.

4. Ranjith Ramasamy et al., "Male Biological Clock: A Critical Analysis of Advanced Paternal Age," *Fertility and Sterility* 103, no. 6 (June 2015).

5. European Society of Human Reproduction and Embryology, "More Than 8 Million Babies Born from IVF Since the World's First in 1978: European IVF Pregnancy Rates Now Steady at Around 36 Percent, According to ESHRE Monitoring," ScienceDaily, July 3, 2018, https://www.sciencedaily.com/releases/2018/07/180703084127.htm.

6. Gabor Kovacs, Peter Brinsden, and Alan DeCherney, *In-Vitro Fertilization: The Pioneers' History* (New York: Cambridge University Press, 2019).

7. M. Kdous et al., "Short vs. Long Agonist Protocols in Poor Responders Undergoing IVF," *Tunis Med* 92, no. 10 (October 2014), 604–609, French.

8. Rachel Gurevich, "The Chances for IVF Pregnancy Success," Verywell Family, September 13, 2019, https://www.verywellfamily.com/what -are-the-chances-for-ivf-success-1960213.

9. F. W. Grimstad et al., "Use of ICSI in IVF Cycles in Women with Tubal Ligation Does Not Improve Pregnancy or Live Birth Rates," *Human Reproduction* 31, no. 12 (December 2016).

10. Duke University Medical Center, "For Women Undergoing IVF, Is Fresh or Frozen Embryo Transfer Best? Some Women Benefit from a Fresh Embryo Transfer While Others Benefit from Delay," Science-Daily, August 21, 2018.

11. Practice Committees of the American Society for Reproductive Medicine and the Society for Assisted Reproductive Technology, "Blastocyst Culture and Transfer in Clinically Assisted Reproduction: a Committee Opinion," *Fertility and Sterility* 99, no. 3 (March 1, 2013).

12. Alan Penzias et al., "Guidance on the Limits to the Number of Embryos to Transfer: a Committee Opinion," *Fertility and Sterility* 107, no. 4 (April 2017), 901–903.

13. Jae Eun Lee et al., "Oocyte Maturity in Repeated Ovarian Stimulation," *Clinical and Experimental Reproductive Medicine* 38, no. 4 (December 2011).

14. "Ovarian Hyperstimulation Syndrome (OHSS)," American Society for Reproductive Medicine, https://www.asrm.org/topics/topics-index /ovarian-hyperstimulation-syndrome-ohss/.

12. So, You're Pregnant! What to Expect Before You're Home Free

1. Jen Juneau and Abby Stern, "Julianne Hough Calls Being Open About Her IVF Journey with Husband Brooks Laich 'Liberating,'" *People,* October 18, 2019.

2. Robert L. Barbieri, MD, "Stop Using the hCG Discriminatory Zone of 1,500 to 2,000 mIU/mL to Guide Intervention During Early Pregnancy," *OBG Management* 27, no. 1 (January 2015).

3. L. Sekhon et al., "Interpreting Early hCG Dynamics in the Era of the Thawed Euploid Single Embryo Transfer: How Important Is Doubling?," *Fertility and Sterility* 106, no. 3 (September 2016), supplement, e341–e342.

4. A BabyCenter Member, "Hope for a Pregnancy with Slow Rising hCG Levels?: Mom Answers," Q&A question posted December 29, 2009, https://www.babycenter.com/400_hope-for-a-pregnancy-with-slow-rising-hcg-levels_6646399_221.bc.

5. Beata E. Seeber, MD, "What Serial hCG Can Tell You, and Cannot Tell You, About an Early Pregnancy," *Fertility and Sterility* 98, no. 5 (November 2012): 1074–77.

6. L. Sekhon et al., "Interpreting Early hCG Dynamics in the Era of the Thawed Euploid Single Embryo Transfer: How Important Is Doubling?," *Fertility and Sterility* 106, no. 3 (September 2016): e341–e342.

7. Amanda Barrell, "Subchorionic Bleeding: Causes, Symptoms, and Risks," Medical News Today, https://www.medicalnewstoday.com/articles/323307.php.

8. "hCG (Human Chorionic Gonadotropin): The Pregnancy Hormone," American Pregnancy Association, https://americanpregnancy.org/while-pregnant/hcg-levels/.

9. "What Is a High-Risk Pregnancy?," Eunice Kennedy Shriver National Institute of Child Health and Human Development, https://www.nichd.nih.gov/health/topics/pregnancy/conditioninfo/high-risk#f6.

13. It's Not You, It's Him: Male Factor Infertility

1. Practice Committee of the American Society for Reproductive Medicine, "Diagnostic Evaluation of the Infertile Male: a Committee Opinion," *Fertility and Sterility* 103, no. 3 (March 2015): e18–e25.

2. Ibid.

3. L. Simon et al., "Paternal Influence of Sperm DNA Integrity on Early Embryonic Development," *Human Reproduction* 29, no. 11 (November 2014).

4. S. E. Lewis et al., "The Impact of Sperm DNA Damage in Assisted Conception and Beyond: Recent Advances in Diagnosis and Treatment," *Reproductive BioMedicine Online* 27, no. 4 (October 2013).

5. Mohamed A. M. Hassan et al., "Effect of Male Age on Fertility: Evidence for the Decline in Male Fertility with Increasing Age," *Fertility and Sterility* 79, supp. 3 (June 2003): 1520–27.

6. E. Callaway, "Fathers Bequeath More Mutations as They Age," *Nature* 488, no. 7412 (August 2012).

7. S. L. Johnson et al., "Consistent Age-Dependent Declines in Human Semen Quality: a Systematic Review and Meta-Analysis," *Ageing Research Reviews,* January 2015.

8. N. Phillips et al., "Maternal, Infant and Childhood Risks Associated with Advanced Paternal Age: the Need for Comprehensive Counseling for Men," *Maturitas* 125 (July 2019).

9. Akanksha Mehta, MD, et al., "Limitations and Barriers in Access to Care for Male Factor Infertility," *Fertility and Sterility* 105, no. 5 (May 2016).

10. Practice Committee of the American Society for Reproductive Medicine, "Diagnostic Evaluation of the Infertile Male: a Committee Opinion," *Fertility and Sterility* 103, no. 3 (March 2015): e18–e25.

11. G. Y. Kim, "What Should Be Done for Men with Sperm DNA Fragmentation?," *Clinical and Experimental Reproductive Medicine* 45, no. 3 (September 2018).

12. C. Foresta et al., "Y Chromosome Microdeletions and Alterations of Spermatogenesis," *Endocrine Reviews* 22, no. 2 (April 2001).

13. "How Can You Reverse a Vasectomy?," WebMD, https://www.webmd .com/infertility-and-reproduction/guide/reversing-a-vasectomy#1.

14. P. J. Turek, "Practical Approaches to the Diagnosis and Management of Male Infertility," *Nature Clinical Practice Urology* 2, no. 5 (May 2005).

15. M. R. Debaun et al., "Association of In Vitro Fertilization with Beckwith-Wiedemann Syndrome and Epigenetic Alterations of LIT1 and H19," *American Journal of Human Genetics* 72, no. 1 (January 2003).

16. Kieron Barclay et al., "Reproductive History and Post-Reproductive Mortality: a Sibling Comparison Analysis Using Swedish Register Data," *Social Science & Medicine* 155 (April 2016).

17. Brent M. Hanson et al., "Male Infertility: a Biomarker of Individual and Familial Cancer Risk," *Fertility and Sterility* 109, no. 1 (January 2018): 6–19.

18. T. J. Walsh et al., "Increased Risk of Testicular Germ Cell Cancer Among Infertile Men," *Archives of Internal Medicine* 169, no. 4 (February 2009).

19. Frida E. Lundberg et al., "Mortality in 43,598 Men with Infertility—a Swedish Nationwide Population-Based Cohort Study," *Clinical Epidemiology* 11 (2019).

20. James F. Smith et al., "Sexual, Marital, and Social Impact of a Man's Perceived Infertility Diagnosis," *Journal of Sexual Medicine* 6, no. 9 (September 2009): 2505–15.

21. Liberty Walther Barnes, *Conceiving Masculinity: Male Infertility, Medicine and Identity* (Philadelphia: Temple University Press, 2014).

14. In Sickness and in Health: How to Preserve Your Partnership

1. Michelle Obama, *Becoming* (New York: Crown, 2018).

2. T. Sujatha, "A Study to Assess the Level of Stress Among Women with Primary Infertility Attending the Infertility Clinic at SRM General Hospital," *International Journal of Pharmacy and Biological Sciences* 6, no. 1 (January–March 2016).

3. B. D. Peterson et al., "Gender Differences in How Men and Women Who Are Referred for IVF Cope with Infertility Stress," *Human Reproduction* 21, no. 9 (September 2006).

4. T. D. Gundersen et al., "Association Between Use of Marijuana and Male Reproductive Hormones and Semen Quality: A Study Among 1,215 Healthy Young Men," *American Journal of Epidemiology* 182, no. 6 (September 2015).

5. A. D. A. C. Smith et al., "Live-Birth Rate Associated with Repeat In Vitro Fertilization Treatment Cycles," *JAMA* 314, no. 24 (December 2015).

6. Lori Gottlieb, *Maybe You Should Talk to Someone: A Therapist, Her Therapist, and Our Lives Revealed* (Boston: Houghton Mifflin Harcourt, 2019).

7. Gemma Hartley, *Fed Up: Emotional Labor, Women, and the Way Forward* (New York: HarperOne, 2018).

8. Leah S. Millheiser et al., "Is Infertility a Risk Factor for Female Sexual

Dysfunction? A Case-Control Study," *Fertility and Sterility* 94, no. 6 (November 2010): 2022–25.

9. Beth Jaeger-Skigen, LCSW, "Sex & Infertility: How to Reconnect Sexually During Infertility," FertilityIQ, https://www.fertilityiq.com/topics /mental-health-and-infertility/sex-and-infertility-how-to-reconnect -sexually-during-infertility.

10. T. Kjaer et al., "Divorce or End of Cohabitation Among Danish Women Evaluated for Fertility Problems," *Acta Obstetricia et Gynecologica Scandinavica* 93, no. 3 (March 2014).

11. Y. Che and J. Cleland, "Infertility in Shanghai: Prevalence, Treatment Seeking and Impact," *Journal of Obstetrics and Gynaecology* 22, no. 6 (November 2002).

12. Mariana V. Martins et al., "Marital Stability and Repartnering: Infertility-Related Stress Trajectories of Unsuccessful Fertility Treatment," *Fertility and Sterility* 102, no. 6 (December 2014).

13. European Society of Human Reproduction and Embryology, "Fertility Treatment Does Not Increase the Risk of Divorce: Huge population study of more than 40,000 women finds no link between IVF and relationship break-up," ScienceDaily, July 5, 2017.

14. L. Schmidt et al., "Does Infertility Cause Marital Benefit?," *Patient Education and Counseling* 59, no. 3 (December 2005).

15. Defending Your Life: How to Have One During Treatment

1. Peter S. Finamore et al., "Social Concerns of Women Undergoing Infertility Treatment," *Fertility and Sterility* 88, no. 4, 817–821.

2. "The FertilityIQ Family Builder Workplace Index: 2017–2018," Fertility IQ, https://www.fertilityiq.com/fertilityiq-data-and-notes/fertilityiq -best-companies-to-work-for-family-builder-workplace-index-2017 -2018.

3. Sara Berg, "AMA Backs Global Health Experts in Calling Infertility a Disease," June 13, 2017, American Medical Association, https://www .ama-assn.org/delivering-care/public-health/ama-backs-global-health -experts-calling-infertility-disease/.

4. *Bragdon v. Abbott,* 524 U.S. 624 (1998), https://en.wikipedia.org/wiki /Bragdon_v._Abbott.

5. Americans with Disabilities Act of 1990, original text, Equal Employment Opportunity Commission, https://www.eeoc.gov/eeoc/history/35th/thelaw/ada.html.

6. Susan Schoenfeld, JD, "Infertility Treatments and the FMLA, ADA, and PDA," HR Daily Advisor, September 3, 2015, https://hrdaily advisor.blr.com/2015/09/03/infertility-treatments-and-the-fmla-ada-and-pda/.

7. "Enforcement Guidance: Pregnancy Discrimination and Related Issues," US Equal Employment Opportunity Commission, June 25, 2015, https://www.eeoc.gov/laws/guidance/pregnancy_guidance.cfm.

8. Merck & Co. Inc., "New Survey Finds Infertility Delivers a Serious Blow to Self-Esteem," PR Newswire, January 21, 2010, https://www.prnewswire.com/news-releases/new-survey-finds-infertility-delivers-a-serious-blow-to-self-esteem-82242177.html.

16. You Gotta Have Faith: How Religion, Prayer, and Community Can Help

1. K. Y. Cha, "Does Prayer Influence the Success of In Vitro Fertilization-Embryo Transfer? Report of a Masked, Randomized Trial," *Journal of Reproductive Medicine* 46, no. 9 (September 2001): 7817.

2. H. Benson et al., "Study of the Therapeutic Effects of Intercessory Prayer (STEP) in Cardiac Bypass Patients: a Multicenter Randomized Trial of Uncertainty and Certainty of Receiving Intercessory Prayer," *American Heart Journal* 151, no. 4 (April 2006).

3. Ibid.

4. John P. Bartkowski et al., "Prayer, Meditation, and Anxiety: Durkheim Revisited," *Religions* 8, no. 9 (September 2017).

5. Harold G. Koenig, MD, "Religion, Spirituality, and Medicine: Application to Clinical Practice," *JAMA* 284, no. 13 (October 2000).

6. Ibid.

7. Harold Koenig et al., "Does Religious Attendance Prolong Survival? A Six-Year Follow-Up Study of 3,968 Older Adults," *Journals of Gerontology Series A: Biological Sciences and Medical Sciences* 54, no. 7 (July 1999).

8. R. A. Hummer et al., "Religious Involvement and U.S. Adult Mortality," *Demography* 36, no. 2 (May 1999).

9. H. G. Koenig et al., "Does Religious Attendance Prolong Survival? A Six-Year Follow-Up Study of 3,968 Older Adults," *Journals of Gerontology Series A: Biological Sciences and Medical Sciences* 54, no. 7 (July 1999).

10. J. Tartaro et al., "Exploring Heart and Soul: Effects of Religiosity/Spirituality and Gender on Blood Pressure and Cortisol Stress Responses," *Journal of Health Psychology* 10, no. 6 (November 2005).

11. Richard V. Grazi, *Overcoming Infertility: A Guide for Jewish Couples* (Jerusalem: Toby Press, 2005).

12. G. R. Weitzman and H. J. Lieman, "Is Testicular Sperm Extraction Permitted by Jewish Law (Halachah)?," *Fertility and Sterility* 88, supp. 1 (September 2007): S393.

13. Ebony Bowden, "California Couple Opens Up About 'Heartbreaking' IVF Mix-Up," *New York Post,* July 10, 2019.

14. "What Does the Church Teach About IVF?," Catholics Come Home, https://www.catholicscomehome.org/what-does-the-church-teach-about-ivf/.

15. Nikita Popov, "Orthodox Pastors on What Should We Do If the Lord Does Not Grant Us Children," Orthodox Christianity, http://orthochristian.com/94626.html.

16. "What Is the INVOcell™ Procedure and Could It Help Me?," Fertility Institute Blog, September 11, 2018, https://fertilityinstitute.com/what-is-the-invocell-procedure-and-could-it-help-me/.

17. St. Paul VI Institute, http://www.popepaulvi.com.

18. Elizabeth Laing Thompson, *When God Says Wait: Navigating Life's Detours and Delays Without Losing Your Faith, Your Friends, or Your Mind* (Urichsville, OH: Shiloh Run Press, 2017).

19. Anonymous, "Infertility Prayer," Beliefnet, https://www.beliefnet.com/prayers/catholic/healing/infertility-prayer.aspx.

20. "Muslim Pregnancy Prayers," compiled by Dilshad Ali, Beliefnet, https://www.beliefnet.com/faiths/prayer/2009/07/muslim-pregnancy-prayers.aspx?p=2#yp3AkpOzcbdG7KuQ.99.

17. Baby Envy: Living with the Green-Eyed Monster

1. K. L. Schwerdtfeger and K. M. Shreffler, "Trauma of Pregnancy Loss and Infertility Among Mothers and Involuntarily Childless Women in the United States," *Journal of Loss and Trauma* 14, no. 3 (2009).

2. Enikő Lakatos et al., "Anxiety and Depression Among Infertile Women: A Cross-sectional Survey from Hungary," *Women's Health* 17, no. 1 (July 2017).

3. "The Psychological Impact of Infertility and Its Treatment," Harvard Health Publishing, May 2009, https://www.health.harvard.edu/news letter_article/The-psychological-impact-of-infertility-and-its -treatment.

18. I Will Survive: Perseverance and How to Keep On Keeping On

1. Linda Graham, *Resilience: Powerful Practices for Bouncing Back from Disappointment, Difficulty, and Even Disaster* (Novato, CA: New World Library, 2019).

19. The Women in Waiting (Room)

1. Sara Reardon, "Genetic Details of Controversial 'Three-Parent Baby' Revealed," *Nature,* April 3, 2017.

2. I. Gurol-Urganci et al., "Impact of Caesarean Section on Subsequent Fertility: a Systematic Review and Meta-Analysis," *Human Reproduction* 28, no. 7 (July 2013).

3. S. Tanimura et al., "New Diagnostic Criteria and Operative Strategy for Cesarean Scar Syndrome: Endoscopic Repair for Secondary Infertility Caused by Cesarean Scar Defect," *Journal of Obstetrics and Gynaecology Research* 41, no. 9 (September 2015).

4. Ethics Committee of the American Society for Reproductive Medicine, "Fertility Preservation and Reproduction in Patients Facing Gonadotoxic Therapies: an Ethics Committee Opinion," *Fertility and Sterility Dialog* 110, no. 3 (May 2018), https://www.fertstertdialog.com/users /16110-fertility-%20and-sterility/posts/33705-26389.

5. K. Oktay et al., "Fertility Preservation in Patients with Cancer: ASCO Clinical Practice Guideline Update," *Journal of Clinical Oncology* 36, no. 19 (July 2018).

6. ASRM Ethics Committee, "Fertility Preservation and Reproduction in Patients Facing Gonadotoxic Therapies."

7. David Sable, "Since When Is Preventive Medicine Elective? Egg Freezing. Is. Healthcare," *Forbes,* August 22, 2019.

8. A quote by Regina Brett, https://www.goodreads.com/quotes/127360 -if-we-all-threw-our-problems-in-a-pile-and.

20: The Whole IVF Toolbox: Trying Everything

1. "Pregnant Molly Sims Opens Up About Her Fertility Journey," *Us Weekly,* November 2, 2016.

2. J. J. Zhang et al., "Minimal Stimulation IVF vs Conventional IVF: A Randomized Controlled Trial," *American Journal of Obstetrics and Gynecology* 214, no. 1 (January 2016).

3. Y. G. Wu et al., "Aging-Related Premature Luteinization of Granulosa Cells Is Avoided by Early Oocyte Retrieval," *Journal of Endocrinology* 226, no. 3 (September 2015).

4. Norbert Gleicher et al., "Older Women Using Their Own Eggs? Issue Framed with Two Oldest Reported IVF Pregnancies and a Live Birth," *Reproductive BioMedicine Online* 37, no. 2 (August 2018): 172–77.

5. Eric J. Forman, "Morphology Matters: Are All Euploid Blastocysts Created Equal?," *Fertility and Sterility* 107, no. 3 (March 2017): 573–74.

6. Zev Rosenwaks et al., "The Pros and Cons of Preimplantation Genetic Testing for Aneuploidy: Clinical and Laboratory Perspectives," *Fertility and Sterility* 110, no. 3 (August 2018): 353–61.

7. Emily K. Osman and Marie D. Werner, "Mosaic Embryos Present a Challenging Clinical Decision," *Fertility and Sterility* 111, no. 1 (January 2019): 52–53.

8. P. R. Brezina et al., "Preimplantation Genetic Testing for Aneuploidy: What Technology Should You Use and What Are the Differences?," *Journal of Assisted Reproduction and Genetics* 33, no. 7 (July 2016).

9. Osman and Werner, "Mosaic Embryos Present a Challenging Clinical Decision," *Fertility and Sterility* 111, no. 1 (January 2019): 52–53.

10. Santiago Munné et al., "Mosaicism: 'Survival of the Fittest' Versus 'No Embryo Left Behind,'" *Fertility and Sterility* 105, no. 5 (May 2016): 1146–49.

11. Final Clinic Summary Report for 2016, Colorado Institute for Reproductive Medicine, https://www.sartcorsonline.com/rptCSR_Public MultYear.aspx?ClinicPKID=1902.

12. Ibid.

13. Jennifer Knudston, MD, and Jessica E. McLaughlin, MD, "Menstrual Cycle," Merck Manual Consumer Version, last reviewed/revised April 2019, https://www.merckmanuals.com/home/women-s-health-issues /biology-of-the-female-reproductive-system/menstrual-cycle.

14. John Zhang, "Luteal Phase Ovarian Stimulation Following Oocyte Retrieval: Is It Helpful for Poor Responders?," *Reproductive Biology and Endocrinology* 13, no. 1 (July 2015).

15. Alberto Vaiarelli et al., "Double Stimulation in the Same Ovarian Cycle (DuoStim) to Maximize the Number of Oocytes Retrieved from Poor Prognosis Patients: A Multicenter Experience and SWOT Analysis," *Frontiers in Endocrinology,* June 2018.

16. Carol B. Hanna et al., "Ovarian Germline Stem Cells: an Unlimited Source of Oocytes?," *Fertility and Sterility* 101, no. 1 (January 2014): 20–30.

17. Elena Labarta et al., "Mitochondria as a Tool for Oocyte Rejuvenation," *Fertility and Sterility* 111, no. 2 (February 2019): 219–26.

18. Mindy S. Christianson et al., "Unleashing the Potential of Stem Cells to Help Poor Responders," *Fertility and Sterility* 110, no. 3 (August 2018): 410–11.

19. Rubina Alves and Ramon Grimalt, "A Review of Platelet-Rich Plasma: History, Biology, Mechanism of Action, and Classification," *Skin Appendage Disorders* 4 (January 2018).

20. Mike Dickson, "Rafael Nadal: How Broken Star Was Rebuilt," *Daily Mail,* October 7, 2013.

21. https://www.nyfertility.org/wp-content/uploads/2017/04/ESHRE -Abstract.pdf.

22. Konstantinos Sfakianoudis et al., "Autologous Platelet-Rich Plasma Treatment Enables Pregnancy for a Woman in Premature Menopause," *Journal of Clinical Medicine* 8, no. 1 (December 2018).

23. E. S. Sills et al., "First Data on In Vitro Fertilization and Blastocyst Formation After Intraovarian Injection of Calcium Gluconate–Activated Autologous Platelet Rich Plasma," *Gynecological Endocrinology* 34, no. 9 (September 2018).

24. D. Obidniak et al., "Randomized Controlled Trial Evaluating Efficacy of Autologous Platelet-Rich Plasma Therapy for Patients with Recurrent Implantation Failure," *Fertility and Sterility* 108, no. 3 (September 2017): e370.

25. M. Farimani et al., "A Report on Three Live Births in Women with Poor Ovarian Response Following Intra-Ovarian Injection of Platelet-Rich Plasma (PRP)," *Molecular Biology Reports* 46, no. 2 (April 2019).

26. Amerigo Vitagliano et al., "Endometrial Scratching for Infertile Women Undergoing a First Embryo Transfer: a Systematic Review and Meta-Analysis of Published and Unpublished Data from Randomized Controlled Trials," *Fertility and Sterility* 111, no. 4 (April 2019): 734–46.e2.

21. Miscarriages: When a Pregnancy Ends

1. Yvonne Butler Tobah, MD, "Blighted Ovum: What Causes It?," Mayo Clinic, August 15, 2019, https://www.mayoclinic.org/diseases-conditions/pregnancy-loss-miscarriage/expert-answers/blighted-ovum/faq-20057783.

2. S. F. Vitez et al., "Preimplantation Genetic Diagnosis in Early Pregnancy Loss," *Seminars in Perinatology* 43, no. 2 (March 2019).

3. B. Refaat et al., "Ectopic Pregnancy Secondary to In Vitro Fertilisation–Embryo Transfer: Pathogenic Mechanisms and Management Strategies," *Reproductive Biology and Endocrinology* 13 (April 2015).

4. Ibid.

5. Amos Grunebaum, "One Ectopic Often Predicts Another," https://www.webpages.uidaho.edu/ngier/ectopicagain.htm.

6. Ariel Levy, *The Rules Do Not Apply: A Memoir* (New York: Random House, 2017).

7. William L. Ledger et al., "Implementation of the Findings of a National Enquiry into the Misdiagnosis of Miscarriage in the Republic of Ire-

land: Impact on Quality of Clinical Care," *Fertility and Sterility* 105, no. 2 (February 2016): 417–22.

8. J. Preisler et al., "Defining Safe Criteria to Diagnose Miscarriage: Prospective Observational Multicentre Study," *BMJ* 351 (September 2015).

9. Ibid.

10. Kavita Nanda et al., "Expectant care versus surgical treatment for miscarriage," *Cochrane Database of Systematic Reviews* 3 (2012).

11. J. Trinder et al., "Management of Miscarriage: Expectant, Medical, or Surgical? Results of Randomised Controlled Trial (Miscarriage Treatment (MIST) Trial)," *BMJ* 332 (May 2006).

12. J. M. Shorter et al., "Management of Early Pregnancy Loss, with a Focus on Patient Centered Care," *Seminars in Perinatology* 43, no. 2 (March 2019).

13. A. N. Lamb et al., "Defining the Impact of Maternal Cell Contamination on the Interpretation of Prenatal Microarray Analysis," *Genetics in Medicine* 14, no. 11 (November 2012).

14. Katherine Zeratsky, "Has the hCG Diet Been Shown to Be Safe and Effective?," Mayo Clinic, October 19, 2019, https://www.mayoclinic.org/healthy-lifestyle/weight-loss/expert-answers/hcg-diet/faq-20058164.

15. J. A. Vázquez-Boland et al., "Listeria Placental Infection," *mBio* 8, no. 3 (June 2017).

16. J. Bardos et al., "A National Survey on Public Perceptions of Miscarriage," *Obstetrics & Gynecology* 125, no. 6 (June 2015).

17. "What Is Stillbirth?," CDC, https://www.cdc.gov/ncbddd/stillbirth/facts.html.

18. K. C. Schliep et al., "Trying to Conceive After an Early Pregnancy Loss," *Obstetrics & Gynecology* 127, no. 2 (February 2016).

22. Repeat Pregnancy Loss: Do You Have Immunological Issues?

1. Katie Price, *You Only Live Once: Heartache, Happiness and New Beginnings* (London: Century, 2010).

2. A. M. Kolte et al., "Depression and Emotional Stress Is Highly Prevalent Among Women with Recurrent Pregnancy Loss," *Human Reproduction* 30, no. 4 (April 2015).

3. Lora Shahine, *Not Broken: An Approachable Guide to Miscarriage and Recurrent Pregnancy Loss* (Seattle: printed by the author, 2017).

4. Kolte et al., "Depression and Emotional Stress."

5. F. Popescu et al., "Recurrent Pregnancy Loss Evaluation Combined with 24-Chromosome Microarray of Miscarriage Tissue Provides a Probable or Definite Cause of Pregnancy Loss in over 90% of Patients," *Human Reproduction* 33, no. 4 (April 2018).

6. A. Bashiri et al., "Recurrent Implantation Failure—Update Overview on Etiology, Diagnosis, Treatment and Future Directions," *Reproductive Biology and Endocrinology* 16, no. 1 (December 2018).

7. Alan E. Beer, "Fetal Erythrocytes in Maternal Circulation of 155 Rh-Negative Women," *Obstetrics and Gynecology* 34, no. 2 (August 1969).

8. O. B. Christiansen, "Reproductive Immunology," *Molecular Immunology* 55, no. 1 (August 2013).

9. "When a Patient Should Consult with Us," BRI Reproductive Immunology & Endometriosis Surgical Center, https://www.preventmiscarriage.com/when-should-a-patient-consult-with-us-.html.

10. R. D. Franklin and W. H. Kutteh, "Antiphospholipid Antibodies (APA) and Recurrent Pregnancy Loss: Treating a Unique APA Positive Population," *Human Reproduction* 17, no. 11 (November 2002).

11. Carolyn Katovich Hurley, PhD, "KIR: Can Anything Be More Complex Than HLA?," Clinical Research Professionals Data Management Conference, San Diego 2012, https://www.cibmtr.org/Meetings/Materials/CRPDMC/Documents/2012/Feb%202012/HurleyC_KIR.pdf.

12. P. Parasar et al., "Endometriosis: Epidemiology, Diagnosis and Clinical Management," *Current Obstetrics and Gynecology Reports* 6, no. 1 (March 2017).

13. "About ReceptivaDx™," ReceptivaDx, https://receptivadx.com/women-families/about-receptiva-testing/.

14. C. Tomassetti et al., "Endometriosis, Recurrent Miscarriage and Implantation Failure: Is There an Immunological Link?," *Reproductive BioMedicine Online* 13, no. 1 (July 2006).

15. C. Pallacks et al., "Endometriosis Doubles Odds for Miscarriage in Pa-

tients Undergoing IVF or ICSI," *European Journal of Obstetrics & Gynecology and Reproductive Biology* 213 (June 2017).

16. S. Lalani et al., "Endometriosis and Adverse Maternal, Fetal and Neonatal Outcomes, a Systematic Review and Meta-Analysis," *Human Reproduction* 33, no. 10 (October 2018).

17. K. Kuroda, "Impaired Endometrial Function and Unexplained Recurrent Pregnancy Loss," *Hypertension Research in Pregnancy* 7, no. 1 (March 2019).

18. Jeffrey Braverman, MD, "Outsmarting Endo—Diagnosing Silent Endometriosis," Endometriosis Foundation of America, 2014, https://www.endofound.org/jeffrey-braverman-md-outsmarting-endo.

19. "Laparoscopic Surgery for Endometriosis," HealthLink BC, https://www.healthlinkbc.ca/health-topics/hw101171.

20. T. Sapir et al., "Intravenous Immunoglobulin (IVIG) as Treatment for Recurrent Pregnancy Loss (RPL)," *Harefuah* 144, no. 6 (June 2005).

21. Lareina, "IVIG Therapy," https://www.cnyfertility.com/ivig-therapy/.

22. Laith Alshawabkeh et al., "Anticoagulation During Pregnancy: Evolving Strategies with a Focus on Mechanical Valves," *Journal of the American College of Cardiology* 68, no. 11 (October 2016), http://www.onlinejacc.org/content/68/16/1804.

23. T. Tang et al., "The Use of Metformin for Women with PCOS Undergoing IVF Treatment," *Human Reproduction* 21, no. 6 (June 2006).

24. "Results of the Survey—Reproductive Immunology Practice in IVF," IVF Worldwide, https://ivf-worldwide.com/survey/reproductive-immunology-practice-in-ivf/results-reproductive-immunology-practice-in-ivf.html.

25. Carolyn Coulam, "Commentary on Current Trends of Reproductive Immunology Practices in IVF: A First World Survey Using IVF-worldwide.com," *American Journal of Reproductive Immunology* 69, no. 2 (December 2012).

26. "Recurrent Pregnancy Loss," Stanford Children's Health, https://www.stanfordchildrens.org/en/service/fertility-and-reproductive-health/recurrent-pregnancy-loss.

27. G. Sacks, "Enough! Stop the Arguments and Get On with the Science of Natural Killer Cell Testing," *Human Reproduction* 30, no. 7 (July 2015).

28. A. Moffett and N. Shreeve, "First Do No Harm: Uterine Natural Killer

(NK) Cells in Assisted Reproduction," *Human Reproduction* 30, no. 7 (July 2015).

29. Aimee E. Raupp, *Body Belief: How to Heal Autoimmune Diseases, Radically Shift Your Health, and Learn to Love Your Body More* (Carlsbad, CA: Hay House, Inc., 2019).

23. Donor, Where Art Thou? Donor Eggs, Sperm, Embryos, and Surrogacy

1. Taryn Ryder, "Lucy Liu Opens Up About Her Journey to Motherhood: 'I Know People Had Opinions About How It Was Done,'" Yahoo! Entertainment, May 5, 2016, https://www.yahoo.com/entertainment/lucy-liu-opens-up-about-her-journey-to-motherhood-233010909.html.

2. Rene Almeling, "The Unregulated Sperm Industry," *New York Times,* November 30, 2013.

3. "Embryo Donation vs. Adoption—What's the Difference?," Embryo Adoption Awareness Center, January 17, 2011, https://embryoadoption.org/2011/01/embryo-donation-vs-adoption-whats-the-difference/.

4. Marna Gatlin and Carole LieberWilkins, MFT, *Let's Talk About Egg Donation: Real Stories from Real People* (Bloomington, IN: Archway Publishing, 2019).

5. Phyllis Martin, "Women, Grief, and the Donor Egg Decision," RESOLVE New England, January 28, 2013, https://www.resolvenewengland.org/2013/01/women-grief-and-the-donor-egg-decision/.

6. "Any experience with donating eggs to family member?," Babycenter (posted by ashleymduncan), https://community.babycenter.com/post/a6365785/any_experience_with_donating_eggs_to_family_member.

7. Christine Barberich, "After 7 Miscarriages, the Surprise I Wasn't Expecting . . . ," Refinery29, September 24, 2018.

8. Alexandra Kimball, *The Seed: Infertility Is a Feminist Issue* (Toronto: Coach House Books, 2019).

24. The End of the Road: Life After No Baby

1. Lena Dunham, "In Her Own Words: Lena Dunham on Her Decision to Have a Hysterectomy at 31," *Vogue,* February 14, 2018.

2. Sigal Klipstein et al., "One Last Chance for Pregnancy: a Review of 2,705 In Vitro Fertilization Cycles Initiated in Women Age 40 Years and Above," *Fertility and Sterility* 84, no. 2 (August 2005): 435–45.

3. Pamela Mahoney Tsigdinos, *Silent Sorority: A (Barren) Woman Gets Busy, Angry, Lost and Found* (BookSurge Publishing, 2013).

4. Lisa Manterfield, *Life Without Baby: Surviving and Thriving When Motherhood Doesn't Happen* (Redonda Beach, CA: Steel Rose Press, 2015).

5. Jody Day, *Living the Life Unexpected: 12 Weeks to Your Plan B for a Meaningful and Fulfilling Future Without Children* (London: Bluebird, 2016).

6. G. L. Lee et al., "Life After Unsuccessful IVF Treatment in an Assisted Reproduction Unit," *Human Reproduction* 24, no. 8 (August 2009), https://www.ncbi.nlm.nih.gov/pubmed/19372145.

7. Ibid.

8. Melanie Notkin, *Otherhood: Modern Women Finding a New Kind of Happiness* (Berkeley, CA: Seal Press, 2014).

9. Jo Jones, "Who Adopts? Characteristics of Women and Men Who Have Adopted Children," *NCHS Data Brief* no. 12 (January 2009), https://www.cdc.gov/nchs/products/databriefs/db12.htm.

10. Farai Chideya, interview with Lulu Garcia-Navarro, "Experiences Attempting Adoption: 'Excuse Me, May I Raise Your Child?,'" *Weekend Edition Sunday,* NPR, July 14, 2019.

Epilogue: Pregnancy and Motherhood After Infertility

1. Pietro Gambadauro et al., "Conception by Means of In Vitro Fertilization Is Not Associated with Maternal Depressive Symptoms During Pregnancy or Postpartum," *Fertility and Sterility* 108, no. 2 (August 2017): 325–32.

RESOURCES

Here's a partial list of information, books, blogs, websites, and podcasts mentioned in this book.

Informational

American Society of Reproductive Medicine (ASRM): www.asrm.org

Centers for Disease Control and Prevention (CDC): www.cdc.gov/reproductive health/infertility/index.htm

CoFertility: Every Fertility Question Asked and Answered: https://cofertility .com/

Endometriosis Foundation of America: www.endofound.org

Environmental Working Group's Online Skin Deep Cosmetics Database

FertilityIQ: The Very Best Information You Wish You Never Needed: www.fertilityiq.com

Parents Via Egg Donation: www.pved.org

PCOS Awareness Association: www.pcosaa.org

RESOLVE: The National Infertility Association: https://resolve.org/

Single Mothers by Choice: www.singlemothersbychoice.org

Society for Assisted Reproductive Technology (SART): www.sart.org

Books

Body Belief: How to Heal Autoimmune Diseases, Radically Shift Your Health, and Learn to Love Your Body More by Aimee E. Raupp, MS, LAC

Conceiving Masculinity: Male Infertility, Medicine, and Identity by Liberty Walther Barnes

Hilariously Infertile: One Woman's Inappropriate Quest to Help Women Laugh Through Infertility by Karen Jeffries

It Starts with the Egg: How the Science of Egg Quality Can Help You Get Pregnant Naturally, Prevent Miscarriage, and Improve Your Odds in IVF by Rebecca Fett

Let's Talk About Egg Donation: Real Stories from Real People by Marna Gatlin and Carole LieberWilkins, MFT

Life Without Baby: Surviving and Thriving When Motherhood Doesn't Happen by Lisa Manterfield

Living the Life Unexpected: How to Find a Meaningful and Fulfilling Future Without Children by Jody Day

Not Broken: An Approachable Guide to Miscarriage and Recurrent Pregnancy Loss by Lora Shahine, MD, FACOG

Overcoming Infertility: A Guide for Jewish Couples by Richard V. Grazi, MD

Silent Sorority: A (Barren) Woman Gets Busy, Angry, Lost and Found by Pamela Mahoney Tsigdinos

The Long-Awaited Stork: A Guide to Parenting After Infertility by Ellen Sarasohn Glazer

The Mind-Body Fertility Connection: The True Pathway to Conception by James Schwartz

The Rules Do Not Apply: A Memoir by Ariel Levy

The Seed: Infertility Is a Feminist Issue by Alexandra Kimball

The Tao of Fertility: A Healing Chinese Medicine Program to Prepare Body, Mind, and Spirit for New Life by Daoshing Ni

When God Says "Wait" and *When God Says "Go"* by Elizabeth Laing Thompson

Your Fertility. Your Family: The Many Roads to Conception by William Schoolcraft, MD

Podcasts

Beat Infertility: https://beatinfertility.co/

Big Fat Negative: https://robynbirkin.com/

Fertility Warriors Podcast: www.samshaber.com

IVFU: www.ivfupodcast.com

Matt & Doree's Eggcellent Adventure: https://art19.com/shows/matt-and-dorees-eggcellent-adventure

The Fertile Nest: www.listennotes.com/podcasts/the-fertile-nest-katie-lynch-licsw-JRMFjHUY_i1/

The Fertility Podcast: www.thefertilitypodcast.com

The Infertile Mafia: https://infertilemafia.podbean.com/

Websites and Blogs

Gateway Women: United By and Beyond Childlessness: https://gateway-women.com/

Life as Dad to Donor Insemination (DI) Kids: http://di-dad.blogspot.com/

Pregnantish: pregnantish.com

Remembyro: Your Source for Evidence-Based IVF Information: www.remembryo.com

The 2 Week Wait Blog: https://wonderwomanwriter.com/the-2-week-wait-blog/

The Broken Brown Egg: http://thebrokenbrownegg.org/

Financial Support

Baby Quest Foundation: www.babyquestfoundation.org

Cade Foundation: www.cadefoundation.org

Carrot: Customized Fertility for Companies: www.get-carrot.com

Fertility for Colored Girls: www.fertilityforcoloredgirls.org

Future Family (Flexible Financing Plans): www.futurefamily.com

Men Having Babies (Unbiased Surrogacy Advice and Support for Gay Men and Beyond): www.menhavingbabies.org

Progny: https://progyny.com/talktohr/

INDEX

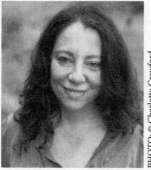

AMY KLEIN is a health journalist and essayist whose work has appeared in *The New York Times* ("Fertility Diary," "Modern Love," and "Draft"), *The Washington Post, Slate, Salon, Aeon, The Forward, Newsweek,* and other publications. Her column, in the *New York Times* Motherlode blog, followed her long fertility journey. She is a Moth slam winner and storyteller. She lives with her husband and daughter in New York City.

ABOUT THE TYPE

This book was set in Minion, a 1990 Adobe Originals typeface by Robert Slimbach. Minion is inspired by classical, old-style typefaces of the late Renaissance, a period of elegant and beautiful type designs. Created primarily for text setting, Minion combines the aesthetic and functional qualities that make text type highly readable with the versatility of digital technology.